SECOND OPINION

SECOND OPINION

**What's Wrong
with Canada's
Health-Care
System**

**and
How to Fix it**

MICHAEL RACHLIS, M.D.
CAROL KUSHNER

Harper & Collins
TORONTO

First Published 1989
by Collins Publishers

This edition published by
Harper & Collins Publishers Ltd.
55 Avenue Road, Suite 2900
Hazelton Lanes
Toronto, Ontario
M5R 3L2

A Peter Livingston Book. Queries regarding radio
broadcasting, motion picture, video cassette, television,
translation, and related rights should be directed to the
author's representative, Peter Livingston Associates, Inc.,
1020 Bland Street, Halifax, Nova Scotia, Canada,
B3H 2S8

Canadian Cataloguing in Publication Data

Rachlis, Michael
Second Opinion

Includes bibliographical references and index.
ISBN 0-00-215441-2 (bound)
ISBN 0-00-215678-4 (paperback)

1. Medical care — Canada. 2. Medical
policy — Canada. 3. Public Health —
Canada. I. Kushner, Carol. II. Title.

RA395.C3R32   1989   362.1′0971   C89-093003-1

Printed and Bound In Canada

Contents

Foreword

It wasn't hard for me to accept the authors' invitation to write this introduction. I've known and respected Dr. Michael Rachlis for more than ten years now; he was one of the first physicians to organize public support in defence of Medicare, through the Medical Reform Group he helped to found. So writing this preamble has been both a pleasure and an honour, especially since I believe that *Second Opinion* is a major achievement, both in terms of its importance and its execution. The chapters that follow analyse every facet of our system in clear language and with precise documentation. The authors don't mince their words when it comes to criticising our system's faults, and yet every page is positive. The truth is, I wish I had written it myself!

Very few people have an in-depth understanding about how our public (and para-public) institutions work. Rachlis and Kushner do. They are well aware of the political, administrative and financial constraints with which ministries of health and hospitals must contend. They know what drives and maintains the current allocation of health resources so that hospitals and doctors get the lion's share and prevention and health promotion get left out in the cold. What's more they zero in on the extraordinary extent of wasteful spending in our system. Much of this waste, it turns out, stems directly from medicine's neglect of science. I couldn't agree more with the authors when they plead for a more rigorously scientific system, one which integrates research evidence into practice. Right now medicine wraps itself in the mantle of science, but the mantle is full of holes. In the pages that follow Rachlis and Kushner expose an inexcusable lack of planning and accountability for quality in our system in ways that should send shivers down your spine. And yet, they also see a way out for us. A way to turn things around.

***

When I was the federal minister of health, working to gain support for the Canada Health Act (1984), it was always clear to me that our efforts were directed at one problem only: the erosion of "free" (pre-paid by taxes) access to health services. When the bill was finally passed into law, it re-inforced one of the original conditions of Medicare — that patients should not be charged "extra" when consulting doctors or going into hospital. That's well and good as far as it goes, but it's important to recognize that that's all it did. That's why I tried very hard, when the Bill was being studied in the House of Commons, to spark a national debate about the future orientation of our health care system. I always hoped that someone, somewhere, would pick up the idea of revamping Medicare and bring it to life. This book has done just that. Michael Rachlis and Carol Kushner have furnished the very document needed to engage consumers, health providers and governments in a process of dialogue and collaboration towards reform.

My own reading of the current situation makes me hopeful about the prospects for reforming our system. The public is not stupid; and there are a number of indications that people aren't quite as happy with Medicare as the polls would seem to show. For example, in the last ten years or so, the millions spent on "alternative" medicines (which for the most part are not covered by Medicare), I take as evidence of a growing dissatisfaction with traditional health care services. And there are other signs of discontent. What does it signify when women's groups lobby for more "well-women" clinics and ask for funding to develop self-care networks? How should we interpret the fact that seniors' associations are becoming more outspoken about how our system is failing to satisfy their urgent health concerns?

I'm not suggesting that these various initiatives represent the majority of users — at least not yet. But they do signal a mounting awareness in the public about the need for change. They are sending out a new message, one that expresses a deep ambivalence about what people really want from their health care system. On the one hand, we want the best medicine has to offer in terms of high-tech sophistication when we fall ill; on the other hand, we want medicine to wear a human face, to treat us with caring and compassion. In other words, we seem to want medicalization and de-medicalization all at the same time. What isn't clear yet, what we haven't figured out, is the right mix. Society hasn't had the opportunity to debate these issues. There's been no forum for such discussions.

From my perspective, what we should really be debating is health — not just medical care. And in doing so, we need to recognize that health is more than just the "absence of disease". For all of us, health, as a goal to be achieved or a state to be maintained, is a lifelong task. It's everybody's business — both individually and collectively. And since health is adversely affected by poverty, unemployment, social stress, inadequate housing, unsafe working conditions and a host of other social and environmental hazards, it is also the business of our politicians. These are public policy issues.

Almost thirty years ago, Canadians gave themselves a great gift: a public health insurance system that ensured access to health care regardless of an individual's ability to pay for it. It didn't happen overnight though. The struggle that began in the twenties and was carried on through the Great Depression and the Second World War, wasn't won until 1971, by which time Medicare was fully established all across the country. During the early 1980s, a determined public made sure that Medicare was saved from erosion by outlawing user fees and extra-billing. Today, public opinion polls reaffirm how highly Canadians value our health care system. Surely by now, we feel collectively secure enough to go a step further. To follow the lead set by Rachlis and Kushner and join in the decisions that will affect our most precious commodity: our nation's health.

The Honourable Monique Bégin,
former Minister of Health and Welfare

Introduction

This is a controversial book on at least two fronts. It challenges conventional wisdom about the importance of health care to our health and it exposes the awesome extent of waste and inefficiency within our beloved Medicare. It does not, however, stop there. For our criticisms lead directly to solutions — fully one third of our text is devoted to discussing opportunities and options for reform.

We set out to write this book in the belief that all of us need to know about these issues and join in the debate. For too long, knowledge about Medicare's troubles has been limited to a small community of academics and health policy experts, from whose work we have drawn our analysis. But for all their erudition, this inner circle is not well poised to turn things around. Only when their understanding is shared by the Canadian community at large will reform of our system become possible. So this is not just a book about health care; this is a *political* book — an appeal to all Canadians to participate in the debate about Medicare's future.

To reach this wider lay audience, we've made every effort to use clear language, and to sustain a logical and analytical argument. Sometimes we resort to strong language to make our points, but only when there's overwhelming evidence for our position. On the other hand, when the evidence is weak, we're much less insistent, content to mention the issue, and encourage further research to clarify its validity.

This brings us to the subject of physicians and our treatment of them in the book. Let's begin by admitting that no reform of our system, however well-motivated, will succeed without the support of the medical profession. A number of prominent physicians have written books about the need for reform; among them, Dr. Howard Hiatt, former dean of the Harvard School of Public Health and a Professor of Medicine there and at

Harvard Medical School, who authored *America's Health in the Balance*;* Seattle cardiologist Dr. Robert Preston, who wrote *The Clay Pedestal,* and Australia's Dr. Richard Taylor who wrote *Medicine Out of Control.* Many Canadian physicians share their concerns about the quality of modern medicine and would like to make it a more accountable science, and a more caring and responsive vocation. This book is a cry for their involvement. A plea for those who agree with us to come forward and help shape that kind of reform.

Our approach, once again, has been to look at the *evidence* of shortcomings in modern medical practice and the undesirable influences and incentives within our system that have made doctors the victims, rather than the villains in the story. Our intention is not to insult physicians or to make them angry, but to highlight justifiable concerns about the quality of care that Canadians deserve and practitioners want to deliver. So this is not a doctor-bashing book; instead it might be described as a hard critical look at medicine and the health-care system.

In the main, we expect that most health and social service professionals will welcome our analysis. For more than fifteen years they've been patiently waiting for provincial governments to act on the recommendations of various royal commissions and inquires into the state of our system. These expert panels have all called for the same two things: a move away from institutionally-based care to community care and a re-orientation of our system so that it focusses on prevention rather than cure. More than anything else, this book consolidates the arguments favouring these policy positions and suggests a strategy for realizing them.

The topics covered on the pages that follow are far ranging — from C-T scanners to affordable housing, from cancer treatment to violence against women, from prescription drugs to poverty. All the same, in our attempt to give a broad overview of our system, we were only able to refer briefly to many vitally important health issues worthy of much more attention. Medical

---

*Howard Hiatt, *America's Health in the Balance: Choice or Chance?,* Toronto: Fitzhenry and Whiteside, 1987. The other two works cited are fully referenced in the notes to our text.

education, bioethics, AIDS, occupational health and safety, the consumer movement — entire books have been devoted to these and many other subjects we do little more than raise. This book is just for openers; interested readers are urged to use our references to explore these areas in more detail.

Now for our bread and butter. To the hundreds of people who agreed to be interviewed — politicians, pharmacists, nurses, physicians, social workers, hospital administrators, civil servants, professors of medicine, journalists, economists, and public health officials — we extend our heartfelt thanks. Their willingness to share their time and expertise with us made our research work a pleasure and a privilege. In particular, we want to acknowledge the contribution of Michael Doleschell, and Drs. John Frank, Debby Copes, and Joel Lexchin, who read all, or portions, of our text and helped to make it more accurate and intelligible. (Obviously, however, the opinions and conclusions expressed in the text are ours and should not be attributed to anyone else.) We are similarly grateful to our editors, Chuck Macli and Matthew Kudelka, for their constructive criticisms and unfailing patience. One of us (MR) owes a special debt to the faculty and staff of the Department of Clinical Epidemiology and Biostatistics and the Centre for Health and Economics and Policy Analysis at McMaster University. And finally, we want to thank our families. This book never would have been written at all, had it not been for their support and forbearance over the past two years.

Michael Rachlis, M.D.
Carol Kushner

This book is dedicated to the memory of two great Canadians: the Honorable Tommy Douglas, P.C., the father of Medicare, and to Dr. Charles Hastings, who between 1910 and 1929 during his tenure as medical officer of health for Toronto made it the healthiest city in the world.

Chapter 1

An Overview
of the
Great Deception

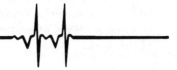

- IF you've ever had to spend hours in an emergency room before getting attention, or had to wait more than two weeks for non-emergency surgery, or had problems trying to get a frail parent into a nursing home, this book is for you.

- IF you're a health or social service professional distressed to see how poorly our system responds to urgent needs, you can't do your job properly until you read this book.

- IF you're a hospital board member who's sick of trying to juggle doctors' competing demands for staff and equipment, here's some ammunition.

- IF you're a minister of health who's fed up with being vilified by the press as a monster who doesn't care if little children die, read on.

CANADA'S HEALTH CARE SYSTEM is in big trouble but hardly anyone — including the public, the media and the medical profession — understands exactly what's wrong with it. A major stumbling block to understanding our system is that its real problems are stubbornly counter-intuitive. For example, how is it possible to have lengthy waiting lists for hospitals and long-term care facilities, and still conclude that there are too many

1

institutional beds? How, when people often have to wait months to see a specialist, can we turn around and say we have too many doctors? Why are emergency rooms so crowded, if hospitals have enough money? Although our health care system is one of the most complex institutions in our modern-day society, its problems *are* understandable. And, what's more, we can resolve them.

To begin: The vital question is not one of underfunding, as you might think, but of quality. Canadians are used to being told they have the best health care system in the world. Surveys of the public's attitudes consistently report a high degree of satisfaction with Medicare. This praise is more than justified when we think of the equal access to medical services all Canadians enjoy. We have been very fortunate in almost eliminating financial barriers to health care, which in the United States still exist and prevent some patients from receiving needed treatment. Equitable access has been an extraordinary achievement, and it's worth bragging about. But now it's time to face up to the fact that in terms of *quality*, we have neither the best health care system in the world nor the best health.

This book looks at why this is so and how we can make reforms for improvement. The first half deals with the complex and subtle problems which are compromising the quality of our medical care; the second, with the kinds of reforms we have to make to turn things around. Some of the problems we identify are shared by health care systems everywhere and are not exclusive to this country; others are specific to Canada. But for both types of problems there are solutions.

Two major themes emerge in our analysis, both of which may come as a surprise to you if you don't work in the area of health policy. The first is that health care is not what makes us healthy. The great equation, the idea that somehow health care equals health, is a delusion.[1]

But the public has been encouraged to grossly overestimate the importance of doctors and hospitals to their well-being. The media play a pivotal role in promoting this misperception. Medical stories have tremendous dramatic appeal, and make for very popular copy. For example, who is not moved by the story of a desperately ill toddler waiting for a liver transplant? Or one about a baby born to barren parents, thanks to *in vitro* fertilization? Combining intense human interest with the latest high-technology solution is a winning formula for a news or feature item.

Yet the overall impression such stories convey is deceptive. Every government official and university researcher we spoke with agreed that medical care contributes only minimally to our health. Other more important factors such as nutrition and adequate income get scant attention by comparison.

Overestimating the importance of health care has had a predictable consequence — a massive misallocation of resources, particularly in social spending. The continued high status of curative medicine has deflected our attention away from the social, economic, and environmental causes of illness. Even though experts everywhere agree that these are what really determine the state of our health, public spending in these sectors is only a tiny fraction of what we devote to the treatment of sickness. In short, we're spending billions of our health dollars in the wrong place, with the end nowhere in sight.

A second theme which dominates our analysis is that our system is outrageously inefficient as a result of mismanagement and a basic neglect of science. An extraordinarily high proportion of the vast resources available to Canada's hospitals and physicians is being squandered on useless or possibly harmful services, and on the misuse of beds within institutions. But the public never gets to hear this side of the story. For example, when you read in the news that hospitals are "dangerously underfunded," does anyone ever mention that 20 to 50% of all patients in acute care hospitals don't belong there? Many of these people are elderly or disabled. Often what they need isn't medical care at all, but personal care — regular assistance with bathing or housekeeping chores. Yet they languish in the most cost-intensive setting we provide, because more appropriate alternatives — nursing homes, home care services, and the like — are unavailable.

A similar situation exists in our nursing homes, where at least 30% of the residents could be released tomorrow if a rational system of home care and elderly day-care services were in place in their communities.* But typically, Canada's home care ser-

---

*An Ontario study for the Ministry of Senior Citizens' Affairs found that 55% of people in nursing homes did not have to be there, as reported in the *Toronto Star*, March 29, 1988.

vices are fragmented and poorly organized. If there's any under-funding within our health care system, home care is perhaps the first place to look for it. Instead, we're asked to look at the serious overcrowding in our institutions, and to give *them* the money.

This is just one example of how the organization of health services in Canada is in a shambles. Having so many people in the wrong care settings is not just wasteful — it also seriously compromises the quality of life for those unlucky enough to be trapped in them. The inadequacy of our current system, to deal with simple human needs, is a national disgrace.

Focussing on Quality

Many people fear that it's impossible to have both quality care and economical care, that somehow quality and efficiency are incompatible. It's possible, of course, to compromise quality by insensitive attempts to control costs. But if quality itself, rather than cost-cutting, becomes the objective, then savings are frequently a spinoff benefit. Alain Enthoven, a professor from the School of Business at Stanford University in California, is quite convinced of this: "It just so happens that quality care, by which I mean getting things right the first time, usually turns out to be more efficient care as well." Of course, the corollary of this is also true — that poor-quality care can be inordinately expensive.

Canada's inefficient use of bed space is an obvious example of how bad medicine can cost plenty. We overhospitalize people all the time, performing unnecessary diagnostic tests and surgeries. Then, once we get people into the hospital, we like to keep them there far longer than the evidence suggests is medically required or even advisable. For example, the average length of stay for Ontario patients following a hernia repair is 4.7 days. Yet doctors at the Shouldice Hospital[2] in Toronto, a world-famous centre specializing in hernia surgery, have found that it's perfectly safe to release patients on the second post-operative day. The Shouldice, it should be noted, has a long-standing record of high-quality care. Its efficiency has *enhanced* quality, not compromised it.

Few incentives within our system ensure either quality or efficiency. Doctors, once licenced, can practice for life. They aren't required to upgrade their skills as medical knowledge expands, and generally, no one monitors what happens inside their offices.* Only licensing bodies in Ontario, Quebec and British Columbia, through their College of Physicians and Surgeons, spot-check doctors' office records to flag substandard care—a program which, though limited, has still been attacked by many doctors. Most of our physicians practice "solo," in isolation from their peers, and have few opportunities to compare their performance with that of their colleagues. Only direct complaints made to the licencing bodies are investigated. We find a similar *laissez-faire* attitude when it comes to hospitals, which enjoy a relative freedom from scrutiny as well. Of course, Canadian hospitals must be accredited, which means they must satisfy certain standards. But these standards refer to processes, not performance — hospitals expend little effort trying to figure out if they're doing a good job as far as patient *health* is concerned. "The patient died, but the operation was a success," is an old and bad joke, but we haven't moved much beyond its cruel irony. Until we do, we stand little chance of improving our standards of care, or reducing wasteful expenditures.

Supplier-Induced Demand

A good part of our rising health care costs can be traced directly to Canada's oversupply of physicians. Canadians may not realize it yet, but we have too many doctors now, and are producing far too many for the future! Over the past 12 years, the number of doctors practicing in Canada has grown by a whopping 41% even though, during the same time period, our population has increased only a modest 13%. This problem is only going to get worse — we are continuing to pump doctors into the system every year at rates two to three times the growth rate of our population. Meanwhile, the overall supply of acute care hospital beds has actually fallen slightly. That means competition among physicians for beds is now intense.**

---

*Some specialist societies do require continuing medical education, but there is little evidence that this is effective.

**Between 1975 and 1986 the number of short-term (acute care) hospital beds in Canada fell by 5.6 percent, from 119,077 to 112,436 (Health and Welfare Canada, November 1987). For more detail, see Chapter 6.

When a new doctor enters the system, he or she begins practice with the expectation of being both useful to society and amply rewarded for the sacrifices clinical medicine demands. The doctor who has more time, and perhaps fewer patients, naturally tries to do more good for them. Physicians can easily ask patients to return for more follow-up or additional tests, without raising any eyebrows. Remember, you can't get a prescription, laboratory tests, or surgery without a doctor's say-so. Since virtually all health care costs are under physician control, having too many doctors is a terrible drain on the system.

Canada's oversupply of physicians has had two effects: a dramatic increase in service intensity in some provinces; and large price hikes for doctors' services in others. People, particularly elderly people, are getting more medical services than ever before, but there's little evidence to show it's doing them much good.

Meanwhile, in a frantic effort to keep the lid on health costs, provincial governments are caught in a bind. The system is open-ended. Governments have few means of controlling the number or type of services provided. They fear being accused of interfering with the practice of medicine. So they've been reduced to blunt cost-cutting exercises which often aren't sensitive to real needs. Thus, in recent years, we've witnessed cuts in hospital beds (Saskatchewan and Manitoba), restrictions on the supply of doctors in particular geographical areas (British Columbia), cutbacks to medical school enrollments or internship and residency programs (almost all provinces), caps on utilization (Québec and British Columbia), and controls on capital expenditures for new technologies in hospitals (all provinces). Alberta even began to tread the dangerous path of *de-insuring* certain types of health services, notably annual eye examinations, family planning counselling, and elective sterilization procedures. (A year later, public pressure forced them to reinstate coverage for sterilization procedures and eye examinations.)

None of these measures, however, addresses the real issue, which is how to improve the quality of medical care we receive. None ensures that we are allocating resources where they will do the most good.

Where Are We Going?

Perhaps the most astounding discovery anyone studying our health care system will make, is that it operates without any overall objectives at all. There is no plan, no vision, no coherent policy. We're running a $46 billion operation with no idea of what we're trying to achieve.[3] Can you imagine any other industry of that size neglecting such a fundamental imperative? Of course not! But in Canada's health care system, long-range planning is at best a sideline occupation. Planning activities are often parcelled out to commissions and institutes, whose recommendations typically are praised (or condemned) and then summarily ignored. Within provincial ministries of health, and around the table at hospital board meetings, the results of such policy exercises — which are vital to making rational spending decisions — become completely overwhelmed by the dictates of crisis management. The result is chaos within complacency.

Where are we trying to go with our health care system? Is good health for everyone the ultimate goal? Many would agree that this is a laudable objective — everyone wants to be healthy. But if health is the target, does it make sense to put virtually all our resources into treating *illness*? In Britain during the 1940s, when the National Health Service (NHS) was introduced, providing medical care to those who otherwise could not afford it was expected to have an enormous impact on the health of the population. Lord Beveridge, who introduced the enabling legislation for the NHS, even predicted that the nation's health status would improve so much that the costs of providing health care would eventually begin to fall. Needless to say, he was overly optimistic. People in England are healthier today than they were in 1948 when the NHS started up. However, as in other countries, it isn't the health care system that accounts for many of these gains, and the costs of British health care have gone up, not down.

We now know, thanks to the work of epidemiologists like Britain's Dr. Thomas McKeown, that medicine has only a minor influence on our health status.[4] We are finally beginning to understand that genetic, environmental, social, and economic factors are far more important. Who we are, where we live, and how we live are the principal determinants of health. It should be a source of pride to us that Canada was the first nation to endorse these ideas officially, when former federal health minister Marc Lalonde's *A New Perspective on the Health of Canadians* was published in 1974. This landmark document won international acclaim, and has had a tremendous influence on health policy throughout the world. It should have placed Canada at the forefront of the reform movement, and yet, perhaps typically, it failed to spearhead much change here at home. In 1986, Minister of Health and Welfare Jake Epp released his *Framework for Health Promotion*, which again thrust Canada into the forefront of health policy reform. But while it was well-received internationally, it is not yet clear how Canada will implement its recommendations.

Barriers to Reform

Why have we been so slow to adapt? Medicare itself is partly to blame. Curiously, our publicly funded, privately run health care system, widely hailed as Canada's most popular social reform, has proven notoriously resistant to change.

Medicare developed in two stages. The first of these, in 1957, put in place coverage for hospital services, and met with relatively little opposition from provider groups. But in order to expand the program so it could cover physician services outside hospitals as well as inside, governments needed the support of the medical community.

Prior to the Second World War, organized medicine actually lobbied for a system of national health insurance, but its enthusiasm for it had waned by the 1960s.[5] Governments had to make a number of concessions to the medical profession to win its cooperation. In return for their support, doctors insisted on guarantees that their professional freedom to act in their patients' best interests would not be compromised by government interference. They made it clear that they would not tolerate government telling doctors how to practice medicine. They wanted assurances that the profession would keep the right to regulate itself. Their argument was that these guarantees were necessary in order to protect the public from the dangers of "socialized" or state medicine. In effect, the government's concessions reinforced the doctors' own professional interests — interests which sometimes conflict with those of their patients.

The most obvious example of this conflict between interests is how we pay doctors. The usual payment system for Canadian physicians offers a fee for every medical service performed. Many critics of health care, from playwright George Bernard Shaw* to Dr. Milton Terris, the American public health advocate, have recognized that "fee-for-service," because of the extraordinary opportunities it offers for maximizing incomes, creates strong incentives to provide more and more services. This is not an inherently bad thing; it could even be a benefit, if it turned out that more health care is better for us. Unfortunately, often the opposite is true.

The Failure to Evaluate

Too much health care can be disastrous for patients; many illnesses are actually caused by the investigations and treatments people undergo on doctors' orders.

This is not an indictment against the good character of physicians, but rather a recognition of something very obvious: medicine is inherently an action-oriented profession. The instinct which motivates the doctor to act usually stems from a genuine desire to help the patient. But the same instinct often induces doctors to intervene even when the potential benefit of doing so has not been established. Good intentions cannot compensate for ill-informed decision-making. For example, by their own admission, doctors are woefully ignorant about the drugs they prescribe. Too many rely on the biased information the drug companies themselves produce to promote their products. There's strong evidence that drug information that comes from the pharmaceutical industry is often misleading.[6] This is a serious problem with serious health consequences; 75% of all office visits to doctors end with a prescription, often for drugs whose properties are poorly under-

---

*Shaw, in the preface to his famous play *The Doctor's Dilemma*, wrote: " That any sane nation, having observed that you could provide for the supply of bread by giving bakers a pecuniary interest in baking for you, should go on to give a surgeon a pecuniary interest in cutting off your leg, is enough to make one despair of political humanity."

stood by the prescriber.[7] Poor prescribing causes a lot of illness — adverse drug reactions account for four to ten percent of all hospital admissions. Particularly at risk are elderly patients — as many as 20% of hospital admissions among those over 65 are for drug-related problems.[8]

Another impediment to quality in clinical practice is that many doctors have a poor understanding of statistics. This is a significant handicap to interpreting many laboratory investigations, and leads to overdiagnosis and overtreatment. Unfortunately, most practicing physicians find it hard to get excited about epidemiology.* Yet it is this discipline which offers the greatest hope for improving medical decision-making, in that it offers the scientific means for studying diseases within populations, and establishing which interventions work and which do not.

Unfortunately, epidemiological research is grossly underused in medicine. Most Canadians would be shocked to learn that most medical therapies have never been rigorously evaluated. As many as 80% of all treatments, including surgeries, have never been scientifically tested to prove their worth. Medical history is littered with abandoned therapies that were once common practice but are now utterly discredited. Not all of these examples hail from the distant past, when leeching, bleeding, and other noxious remedies were part of every doctor's stock in trade — we've had to drop a number of modern treatments as well. As just one of many examples, freezing the stomach was used for years as a therapy for ulcers, until it was finally evaluated and found useless.[9] Despite a dismal record of embracing and then discarding useless interventions, evaluation still meets with a lot of resistance.

Episodic Meddling and Heroic Salvage

Facing up to the limitations of medicine is both frightening and compelling. Each of us is afraid of illness, pain, and death. Our vulnerability to all three makes us receptive to the promises of medicine. We cling with confidence to the expectation that the

---

*Epidemiology comes from three Greek words: *epi*, "about," *demos*, "people," and *logos*, "science."

operation will be a success or that the pills will work; in short, we have faith that the doctor will cure us.

The expression of this modern faith can be seen all over North America. A century ago, people rarely went to see a doctor; they feared, with some justification, that the cure was likely to be worse than the disease. Hospitals were little more than death houses for the destitute, places to be avoided at all cost.[10] Since then, however, public attitudes toward medicine have made a complete turnaround. Modern cynicism aside, the fictional physicians we see on television are still usually portrayed as heroes. Even though their real-life counterparts may fall short of that ideal, doctors remain the most highly respected professionals in our society. And our hospitals, boasting undreamt-of technological marvels, have become like modern-day temples — sources of pride and hope within their communities.

Sadly, our great expectations of medicine are largely based on a delusion. Health care, despite some remarkable successes, is extremely limited in its ability to address our most pressing health problems. Dr. Richard Hudson, a high-spirited family doctor from the James Bay Community Health Centre in Victoria, British Columbia, shares this perspective. In his view, "Modern medicine is little more than episodic meddling and heroic salvage." This rather unflattering description confronts squarely the gap between perception and reality. There are, alas, only a few truly curable diseases; cures for most illnesses will likely elude researchers for decades to come. This is particularly true of the chronic diseases, like heart disease and cancer, from which most of us will die. Experts everywhere admit that prevention is the only answer.

All the same, our system remains heavily tilted toward treating illness. That's where the money goes. "We don't have a health care system," says Dr. Trevor Hancock, a Canadian physician and consultant to the World Health Organization, "we've got a sickness treatment system. There's a world of difference." Perhaps an analogy will illustrate the point more clearly. The Autobahn, Germany's most famous expressway, has no speed limit, and motor vehicle accidents are frequent and often result in loss of life. All along its length, Germany has established trauma centres to deal with the carnage.[11] Air ambulances are stationed in between these centres so that at no point along the Autobahn is an injured person further than 50 kilometres from treatment. This "solution," in short, requires enormous resources to maintain, even though the problem could be handled more effectively by a simple preventive measure — establishing and enforcing a safe speed limit.

Prevention should be a major health priority, but it's not. The current emphasis on altering individual behaviour to improve health is too narrow — it doesn't address the real problems. While more affluent Canadians are eating more carefully, exercising more often, and kicking the tobacco habit, those trapped by poverty, illiteracy, and environmental and occupational hazards continue to fall prey to illnesses beyond their individual control. Expecting medicine to "fix" the casualties from these conditions of life is unrealistic and unfair.

Canada's Victims

It's distressing to discover that although Canadians have equal access to health care, they don't share equally in health. Poverty is a potent health risk. Canadians with the lowest incomes die years sooner than the rest of us, and have more disability. Poverty is particularly tragic for children, who experience, through no fault of their own, a disproportionate share of the nation's ill health. Current Canadian statistics indicate that one child in six lives below the poverty line. Surveys have shown these kids have more medical and social problems than their wealthier counterparts. Does anyone care?

Dr. Fraser Mustard, who heads Canada's Institute for Advanced Research,* challenges this neglect: "A nation that isn't interested in the health of its people, particularly its young people, has no future." Most of us now are well aware that our nation is "greying," but few realize that the proportion of school-

---

*The Canadian Institute for Advanced Research is our most prestigious "think tank." Originally established to prevent the "brain drain" to the United States, it operates essentially as a university without walls; it funds researchers in science and the humanities from all over Canada, who then work together on projects of national importance. CIAR's current activities include projects on cosmology, artificial intelligence, and population health.

age children in our population has already dropped by almost 50% in the past 15 years, and is continuing to fall.[12] "A nation concerned about the future would do everything possible to maximize the productivity of these young people," says Dr. Mustard. "They'll need to become outstanding performers in producing tradable goods and services in a climate of intense competition." His point is that only a healthy economy can afford to pay for universal services like health care and education. And to maintain a healthy economy, we must have healthy people.

Canada's priorities as a nation are self-evident from our spending record. Clearly, we are willing to pay top dollar for medical care — hospital and physician services are the largest single item in every province's budget. But how important is "health" to our nation?

Fortunately, the bleak picture we've just painted of Canada's health care system can be redrawn; we can improve the quality of sickness treatment and, at the same time, reduce our dependency on it by expanding preventive efforts. We will look at opportunities for reform in the second part of this book. But first, we need to investigate the problems we've just sketched, beginning with the misallocation of health care funds under Medicare.

Chapter 2

Dollars and Sense

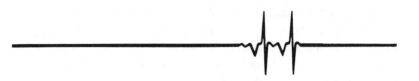

The Price Tag

THIS YEAR CANADIANS WILL spend $46 billion on health care.[1] If you're like most people, a figure as large as this is utterly incomprehensible, so let's put it into understandable terms. Assuming you have a stack of $1,000 bills, with about 300 to the inch, the average person could reach in and grab a couple of handfuls totalling more than a million dollars without any trouble at all. But $46 billion stacked this way translates into a pile of money nearly four kilometres high! Put another way, it represents almost $2,000 for every man, woman and child in the country — enough to feed a family of four for a year, or to purchase a new 20-inch colour TV every three months. Get the picture?

Approximately $35 billion, or three-quarters of total health spending, is publicly funded through taxes, as well as revenues from the health insurance premiums Ontario, British Columbia, and Alberta impose. (The other provinces don't charge premiums.) To put the level of publicly funded health care in personal terms, this means that about one dollar out of every four you pay in taxes goes toward health care.[2]

The remaining $11 billion spent on health also comes from you. It represents the money you pay privately for additional insurance benefits (dental coverage, extended care insurance, and so on), as well as other items not covered by provincial health plans (non-prescription drugs, visits to alternative medical practitioners, eyeglasses, and the like).*

At this point all we have said about our health care spending is that the total amount is significantly high; we're sure you'd agree that $46 billion is a lot of money in anyone's books. But the real issue is whether this level of funding is appropriate. Are we spending too little, just enough, or too much? That is the question this chapter will begin to answer. But first you need some background about how Canada's much-praised health care system came into being.

How Did We Get Here?

Mackenzie King first promised Canadians national health insurance way back in 1919, but it didn't really get off the ground until Saskatchewan's Tommy Douglas led the way.[3] Douglas's commitment to public health insurance stemmed from an experience he had when he was a boy in Winnipeg. He'd developed a bone infection in his leg (osteomyelitis) and a doctor recommended amputation. Fortunately, young Tommy improved, so there was no need for this surgery. All the same, he was left with the impression that his treatment had been second-rate because he was a public rather than a private patient.

Douglas never forgot this experience, and two years after his Cooperative Commonwealth Federation (CCF) came to power in 1944, the province passed the Saskatchewan Hospitalization Act, which provided public insurance coverage for hospital care. The federal government dipped its toe in the water in 1948 by instituting the National Health Grant Program. Most of the grants under this program went to build hospitals. Then in 1957, Parliament passed the Hospital Insurance and Diagnostic Services Act, which offered federal funds to any province that established a hospital insurance program. To qualify for federal money, a provincial program had to meet certain conditions:

---

*Individual provinces vary in terms of what they cover; coverage for practitioners of alternative medicine (*medicine douce*) is much more generous in Québec, for example.

1. The services had to be *comprehensive*, that is, the province had to insure all the services listed in the Act.
2. The services had to be reasonably *accessible* to all provincial residents.
3. The province had to provide *universal* coverage.
4. The coverage had to be *portable*, meaning that a resident of one province had to be covered for services received in any other province.

Eventually, every province in Canada joined this program, in which the federal government agreed to pay half the cost of services provided in hospitals. But only services performed *within* a hospital's walls were eligible for reimbursement under this Act — costs for treating patients in the doctor's office were not. As a consequence, many people were needlessly hospitalized for tests and procedures that could have been performed outside an institution. Coverage depended on *where* they were done.

When it came to establishing public insurance for medical services performed *outside* hospitals, Saskatchewan again led the way — though not without opposition. In 1962, 90% of Saskatchewan's doctors protested the implementation of the Saskatchewan Medical Care Insurance Act by going on strike. But the government prevailed, and Saskatchewan became the first jurisdiction in North America with a tax-supported universal insurance program for medical care. Once again, the federal government followed suit with its own legislation — it passed the National Medicare Insurance Act in 1966, and implemented it in 1968. This Act offered the same cost-sharing arrangements as the 1957 Act, and carried the same four conditions. Provided the provinces met them, whatever they spent on physician services, the federal government agreed to pay half.

As the economic boom of the 1960s gave way to the stagnation of the 1970s, the federal government grew concerned about its open-ended liability for health costs. Health policy analysts pointed to the folly of stimulating the construction and use of hospitals (the most expensive part of the system), while leaving out coverage for home care and outpatient nursing. Besides, some provinces wanted to experiment with these new delivery systems. So in 1977, Parliament passed the Established Programs Financing Act (EPF), which abolished 50-50 cost-sharing and instead provided "block funding" for health and post-secondary education programs. This meant that federal funding was no longer tied to what these programs were actually costing. Finally, mounting concerns that financial barriers were limiting poorer Canadians' access to doctors, led Parliament to pass the Canada Health Act in 1984. This legislation penalized any province that allowed user charges for hospital or physician services, but its main intent was to eliminate extra-billing* by doctors.

While Canada's achievement is outstanding, in that we've created such an equitable Medicare plan, the order in which the various program components were put in place has had unfortunate consequences. This "from the top down" pattern of development created an overreliance on hospitals, other institutions, and doctors. As you will see, we might have ended up with a more balanced system had we covered community nursing care first, and then built the system "from the ground up."

Now that you have some background about Medicare's evolution, it's time to return to our original question about health funding. Are we spending too little, just enough, or too much?

Muddying the Waters: Media Confusion

It's virtually impossible to pick up a newspaper in Canada without reading one or more items dealing with our health care system; health care *costs* in particular are a favourite preoccupation. But journalists and newscasters confuse the public with the mixed messages they offer. Indeed, the two most frequently seen headlines about health care costs actually contradict each other.

First we are told HEALTH CARE COSTS ARE SPIRALLING OUT OF CONTROL. That's the message governments want to get across, as they see one-quarter of their provincial budgets draining directly into the health sector.**

---

*Doctors used to be able to charge fees over and above the level negotiated by their own medical association and the provincial government. They passed on this "extra-billing" to their patients as a user fee.

**Actually this is an average; provincial spending on health as a proportion of total provincial expenditures varies greatly from province to province, with Newfoundland at the low end spending one-fifth of its budget (19.5 percent) in 1987/88, and Ontario at the high end devoting almost one-third (32.2 percent). (Health and Welfare Canada, Policy, Communications and Information Branch, 1988)

Then we are hit with HEALTH CARE IN CANADA IS DANGER-OUSLY UNDERFUNDED. That's the message doctors and hospitals want the public to understand, as they complain about hospital bed shortages and the need for more chronic-care facilities.

Which view is the correct one? Surely both can't be true. We can't simultaneously be spending too much *and* too little! As you will learn, widespread inefficiencies within our health care system lie at the heart of the problem. We're so wasteful that virtually no amount of money could ever satisfy our system's proclaimed needs.

Too Little? Just Enough? Or Too Much?

Let's look at the facts. By the time all the provinces were fully participating in Medicare back in 1971, health care was costing the country around $7 billion a year.[4]. Since we're now spending $46 billion a year, that means costs have gone up 550% in the past 16 years!

But using current dollars obscures the fact that the purchasing power of money has declined over time. Think of your own expenditures — you may be spending twice as much on clothes today as you were in 1971, but that doesn't necessarily mean you're buying twice as much clothing. If you use constant dollars to eliminate the effects of inflation, you might discover that spending on your wardrobe has only gone up by 25%. By using constant dollars to analyse health care costs, you will see that Canada's health spending has doubled since 1971.[5]

But economists prefer yet another method for analysing expenditures. They like to express health care costs as a percentage of our national wealth (Gross National Product, or GNP). This accomplishes two things: it eliminates the effect of inflation, and it puts spending in the context of affordability. As wealth increases, the ability to spend goes up as well. To return to our analogy, expressing your clothing purchases as a percentage of your income might show that you are spending about the same proportion of your wealth on clothes today as you were in 1971. Even the effects of price increases above inflation are softened because your income has gone up as well. If, however, you've become a slave to fashion in the meantime, such an analysis would

Health Expenditures as a % of GNP
Canada and United States

Figure 2.1

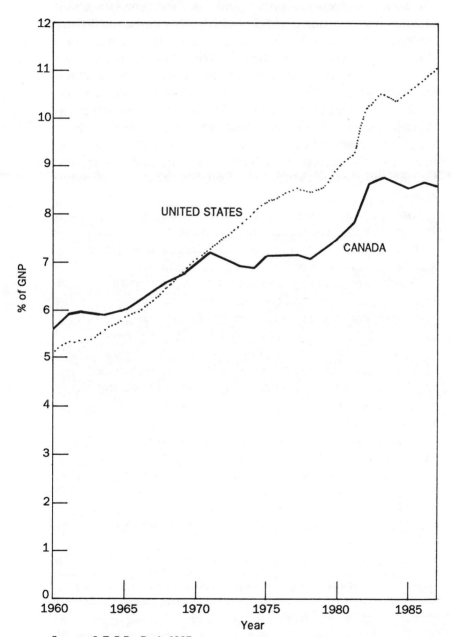

Source: O.E.C.D., Paris 1987

reveal it, by showing that you now spend a greater proportion of your wealth on clothing.

Figure 2.1 expresses health care costs in Canada and the United States as a proportion of GNP. Health economists, like Professor Robert Evans at the University of British Columbia, and Professor Richard Plain at the University of Alberta, argue that this shows that health costs in Canada have been relatively well controlled since Medicare was introduced — that an increase from 7.4% of GNP in 1971 to 8.5% in 1987 simply isn't large enough to support the contention that spending is out of control. To quote Evans, "We should be proud that the overall share of health care in the nation's resources in Canada has been roughly stable [since the introduction of Medicare]. Runaway costs are nonsense statements."[6]

Some provinces, however, find it difficult to take much comfort from such reassurances. From their perspective, health care costs are skyrocketing out of control; some premiers, treasurers, and health ministers are sounding the alarm bell.

They're worried not just because health is the costliest "envelope" in provincial budgets, but especially because in some provinces, per capita spending on health care has gone through the roof! For example, from 1983 to 1987, per capita health spending in Ontario has ballooned by 41%; in Nova Scotia, by 33%; and in Saskatchewan, by 29%. Other provinces have been much more effective in controlling costs: Alberta and British Columbia only increased their per capita health spending by 13% and 18% respectively over the same period.*

A second source of concern to provincial governments is their ability to pay for health care; they realize it is very much affected by the state of our economy. Health care is their responsibility; they have legal, political, and historical commitments to it which must be met. Dr. Fraser Mustard reminds us that spending on

---

*This leaves aside for the moment any analysis of the methods used to control costs in these provinces, as well as the fact that Alberta has historically spent more per capita on health than any other province ($1,230 in 1983/84 and $1,387 in 1987/88). (Health and Welfare Canada, Policy, Communications and Information Branch, 1988.)

services such as health and education is utterly dependent on the nation's wealth. It doesn't matter which political party is in power — Liberal, Conservative, Social Credit, Parti Québécois or NDP — only provinces that *have* money can spend it on their social programs.* But, says Dr. Mustard, "People forget that our wealth is determined by our ability to generate income by producing tradable goods and services." In other words, our economic health must be nurtured in order to afford all those programs that generate no income from trade themselves. Canada's economy has put in a particularly strong showing in recent years, growing faster than that of any other industrialized nation, but the disparities among provinces tell a different story. When it was boom in Alberta, it was bust in the rest of the country. Now that it's boom in Ontario, it's bust in Alberta and the Atlantic provinces. In this light, it's easy to see why individual provinces may view the trends in health care costs with apprehension.

A third source of anxiety is that, although the provinces have to pay for health care, they really don't have very much control over how much it's going to cost them in any single period. They may pay the piper but the tune is very much determined by hospitals and physicians. Larry Grossman, who's held both the health and finance portfolios in Ontario, says there's no question that budgets for hospitals and OHIP (Ontario Health Insurance Plan, which pays for physician services) are uncontrolled. "The fact is when hospitals go over budget, you don't close them down, you pay them. Remember as well that the major portion of hospital expenditure is for labour costs, over which government has little influence. In real terms it's an arbitrator who decides what next year's budget will be — not the minister of health or his deputies or the chairman of the hospital board, but an arbitrator."

But these are only a few of the more obvious reasons why health care costs are so high and so poorly controlled. To give you further insight, we'll leave the complexities of health economics aside for the moment, and offer the following anecdote, which though fictional, is based on some astounding facts!

---

*They can of course borrow it, but they'd far rather not, as you can understand.

No Room at the Inn

John D. woke up early one frosty March morning bathed in a cold sweat. He was in terrible pain and feared his ulcer was bleeding again. He called Dr. C., his trusted family physician, who told him to get to the hospital right away, and that he would call ahead to arrange a bed. But when John arrived, there wasn't a bed available for him. So he was placed on a stretcher in the hallway of the emergency department.

When Dr. C. arrived he felt terrible about having to tell John that there probably wouldn't be a free bed on the ward for at least another three days. Bed shortages were a continual source of frustration to Dr. C. and he couldn't hide his exasperation from his patient: "It's government underfunding, John, that's the problem. If we had adequate money for this hospital, there'd be a bed for you tonight, and for as long as you needed it. But as things are . . . ."

John was angry too, but the medication he'd been given was beginning to take effect. Relaxed, free from pain, and pleasantly drifting in and out of sleep, John began to experience an odd, floating sensation. He opened his eyes and was astonished to find himself hovering over his sleeping body on the stretcher. "I must be having one of those 'out-of-body' experiences you always read about," he thought. John was about to make a journey, a magical mystery tour of the hospital. It would prove to be an insider's look, one that TV never shows us.

Lengths of Stay   First stop on the tour was the obstetrics ward. He found himself in the centre of a flower-filled room occupied by four mothers happily nursing their recently delivered babies. This was Monday and John learned that since all of these women had delivered their babies on Saturday, they'd be going home on Wednesday or Thursday. In Canada, a nurse reminded him, it's standard practice to keep mothers who have uncomplicated natural deliveries in hospital for four or five days. This was a great improvement, he was assured, over the standard of a bygone era, which insisted women stay in for ten days. John was impressed until she informed him that American hospitals usually release women 24 to 48 hours after birth, provided there are no complications. Early discharges there are routine. Most American health plans follow mothers at home with nurses and homemakers, so there is no compromise to the health of mothers or their babies.

Thinking this over, John barely noticed that he had moved on to another part of the hospital. This was the coronary care unit (CCU) and it fairly buzzed and twinkled with lots of fancy equipment. There were plenty of nurses bustling about too, busily checking dials and reading monitors, obviously intent on healing. But the atmosphere in the CCU was hardly conducive to recovery — you could almost taste the tension. Almost all of the patients were men, lying flat on their backs with worried expressions. Most had suffered an uncomplicated heart attack, and were expected to stay in hospital for two weeks. John was reminded, this time by an intern, that even as recently as 1974, victims of heart attack were kept in hospital for six weeks. Bed rest was believed to be vitally important to recovery. In retrospect, we now know that 10 to 20% of deaths among heart attack patients in the 1950s and 1960s were caused by blood clots, a direct consequence of this enforced bed rest, once thought so therapeutic.[7] Then John was handed the results of an experiment in Britain. It showed that patients with uncomplicated heart attacks did as well at home as they did in hospital.[8] Somewhere between 48 and 72 hours of close observation in the hospital is probably more than enough time to identify any possible complications. After that, patients without complications can be discharged back to the comfort of their own homes, with help coming in as required. John was amazed, and wanted to ask the intern a few questions, but he was beginning to "float" again to another part of the hospital where even more surprises were in store for him.

Elective Surgery Next stop was the surgical ward, where John took note of how many elective surgeries* were being performed. Beds were really at a premium here, and one fellow

---

*Elective surgery means non-emergency surgery, in the sense that it can be scheduled. It does not imply that patients are given much choice about whether to have the operation, although depending on the nature of the surgery, and bed availability, patients may have a say in *when* it takes place.

patient confided that he'd had to wait months to have his gall-bladder out because of the demand for hospital beds. John was very sympathetic until he learned, from a mysterious fellow in a white coat, that for some reason Canada does ten times more gallbladder operations per capita than Denmark.[9] He first thought that perhaps this was because Canadians as a group had more gallbladder disease than the Danes, but was assured this was not the case. Puzzled, he crossed the hall with the white-coated stranger, and found a room full of women recovering from hysterectomies. Surely these were all necessary surgeries, weren't they? Once again John got a shock. The Canadian hysterectomy rate is twice that of Great Britain and continental Europe.[10] At the same time he discovered that many Canadian surgeons are performing radical mastectomies for breast cancer, despite evidence that less invasive surgery is just as effective.[11]

"What's going on?" he wondered. "Are we sicker than the rest of the world, or is it just possible we're doing more than is really necessary?"

Bed Blockers   John had barely had time to consider this disturbing conjecture when he was whisked off to the internal medicine ward. There he found himself next to an elderly patient, who looked terribly unhappy.

"My name is Sarah, do you have a minute to talk?"

"Sure," John said, pulling a chair over to her bedside.

"I've been here for months," the woman sighed. "Last November, I fell and broke my hip. I don't like to complain but it'll be Easter soon and I'm still here. I'd really like to go home but I don't see how I'd manage. My walking is just terrible — I could never handle the stairs. My doctor thinks I should go into a nursing home, but there's no room for me." She paused to take a breath before continuing. "So I've been stuck here waiting all this time. I hate the idea of going into an institution but what else can I do?"

John tried to comfort her by changing the subject. He asked about what treatment she was getting.

"Well, not much really. They explained to me that this is an acute care hospital — they don't do rehabilitation here. Every week that passes, I just seem to go further downhill." She lowered her voice to almost a whisper. "But what really gets me down is the feeling that the nurses don't like me. I know they're busy and all, but it seems that they never come in unless they have to, you know. And when they do, they're just not as friendly as they used to be. I get the feeling they'd love to be rid of me so they could use the bed for someone who's *really* ill.''

John was feeling very sorry for this lady, and wondering what on earth could be done for her, when he learned from her companion in the next bed that Canada institutionalizes its elderly at a rate almost 80% higher than the United States, and 90% higher than Britain.[12] This was one of the biggest shocks of all — there must be thousands of Sarahs in Canada. Were they all going to end up in institutions? As a society, are we Canadians really that intent on warehousing our elderly? Shaking his head and murmuring a goodbye to Sarah, John emerged into the long corridor again.

Drug Abuse   As he meandered along, negotiating a series of twists and turns, he suddenly heard a ''Psst'' from behind a partly open doorway. Moving closer, he noted a sign on the door that read PHARMACY SERVICES — AUTHORIZED PERSONNEL ONLY. John furtively looked both ways, pushed the door further open, and went in. ''I'm glad I caught you,'' said a quiet-spoken gentleman in a lab coat. ''Come in, please, and let me introduce myself. My name is Mr. Potion, I'm in charge of the pharmacy. Won't you sit down? I have a few things I'd really like to get off my chest.''

''About what?'' asked John, fearing the worst as he inched onto a stool in the dispensary's stockroom.

''Well, to begin with, I think there are a few things you ought to know about this part of the hospital, if you're interested in efficiency. For one thing, the doctors around here routinely prescribe expensive drugs when cheaper ones would work just as well. Sometimes the ones they pick are a hundred times more expensive than their therapeutic equivalents, and I can't do anything about it.''* Mr. Potion's voice grew louder as he continued. ''And there's another thing — I spend half my day filling

---

*A few hospitals in Canada do have policies which favour the substitution of therapeutic equivalents, but most do not.

prescriptions for drugs of all kinds that weren't indicated in the first place.''

"What do you mean, not indicated?" asked John.

"I mean not necessary, not suitable, a waste of money, and a possible source of harm to the patients," retorted the pharmacist, his face reddening visibly. "Let me give you an example. Antibiotics are doled out in this hospital almost like candy, and for inappropriate, trivial reasons. At the first sign of fever, down comes the prescription. In fact, so many of our patients are put on antibiotics for no reason, that if and when they really *do* get an infection requiring antibiotic treatment, the microbe often turns out to be resistant.''

"You mean the drug won't work?" asked John.

"Maybe," answered the pharmacist, "or maybe you just have to up the dose to levels that cause more side effects.''

John could feel that his medication was beginning to wear off; his attention was increasingly being drawn to his own returning discomfort. Given the pharmacist's tirade on "drug abuse," he didn't think he wanted to ask *him* for more painkiller, but as it turned out he didn't have to. In the blink of an eye, he found himself once again languishing on the stretcher in the emergency-room corridor.

Even though his insider's glimpse of how the hospital operated was only very brief and incomplete, he had a much better idea now why it was so overcrowded. Much that he had learned frightened him. He was haunted by the spectre of unnecessary surgeries — the very idea gave him the willies. Information about the wide differences between Canada's standard practices and those of some other nations made him nervous, too. And Mr. Potion's outburst only added to his growing doubts about the quality of care in the hospital. But John was first and foremost a practical man, so what distressed him most of all was the appalling waste and inefficiency he saw at virtually every stop on the tour.

"I can't understand it. Who's in charge here, anyway?"

Painfully he rolled over, only to see a friendly nurse ready with his injection. It took effect almost immediately, so John only had time to ask one more question before he dropped off to sleep:

"Before we can say hospitals need more money, don't we first have to question how they're spending what they already have?''

Perverse Incentives

You don't need a background in economics to understand that financial policies can influence decisions. If something's on sale, you're more likely to buy it. If you had a year's worth of two-for-one passes to the movies, you'd probably spend a lot more time at the cinema. A bargain's a bargain.

Provinces viewed the federal government's National Health Grants Program as a great bargain, and responded by building many new hospitals, which often duplicated existing facilities. The late Duncan Gordon, who chaired the board of Toronto's Hospital for Sick Children, identified this expansion as an important source of waste. "Look at the number of communities we have in Canada which have a Catholic hospital on one block and a Protestant one on the next. Each trying to outdo the other, to keep its grip on the community. No one ever [questioned] whether a town of 50,000 really [needed] two hospitals."

Medicare represented yet another bargain to the provinces. The total package was cost-shared 50-50 with the federal government. As long as the money went either to hospitals or doctors, every dollar the province spent was matched by another federal dollar. "This was a tremendously seductive enticement to provincial governments and it totally skewed the way provinces decided to spend money on health," says Evelyn Shapiro, a professor at the University of Manitoba's medical school and the chairperson of the Manitoba Health Services Commission. "We've had rapid expansion in the institutional sector as a result, because it could be cost-shared, and very little movement in health promotion, home care support, and other terribly important health areas because, for the most part, they were not eligible for federal funding."

With the demise of the 50-cent health dollar under EPF, the gravy train came to a dead stop. The switch to "block grants" upped the burden on provincial purses.* But current health

---

*For example, in 1977/78, prior to the implementation of EPF, federal contributions amounted to almost 45 percent of total health and social service expenditures in Québec. This figure had fallen to 39.7 percent by 1987/88. (Rapport de la Commission d'enquête sur les services de santé et les services sociaux [Rochon Commission], 1988.)

spending patterns in Canada still reflect the legacy of 50-50 cost-sharing. To see what we mean, look at the percentage breakdown of health spending for 1987 in Figure 2.2.

Figure 2-2: Health Spending In Canada 1987

Hospitals	40%
Other institutions*	11%
Physician Services	16%
Drugs	11%
Dentists' Services	5%
Capital Expenditures	4%
Public Health	4%**
Appliances	2%
Other	7%

100%

(*Source:* Health and Welfare Canada, 1987)

*Other institutions include nursing homes, homes for the aged, and facilities referred to as "homes for special care."

**Estimate.

And the Winner Is . . . Hospitals

As you can see, hospitals are by far the largest consumers of our health care dollars, gobbling up 40% of the budget. The fastest growth in the hospital sector in Canada occurred in the 1950s, when the federal government offered grants to encourage hospital construction. By the 1970s, once restraints on expansion were in place, the situation had stabilized. But these restrictions on capital funding were not enough to control hospital costs, since the major source of expenditure comes from what hospitals *do*, not what they *have*. Professor Robert Evans points out in his book, *Strained Mercy*, that "the most prominent growth pattern in the hospital sector has been the increase in costs per patient-day, adjusted for general inflation." For the 30 years preceding 1976, we had average increases in costs per patient-day of over seven percent.[13] Evidence from Québec suggests that growth in the number of services accounted for as much as one-quarter of the spending increase hospitals there experienced between 1975 and 1984 — and this was during a period when occupancy levels in Québec hospitals were actually falling.[14]

Evelyn Shapiro confirms that the increased number of services provided has had a tremendous impact on costs. "Our hospital budget in Manitoba has grown by 70% in four years [1982/83 to 1986/87]. This was not a period of high inflation, nor were huge increases in labour costs a factor. Our population didn't grow. The number of hospital beds didn't increase. But the number of *services* skyrocketed. I find that hard to explain."

Martin Barkin, former president of Toronto's Sunnybrook Hospital and now deputy health minister for Ontario, says that Canadians annually use 1,200 hospital bed-days for each 1,000 in our population. The rate in the United States is 800 bed-days per 1000.[15] Since there's no evidence to suggest we are 50% sicker than Americans, the explanation must lie elsewhere.

Hospitals may be the biggest spenders in our system but they are also the least accountable to us in terms of how they spend that money. A curious feature of hospitals is that they are not funded on the basis of what they do, or even on how well their patients do. On top of that, a hospital's decisions about how and where to spend its budget are almost totally within its own control.

Hospitals are funded mainly by global budgets, based on their own forecasts about how much will be needed to run their operations. These lump-sum grants are then divided up according to internal hospital priorities and pressures. Typically, over 70% of hospital operating budgets go to fixed costs, and most of these are for labour. Other operating expenses — pharmacy, and laboratory and other diagnostic activities — account for most of the remainder. For hospitals wishing to expand their programs, the margin for manoeuvring is usually quite limited, particularly in provinces which have instituted tough restraint policies. Capital funding for new equipment or other facilities has been severely curtailed in most provinces.

Given the high proportion of health spending they control, it is unfortunate that hospitals in our system are given few incentives to use their resources wisely. On the contrary, the funding mechanisms now in place offer every incentive for them to overspend and exceed their budgets. Ted Ball, a Toronto health-care consultant, explains with an example from Ontario: "You get some doctor arguing that his hospital needs to have a better cardiac care capability than the one around the block. And if the board argues, the doctor says that without this new unit people will die. So the board crumbles. And lo and behold, at the end of the year, the hospital is facing a $5 million deficit. This is labelled government *underfunding*."

When enough hospitals accumulate large deficits, they collectively turn around and demand a provincial bailout. This can cost taxpayers additional millions, all because there is no rational planning taking place, and no incentives for efficiency. Ball continues, "Hospital boards don't think beyond the confines of the bricks and mortar of their own institutions, they don't look at the health needs of the population they serve, or at prudent, low-cost methods of meeting those needs. They look at ways they can increase their share of the pie."

In September of 1988, 117 of Ontario's 222 hospitals were operating in the red.[16] For example, the Cambridge Memorial Hospital, which had a $1.4 million deficit in 1987, has predicted a $3 million loss for this year, and is threatening to close beds, lay off staff, and charge user fees if the government fails to come to its aid.[17]

Unaccountable Accounting

But when hospital administrators say they need more money, it doesn't mean they have a good idea about where the funds they already have are going. Hospitals vary greatly in size but the larger ones have annual budgets of over $100 million. Can you imagine any other industry of this size lacking this fundamental financial knowledge? How can we expect rational planning and coordination to take place in this information vacuum?

Sunnybrook Hospital's president, Peter Ellis, says a hospital is just about the only "business" you'll ever find that has no idea what its product — "a healthy patient" — costs to produce.[18] He's working to change that at Sunnybrook with the help of a newly designed computer information system, which will be able to track patients — along with the services they use, and their costs — throughout their hospital stay. As well, the

Canadian Hospital Association has initiated a project, a new Management Information System, that will match clinical services and their costs to individual patients. But it's not going to be implemented for another ten years.

Despite these promising beginnings, it's still fair to say that most hospitals in Canada have virtually no handle on what it costs to run their services. Michael Dector, a former cabinet secretary in Manitoba, now a health care consultant in Winnipeg, shows how this lack of concern about costs permeates the hospital system: "When national hospital insurance was introduced, one of the first things hospitals did was to get rid of their cost accountants. They didn't need to know anymore what their programs were costing since someone else was paying the shot. So they lost the ability to find out what was driving costs upwards."

Since we don't really have a handle on how much, say, an intensive care unit costs each year, we don't have any basis for determining whether it is or isn't being efficiently operated. We have no way of comparing its operation to others. And when that unit requests more resources, we have no way of knowing whether putting more money in will achieve desired results.

This type of comparative information is important within the hospital as well. Hospitals are traditionally organized by department: internal medicine, cardiology, obstetrics and gynecology, and so on. The daily operating costs for a bed can vary greatly from one department to another. Peter Ellis says that without a detailed understanding of these differences, the arbitrary decision to reallocate three beds from one kind of care to another can have unforeseen consequences. "You could easily have tripled your costs without even realizing what you'd done or how you'd done it."[19]

Hospital boards are well aware that their operating costs are primarily controlled by physicians, who have a virtually unlimited capacity to generate services for their patients.* Boards which fail to address this fundamental issue inevitably run into financial difficulty.

---

*For more details about how physician behaviour can generate demand, see Chapter 6.

Governments Cop Out

Duncan Gordon made the point that ministries of health haven't been much help to hospitals in the planning process. "Nobody ever tells us what services we should be providing. When a specialist moves to a new area and the hospital takes him on staff, what does he do? Right away he starts building up his specialty. He's going to do everything he can to get more space, equipment, and support staff. Nobody looks at whether there's a requirement for that specialty. And the poor hospital board doesn't know whether to say yes or no. We have to eliminate this kind of empire-building and encourage governments to accept some responsibility for setting guidelines and standards."

Indeed, most provincial governments seem to have completely abdicated their duty when it comes to seeing that our health dollars are well spent. Part of the reason is that health ministries have only recently had to administer our system as a whole. Prior to Medicare, these ministries functioned as the administrative arm for the public health departments — they never ventured into the hospital sector, except for mental health. Health ministries have very few people with training in clinical epidemiology or economic evaluation. As a result they have a great deal of difficulty determining whether things work, and if they do, whether they are cost-effective. Ted Ball comments, "The hospital branch in Ontario only employs about 50 non-clerical people, and yet they are responsible for a $6 billion budget! They don't have nearly the capability they require for strategic planning or good resource management. They're too busy writing cheques!"

A further obstacle to government action is the sheer complexity of our system. Managing it wisely requires a broad background in a number of disciplines. Few ministers have time to develop this expertise before they're switched to another portfolio. At the very least, it requires clear thinking — a quality not always evident among our elected representatives. As an example, one senior civil servant shared the following conversation he'd had with his health minister about a decade ago. (He agreed we could use it provided no names were revealed.)

CIVIL SERVANT: Minister, I'm concerned about hospital deficits. The way things are now, we penalize those few hospitals which manage to come in below budget by taking away their surpluses. But the vast majority wind up with huge cost overruns, which we then reward by covering their losses. The system we have now actually encourages waste because the easiest way to get a bigger budget is to overspend. Why don't we try rewarding good management by allowing hospitals to keep their surpluses?*

> MINISTER: But we can't do that! If we allowed well-managed hospitals to keep their surpluses, how would we ever be able to cover the deficits of the poorly managed ones?

The muddy thinking reflected in this conversation is still only part of the problem. More important by far are the political consequences for governments who try to limit hospital spending. Civil servants are stymied by conflicting mandates: they are obliged to come up with a rational accounting of how public monies are being spent, but at the same time, must protect their minister from criticism and public embarrassment. The latter mandate represents by far the most pervasive obstacle, for when hospitals gang up to get more money, they really know how to turn on the pressure. Their tactics? They use the same time-tested strategy on governments as their own doctors use on them. And governments don't find it any easier to resist the "people are going to die" arguments than hospital boards do.

In summary, hospitals are very astute lobbyists. For example, when a hospital board chairperson comes to see a minister of health, he delicately but firmly makes it very clear that if government isn't willing to cough up the money, the board will just have to close the obstetrics ward, or maybe the emergency department. Implicit or explicit threats of this kind add fuel to an already smoldering antagonism between provider groups and health ministers, but they can be very effective. As well, most hospitals have fully developed public relations departments whose sole

---

*Some provinces nowadays do allow hospitals to retain part or even all of their surpluses, but as Robert Evans points out in *Strained Mercy* (Butterworth, 1984), "hospital administrators tend to believe that such surpluses may be removed from next year's budget." Considering the powerful incentives to overspend which derive from the high probability that governments will step in and cover all losses, the promise of retaining surpluses is far too weak an instrument to encourage good management.

function is to promote their institution to the public. And of course the press delights in the drama of such stories.

Hospitals are also very successful entrepreneurs, always on the lookout for new sources of funding. When, for example, Ontario was trying to expand community mental health services, much of the money slated for the community somehow found its way back into the hospital system. Hospitals have found they can word their funding proposals so that the prospective service sounds convincingly like a community program. In one Ontario hospital, for example, the psychiatric department decided to go after these "community" dollars by proposing a ten-bed supportive-housing project for mental health patients. Included in their proposal was a budget item for $150,000 for sessional fees for a physician. "Now maybe if that program had actually been run out of and by the community, some of those funds would have been used to purchase psychiatric treatment," says Ted Ball, "but the rest would have gone to activation programs, drop-in centres, training, and a host of other badly needed options."

Doesn't it seem like a cruel hoax to suggest that life on a mental-health ward in a hospital is anything remotely like the "supportive community-living arrangements" these monies were intended to fund? What's particularly frustrating is that government bureaucracy plays the "dupe" in this farce. They lack faith in low-cost, community-based activities. According to Ball, they would rather "hyper-fund" professional groups than provide money where it's really needed.

Bigger Isn't Necessarily Better

Our saying all this doesn't mean we blame hospitals for going after as much as they can get. Who wouldn't? But we're still left wondering why their success is not measured in terms of patient outcome. How much difference does a hospital make to the health status of the people living in its community? We neither know nor seemingly care. Instead, within their own corporate culture, the most successful hospitals are those with the biggest budgets, the most high-tech technology, and the most prestigious medical staffs. As long as governments fail to provide different incentives, and continue to offer program money without establishing tight criteria for its use, hospitals will keep on expanding their empires.

The next time you hear about waiting lists for elective surgery, or how hard it is to get into a chronic care or nursing home bed, or how overcrowded the emergency department is in your local hospital, remember John D. Unnecessary surgery, over-long hospital stays, and the inappropriate use of institutions may have more to do with explaining the problem than lack of funds.

Priming the Pump: Doctors

To understand why our health system costs as much as it does, you need to understand who controls it. Government, as the paymaster of our system, theoretically has ultimate control — they do, after all, approve the budgets and write the cheques. But it's important to remember that doctors are the gatekeepers to our system and, as such, control access to all hospital and medical services. They hold the real power: you can't be admitted to a hospital, see a specialist, have a test done, or get a prescription, without first seeing a physician. Doctors, and doctors alone, make the decisions about what services their patients receive.

Most doctors in Canada are paid by government on a fee-for-service basis. The more they do, the more they make. On the face of it this seems very fair; medicine is a profession we all rely on, and most would agree that doctors have a right to reasonable compensation for their expertise. Medical practitioners, intent on protecting their professional freedom, argue that they must remain in charge of deciding what their patients need, and further, that the system must have the flexibility to provide whatever services they deem "necessary" to meet those needs.

This implies that the *only* influence on doctors' decision-making is their objective assessment of patient needs. It completely ignores the possibility that professional judgment may be swayed, consciously or unconsciously, by the economic incentives inherent in the fee-for-service system. Further, it implies that the services doctors decide are "necessary" are in fact the best way to meet patient needs. And finally, it assumes that when the health care system fails to provide enough resources to meet those needs, it is a clear indication of "underfunding."

Physicians today enjoy high incomes, but this wasn't always the case. In the old pre-Medicare days, getting paid was a big problem for many doctors, and bad debts were a common complaint. For example, during the Great Depression, the government of Saskatchewan had to pay stipends to physicians just to keep them in business. But national public health insurance put an end to bad debts once and for all, and today, the average physician can look forward to an income 400% higher than the average industrial wage.

Governments face a dilemma when it comes to fee-for-service reimbursement. They fully understand the extent to which doctors are responsible for the high cost of health care, but they shy away from the prospect of being accused of interfering in the way physicians practice medicine. At the same time, governments recognize that fee-for-service is extraordinarily flexible in its ability to generate income for any number of physicians. That wouldn't be so bad if the rest of us didn't have to pay for all that flexibility.

One of the best-documented examples of this phenomenon comes from Manitoba, which like the rest of the country has too many doctors. (See also Chapter 6.) The problem is most severe in Winnipeg, where between 1971 and 1981, the number of general practitioners increased by two-thirds.[20] This explosion in the physician population resulted from a disastrous government decision in the late 1960s to expand existing medical schools and build new ones. At the time, governments expected that our population would continue growing as it had during the baby-boom years. But the boom became a barely audible peep; indeed, Winnipeg's population remained virtually the same through the 1970s.

In any normal market economy, a drastic increase in the number of providers without any similar increase in the number of consumers would produce fierce competition for customers. You would expect this competition to bring down prices. But this didn't happen in Winnipeg. Particularly fierce competition usually also implies that some providers will be edged out of the market altogether. But this didn't happen in Winnipeg, either. At the very least, one would expect physicians' overall incomes to drop. Nope, not in Winnipeg. In their book, *Manitoba and Medicare*, the authors report that "in aggregate, adjusting for fee schedule increases, there was little significant difference between the gross revenues generated by a physician in 1971/72 versus the gross revenues generated by a physician in 1981/82 . . . . This illustrates the flexibility with which the fee-for-service system can accommodate an increase in physicians,'' even with no increase in population.[21]

Unhealthy Health Care

Fee-for-service also seems to encourage doctors to become workaholics. The financial rewards to those who see more patients, and work longer hours, are there for the taking and provide a strong temptation to go overboard, even to the detriment of the physician's own mental and physical health. Dr. Leo-Paul Landry, executive director of the Canadian Medical Association, asks, "Why is it that doctors have a higher suicide rate, take more drugs, divorce more frequently, and die sooner than others at the same socio-economic level?" In his opinion, the straight-jacket of fee-for-service medicine is a contributing factor to physician illness. The temptation to maximize income is very strong. For example, if an Ontario physician who normally works five days a week, decides to go into the office on Saturdays too, that additional eight hours a week can generate an extra $45,000 a year in net income!* Even if this means doctors have less recreational time to spend with their families, economic gains of this magnitude are hard to pass up. The point is, fee-for-service medicine may be just as unhealthy for doctors as it is for their patients.

The Fee Schedule: Ticket to Prosperity

The fee schedule establishes a price for each medical service or procedure covered by public insurance. People frequently have the mistaken idea that fee-schedule increases for doctors are imposed on them by government. This is not the case. Medical associations and provincial governments *together* negotiate the overall increase in the fee schedule. And it is the medical associations, not the governments, that decide how the money should

---

*This calculation assumes the doctor receives an average per-visit billing of $20 and sees six patients an hour. Both are low rather than high estimates of actual earning potential.

be allocated to different specialties and services. Once government has agreed to the percentage increase in the fee schedule, its role in controlling physician costs is over.*

Most of the doctors who serve on the executive councils of medical associations in Canada are specialists. Perhaps because of the demands on their time, general practitioners find it more difficult to participate in this important political function. Similarly, when the associations establish committees to allocate the fee schedule's new resources, most of the participants on these committees are specialists too. Consequently, performing a procedure, especially a surgery, pays much better on a per-hour basis than taking a good history or just listening to how someone feels.

As one doctor reported, "As long as it involves operating on someone, or sticking something into them, like a needle or a probe, it pays well. Over time, we've seen fee schedules gradually expanding the earning potential of specialists, while general practitioners have been left out in the cold."

In this way, the fee schedule may actually promote the overuse of some of the most expensive medical therapies, while at the same time discouraging many other types of treatment that might be equally effective (if not more so). Disease prevention, patient education, and health-promotion activities don't pay the physician nearly as well as other more intrusive therapies. For example, doctors can and should encourage their patients to quit smoking. In Ontario this kind of counselling pays less than $90 an hour. A doctor can easily make $140 in that same hour merely be seeing seven people with colds, who don't really need a physician's care at all. Which would you do?

It would be naive to assume that these biases in the fee schedule have no influence on the way doctors practice medicine. It's quite possible that Canada's higher rates for various surgeries and diagnostic tests are a reflection of the perverse economic incentives inherent in our fee schedules. Nick Poushinski worked as an advisor to a former minister of health in Manitoba. He says there's no problem with fee-for-service, as long as you believe

---

*This is changing. In British Columbia, for example, the government and the medical profession have negotiated an overall utilization cap. In 1987, the government required BC doctors to pay back $12 million because this cap had been exceeded.

that more medical interventions are likely to produce better health. But, he cautions, that's simply not the case.

Does this mean doctors deliberately overservice their patients just to make money? We think that's unlikely. As Michael Dector points out, "A lot of overservicing is quite unconscious."

The Myths about America

Doctors often argue that the high cost of health care in Canada is the direct result of "socialized medicine." They say that if we returned to a more private system, such as they have in the United States, we could add much-needed billions to our health care budgets. This argument stems from several misconceptions about both systems, which need debunking. To start with, Canada does *not* have socialized medicine; in point of fact, 95% of our doctors work for themselves, not for the state, and 90% of our hospitals are private, non-profit corporations.* What we *do* have is a publicly funded system which pays private providers, as opposed to a largely privately funded system, which is what the Americans have.

In fact, many Americans envy Canada's system, and some politicians, like Senator Edward Kennedy, would like to see something like it evolve there. The reasons are economic as well as humanitarian. A recent *New England Journal of Medicine* article pointed out that the administrative costs of private insurance in America represented 10% of expenditures on health. In Canada, which has public insurance, the figure is 2.5%.[22] Similarly, hospital administration and accounting costs are much higher in the United States, as is the proportion of a physician's gross income that goes toward overhead expense. The authors concluded that if America were to adopt a Canadian-style system, they could *save* over eight percent of their total health spending.[23]

As a further proof of the economic advantages of our publicly funded system, let's return to the graph showing health spending as a proportion of GNP. In 1987, Canada spent 8.6% of its GNP on health, while the United States spent 11%.[24] And

---

*Major exceptions are federally owned and operated veterans' hospitals and provincial psychiatric hospitals.

although our costs have increased over time, we haven't experienced nearly as rapid a rate of increase as the United States. There's no question that national health insurance has saved us billions of dollars.

There is also a political argument against the American system. We Canadians view access to needed medical services as a right, and reject the notion that greater ability to pay automatically entitles someone to better health care. The public insurance scheme we know as Medicare was set up to guarantee that every Canadian could see the doctor or receive hospital treatment without worrying about crippling costs.

Meanwhile, nearly 40 million Americans are not so fortunate; they have no health insurance coverage at all.[25] Without it, of course, one major illness can wipe out a person's life savings. Many Americans belong to the working poor — too "wealthy" to qualify for public assistance under Medicaid, but too young to take advantage of U.S. Medicare, which covers hospital and doctors' services for seniors — and simply cannot afford to pay for a private health plan.

To give you some idea of how expensive health insurance is in the United States, a family of four living in Bethlehem, Pennsylvania, pays $2,200 [U.S.] a year just for hospital and drug coverage. Office visits to the doctor are not covered. And there's a $1,000 deductible which must be paid out-of-pocket before the insurance coverage begins. In the local hospital there, a sign is prominently displayed over the admitting desk in the emergency room: IF YOU CAN'T PAY, WE CAN'T TREAT. Other signs in evidence would be much more familiar to the average Canadian, though not in a hospital setting. We mean, of course, credit-card acceptance plaques assuring customers that WE TAKE VISA OR MASTERCHARGE. Such a cold-hearted, all-business approach, whenever they encounter it, tends to shock Canadians into blessing parliamentarians like Tommy Douglas and Monique Bégin for their commitment to a more equitable system.

Separate Agendas

In 1983/84, the Canadian Medical Association (CMA) spent $500,000 on a study they thought would prove that our health care system was underfinanced.[26] Chairing the task force for this study was Joan Watson, the noted consumer reporter and former host of CBC's "Marketplace." The other members of the task force were equally prestigious: Pauline McGibbon, former lieutenant-governor of Ontario; Roy Romanow, former attorney general of Saskatchewan; Dr. John O'Brien-Bell; and Dr. Leon Richard. Both physicians have been presidents of the CMA.

The task force travelled the country and heard briefs from hundreds of individuals and organizations. Woods Gordon, the consulting firm, investigated what impact the aging of our population would have on future demands for health services. Their report led the task force to conclude that for economic as well as humane reasons, we need to shift the focus away from institutional solutions, toward "a new program of care . . . which emphasizes independent and productive living at home."

The task force also contracted McMaster University to study how the rapid introduction of new medical technology has affected medical practice and costs. This research found that "although some modern technologies can indeed achieve remarkable results, it would appear that there are others which may in fact be useless or even harmful." The task force therefore recommended establishing a National Health Technology Assessment Council to formulate a set of uniform guidelines "for evaluating, acquiring, operating and funding high technology."

As for underfunding, the task force in its final report concluded: "We cannot assess the extent of existing *inefficiencies*, and because there is no guarantee that putting more money into the system is necessarily the best way of improving health, the Task Force cannot make a clear-cut recommendation."

In essence, this report confirms what John D. learned on his hospital tour: our system's inefficiencies have to be assessed and resolved before any decision can be made about whether it actually needs more money. But clearly this was not the conclusion the CMA hoped for.

The task force tabled its report in August 1984, and the CMA's council promptly referred it to the board of directors for "more study." Since that time, no action has been taken. As recently as March 1986, the CMA issued a policy statement warning that the system was "dangerously underfunded."[27]

Among people in the know, few agree with this diagnosis. Even within Canada's medical and hospital establishment, a number of prominent players prefer to hedge the question. When asked if he thought the system was underfunded, Dr. John Evans, who chaired an Ontario commission on health care, responded obliquely, "Compared to what?" When the same question was put to J.C. Martin, executive director of the Canadian Hospital Association, he said the issue of money was secondary to establishing goals. He believes we can't assess whether the system is underfunded "unless we know what we want to achieve, and set some objectives." The CMA's executive director, Dr. Leo-Paul Landry, claims the whole issue is a political one, and can't be deduced from the facts.

In contrast, there is a high level of consensus among academics and government officials that the current level of health funding is, at the very least, adequate, if not over-generous. "I'm one of those who comes right out and says that our system is actually overfunded," says Professor Pran Manga, who teaches health administration at the University of Ottawa.

Professor Manga is a well-known critic of our health system. He achieved considerable notoriety when he was called as the first witness for the parliamentary hearings on the Canada Health Act in 1984. Flora Macdonald had been very vigorous throughout the questioning period, and although Manga believes he gave "very good answers," she didn't seem to like what he had to say. At one point she went so far as to suggest he was nothing more than a "cold-blooded economist." Manga waited for an opportunity to retaliate, and didn't have to wait long. They were discussing what to do about the oversupply of physicians when he told Macdonald that one solution would be to close one or two medical schools. Right away she asked, "Which ones?"

"Well," he replied, "you could start with Queen's."

All hell broke loose then, remembers Manga. "She got out of her chair and came menacingly towards me and [gesturing a mock kick] went with her foot, like so." With a puckish smile, he adds, "Queen's was in her riding."

Turf Wars

Doctors may exert the most influence over our health care system, and the costs it generates, but they aren't the only players in the field. A host of other providers from as many as 40 different occupational groups are constantly jockeying for position. Relationships within and among these groups are often strained and even acrimonious. Name-calling, professional disparagement, and even censure have not been at all uncommon in the past, and even today, certain groups seem to attract more than their share of abuse.

We've already talked about how the dominance of specialists in the medical associations has tended to improve that sector's income potential at the expense of general practitioners. But that's only one example of struggle within the hierarchy. Meanwhile, nurse practitioners — professionals who can deliver quality patient care at lower cost — aren't allowed to bill our system directly. Nurse practitioners face formidable resistance from doctors, who view their scope of practice as a direct threat to their own territory.

At the same time, nurses are demanding wider recognition of their particular skills, and their professional associations are busy trying to convince doctors and government that nursing is a profession "separate and distinct from medicine, but equally important." The Canadian Nurses Association is lobbying for all new nurses to have university training by the year 2000. These "baccalaureate" nurses are now a minority in the profession, but won't be for long if this policy becomes reality. Most Canadian nurses joining the profession today have been trained in community colleges; they see this move as a threat and wonder whether our system will still have room for them in the future.

All told, there are dozens of different health professionals and para-professionals, each with their own agenda. Bogna Andersson, executive director of the Ontario Speech and Hearing Association, cites one example of territorial squabbling, in this case between audiologists, who evaluate hearing, and the group of physicians most affected by their work — the ear, nose, and throat specialists (ENTs).

"It's provincial policy that audiologists be supervised by and work in association with ENT physicians," Andersson says. "Audiologists are not even supposed to own their equipment. The fact remains that the expertise for testing and evaluating individuals with hearing loss rests with audiologists. They have the training for it, not doctors. But physicians insist on retaining control in this area of health care, as in every other one."

We could document similar turf battles involving many other provider groups, like midwives, chiropodists, chiropractors, naturopaths, and homeopaths. Each wants a piece of the action but remains for the most part outside our publicly funded system. If we have evidence to show that these practitioners can deliver effective, high-quality care at a lower cost, their participation should be actively encouraged, not locked out by vested interests.

Cost Containment

Governments fully recognize the power that doctors and hospitals have, and know only too painfully that trying to exercise authority over them can have nasty side effects. All the same, provincial health ministries have made some attempts at containing costs, mainly by squeezing hospital budgets wherever possible, and by controlling the supply of doctors.

Several provinces have gone the route of reducing enrollments in medical schools, or lowering the number of internship and residency positions funded, or both. While he was Ontario's health minister, Larry Grossman questioned the wisdom of producing more and more pediatricians when the proportion of children in the population was falling, and asked why the demand for other more urgently needed specialists — geriatricians, oncologists,* and so on — was being left unmet.

"It made absolutely no sense," Grossman observed, "so I started with a five percent cut in residency positions and then tried to return them to areas where there was a shortage. But I learned there was enormous resistance from physicians in hospitals, who said, 'I can't carry out my surgical work without resi-

---

*Specialists concerned with aging and cancer respectively.

dents to help run the place.' Well, that's not a reason to graduate a specialist who's going to practice for 30 years — because you need him for twelve months as an extra hand to hold a retractor. So I ignored them and made the cuts.''

British Columbia has attempted to gain some control over its ballooning physician population by placing a cap on the number of doctors who can bill the insurance scheme in certain geographical areas considered to be over-doctored. But restricting billing numbers was ruled unconstitutional in BC and the Supreme Court of Canada has refused to hear an appeal of the decision.

Manitoba has taken a hard line on hospitals by categorically refusing bail-outs to institutions that have gone over budget.* In December 1987, then-Minister of Health Wilson Parasiuk announced that 114 acute care beds would be closed to eliminate hospital deficits. He also announced that Manitoba would put $50 million into a trust fund to develop more community programs — programs expected to reduce demand on acute care facilities. The second of these initiatives was short-circuited by the defeat of the NDP and the election of the Conservatives in the spring of 1988.

Alberta took a new tack (some might say, a politically courageous one) and actually de-insured certain types of services; in 1987 they announced that the province would no longer pay doctors for family planning counselling, tubal ligations, vasectomies, or periodic eye examinations.** Professor Richard Plain, among others, criticized the choice of services Alberta decided to exclude from coverage. Sterilization, contraceptive counselling, and eye exams are important preventive measures of long-proven effectiveness. Why pick on these when there are so many richer sources of wasteful spending? In the face of mounting criticism, Alberta was forced to back off partway; in the spring of 1988, the province announced that it was re-insuring sterilizations, and by July, eye examinations were back as an insured service too.

---

*Québec and recently Ontario have instituted the same "no bail-out" policy.

**Only *non-medically necessary* sterilizations were de-insured. It's hard to say exactly what this meant — whether, for example, it considered the potential damage to mental health as an indication of "necessity" for either procedure.

Usually governments try to enlist support from provider groups before introducing cost-control measures. But since these groups rarely agree on solutions, a consensus is hard to come by. Governments also know from experience that bitterness and poor morale are sure to follow any unilateral action. The instruments provinces have at their disposal are too blunt for problems of such complexity and subtlety. Using them injudiciously can affect quality and undermine the cooperative climate so essential to the development of a more efficient and rational system.

Canada's health care system is like an orchestra without a conductor. Without someone to lead, there's no common vision — no agreement even about what should be played, let alone *how* it should be played. Think how an orchestra sounds before the concertmaster calls its players to tune up. Total cacophony — sound without meaning. The players go their own way, and the loudest and shrillest instruments tend to rise above the general chaos to get our attention, even though the parts they play may be small.

But when a conductor steps onto the podium and signals his readiness to begin, the most wonderful transformation occurs: chaos becomes order, selfishness gives way to cooperation, distractions dissolve into concentrated attention on a common goal, and the music in the score comes to life.

Surely, $46 billion is more than enough money to provide all Canadians with quality health care. But until we find ways to eliminate the system's chronic waste and inefficiency, and until we can dispense with the internal wrangling among health professionals, and the external tug-of-war between governments and providers, no amount will ever be enough.

Chapter 3

Medicine, the Un-Science

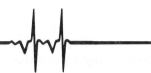

WITH BILLIONS OF DOLLARS squandered every year on useless or inappropriate medical services, it's fair to diagnose waste as health care's chronic illness. Why is there so much waste? Much of it stems from the unscientific way doctors practice medicine.

Criticizing medicine carries the two-fold risk of offending practitioners and alarming the public. Neither is our intention. Even though "doctor-bashing" has become a popular sport among journalists, the analysis presented in this chapter is not meant as an attack on the personal integrity of physicians, most of whom are dedicated and hard-working professionals. Nor, by exposing some of the inadequacies of current practice, do we wish to scare readers so much they avoid seeking needed treatment. Nevertheless, public debate on the issues we raise is long overdue and urgently required. There remains little doubt that the lack of "science" in medicine leads directly to a lot of unwarranted intervention, which not only wastes scarce resources but risks harming patients as well.

Admittedly, it sounds preposterous to suggest medicine is unscientific. Doctors are scientists, aren't they? Look at the enormous amount of biological knowledge they have to cram in at medical school. And what about all the miraculous medical advances made possible thanks to science — the new sophisticated surgeries, revolutionary drugs, and high-tech equipment we hear about every day? Doesn't the connection between science and medical progress prove medicine is scientific?

In a word, no. Doctors routinely make decisions about how to diagnose and treat patients without regard to scientific evidence. Most of the time it's not their fault, because there isn't any solid evidence to go on. But even when there *is* good scientific research, doctors may discount it, if it fails to coincide with their own intuition.

Medicine is all about decision-making: physicians have to decide what questions to ask the patient, what tests to order to establish a diagnosis, what treatment to recommend. Most people assume that these decisions are clear-cut, but very often they aren't. Medicine is full of uncertainties:

> Doctors are confronted with patients who have symptoms and syndromes, not labels with their diseases. A set of symptoms can be associated with any of several diseases. The chest pains produced by a gall bladder attack and by a heart attack can be confused by excellent doctors.[1]

Many times doctors are able to establish a diagnosis on the basis of the patient's history and a physical examination, but sometimes finding out exactly what's wrong with a patient can be very difficult. Two research studies comparing the cause of death listed on death certificates with the autopsy reports that followed found that up to 40% of the diagnoses were incorrect![2] This only goes to show that doctors are not infallible. Medicine is tough. Even with modern diagnostic technology, gross errors are quite common.

Even when the diagnosis is reasonably certain, for many medical conditions there are several possible treatments. Should the person with chronic back pain be given surgery, or bed rest and medication? Will a cancer patient do better on chemotherapy, radiation, surgery, or a combination of two or more of these? What's the best way for doctors to choose among these alternatives? How can they weigh the risks versus the advantages?

Science has provided useful tools for resolving some of these uncertainties, but usually medicine has ignored them. This harsh assessment is based on three observations.

1. We don't know what works: Most medical therapies have never been rigorously evaluated to see whether they work or not.

Testing new ideas — the very core of scientific inquiry — is the exception in medicine, not the rule. Even when it is done, it's usually carried out too late, long after the innovation has been adopted by professional groups, endorsed by insurers, and accepted by the public. History shows how often we've been deceived by failing to test. What's more, there's no guarantee that what evidence we do have is incorporated into clinical practice. There are thousands of medical journals published today, although only a few dozen are truly prestigious. The physician with a busy practice is at a disadvantage when it comes to selecting those studies which have clinical relevance to his or her work. Although computer information systems are now helping to link the doctors' office to the world of academic medicine, there's little doubt that physicians continue to employ many therapies even when research has shown them to be of no benefit.

Here are two examples. Many surgeons are still doing radical mastectomies, even though it's been known for some time that this operation for breast cancer is no more effective, and a lot more disfiguring, than a partial mastectomy.[3] Also, one leading American cardiologist has suggested that many of the 350,000 patients who have heart bypass surgery every year in the United States would do as well on medication.[4] We don't know how many unnecessary bypass operations occur in Canada* — we've never researched the question. In fact, Canada has no coordinated policy to make sure innovations in diagnosis and treatment are rigorously evaluated. The vast majority of medical technologies, which are foisted on an unsuspecting population and paid for out of the public purse, have never been proven as to their safety or effectiveness.

2. We don't train doctors in critical appraisal: Although doctors use the fruits of science, they don't know how to apply them scientifically. Medical training places very little emphasis on teaching doctors how to think in a scientific way. Instead, students are required to master a body of scientific "facts," without being given the analytical tools that would help them apply this information.[5]

---

*As of 1980, Canada's per capita rate of bypass surgery was about half that of the U.S. (OECD, *Measuring Health Care,* p. 118.)

Human beings differ very widely in the ways they respond to disease and therapies; medicine is full of uncertainties. A physician, based on his own limited experience, has no way of predicting accurately how an individual patient will respond to a particular intervention. The responses of thousands of patients must be analysed to establish probable outcomes. That's why interpreting medical information requires knowledge of both statistics and proper research design. Yet most graduates emerge from medical school without even a rudimentary understanding of either. As a result, they have trouble judging the quality *or even the meaning* of what little evaluation research has been done. Inadequate training has robbed doctors of the very skills they need in order to make good decisions about how to diagnose and treat patients.

3. The quality of medical research is highly variable: Much of continuing medical education displays a woeful lack of scientific rigour. To update their knowledge and skills, doctors must rely on the information they get by reading journals and attending conferences. But the quality of both information sources is highly variable. A review of research studies in medical literature revealed that almost 75% of the reports drew conclusions which were either unsupported by the evidence or invalid.[6] Dr. David Eddy has reviewed the published literature on drug treatment for glaucoma, a major cause of blindness.[7] Treatments for glaucoma include laser therapy and surgery, or both, but usually drugs are tried first in an effort to reduce high pressure within the eye, a sign associated with the disease. Dr. Eddy discovered that there have been many randomized controlled trials comparing various drug treatments, and that the drugs differ mainly in their side effects, many of which can be quite severe. In terms of effectiveness, no drug was shown to be better than any other in stopping the progression of field defects and blindness. But Dr. Eddy was unable to find any high-quality research comparing drug treatment with doing nothing at all. The few studies which did make this comparison were flawed, but if anything, they suggested that drug treatment did more harm than no treatment at all.

Another cause for concern about the quality of medical evidence is that reports of case studies, which are subjective and therefore inherently unscientific, by far outnumber scientifically valid investigations. This is the case in both the literature and the conference hall. No doubt, studies based on such anecdotal evidence are more interesting — and, given the orientation of medical education, much easier to understand — but that doesn't make them valid. Unsubstantiated research has had too much influence on medical practice for too long.

In combination, these three factors — the failure to test its own practices, inadequate training, and the prevalence of poor-quality research masquerading as good evidence in continuing medical education — cast serious doubt on medicine's claim to be considered a science at all.

It might help to remember that the historical link between science and medicine is a recent one, dating only from the last decades of the 1800s. The traditions of these two fields evolved quite separately, which perhaps explains why medicine, by far the older, still resists the scientific method.

Science: The New Magic

Throughout its five centuries of development, science was slowly but relentlessly displacing the non-rational ideologies which had prevailed in the West for thousands of years. By the late 1800s, science finally won out over magic and mysticism to become the dominant belief system. Science was "hot" — the wave of the future. It didn't take long for society to realize what a powerful tool it had adopted. The new technologies science made possible would affect almost every aspect of life — transportation, agriculture, manufacturing, communication, and of course medicine.

What made science such a powerhouse then and now is its method of obtaining information. The word *science* means "knowledge," but a more accurate definition would be "knowledge obtained through the *scientific method*." Briefly, this method involves identifying a problem, suggesting a solution (the hypothesis), designing and conducting a test to see if the solution works (the experiment), recording the results of the test (the observations), and finally, drawing conclusions based on the results. If this process upholds the solution, the hypothesis becomes a new theory. If it fails, it's back to the drawing board to do more thinking.

Objectivity is a critical component of the scientific method, but one which is very difficult to achieve and maintain. People have a personal investment in their own ideas — it's part of being human — and scientists are no exception. Naturally, when they test their own ideas they don't set out to disprove them. They're hoping for positive results. But this quite understandable desire can lead to all sorts of errors and make the test invalid.

To ward against bias*, science first insists that testing be rigorous and conform to accepted standards. The research must be well designed, the observations accurate, and the conclusions fully supported by the test results. In addition, the test results must be repeatable; by following the "recipe" or methodology of the experiment, a researcher other than the original investigator should be able to come up with similar results. It is the replication of research findings that gives science credibility as an objective discipline. Finally, hypotheses, even ones that look very promising, are never accepted at face value. Every new idea, before it can be added to the body of scientific knowledge, must be tested according to the scientific method.

In this century, science has developed a tool which is particularly useful for testing medical innovations. It is called the randomized controlled trial (RCT). Controlled trials were first used in agriculture to develop better grain products. Adjacent fields were planted with different types of seeds, which were allowed to grow under identical conditions, and the resulting plants were compared.

In medicine, this technique allows scientists to compare the results for patients who receive a particular therapy (the treatment group) with the results for those who do not (the control group). Because people can vary so widely in the ways they respond to disease and therapies, enough people must participate in the test to even out these variations. Also, the groups must be similar to one another, otherwise different results between the groups might be due to factors other than the new treatment being tested. It's been shown that the best way to ensure that groups

---

*The word "bias" in science means the systematic distortion of the truth. As such, personal bias on the part of researchers is only one of many possible sources of error.

are comparable is to establish them using a random process. That way, everyone participating in the trial has an even chance of being assigned to the treatment group or to the control group, and individual differences are equally divided between the groups.[8] As a further precaution, researchers prefer "double-blind" experiments. In these, patients have agreed to participate in a trial but neither they nor their physicians know who is slated to receive the active therapy being tested.

Can we ever be sure a new treatment works *without* doing an RCT? Only when the more traditional therapy is *invariably* followed by a bad outcome. For example,

> Prior to 1946, the outcome of tuberculous meningitis was invariably fatal. Then when small amounts of streptomycin became available for use in humans, a few U.S. victims treated with the new drug survived. This remarkable survival following streptomycin was repeated shortly thereafter in the United Kingdom. Thus the ability to show, with replication, that patients with previously universally fatal disease can survive following a new treatment constitutes sufficient evidence, all by itself, for efficacy.[9]

Even though RCTs in medicine are both expensive to conduct and difficult to organize, they are the most accurate way to determine whether a treatment works or not. It's disappointing how rarely medicine makes use of them, but hardly surprising. The RCT is an example of a scientific methodology. Medicine's methodology is pre-scientific; its roots are in antiquity.

Medicine: The Old Magic

Medicine predates science by thousands of years. Its own development was fostered by the very belief systems which science ultimately displaced. In ancient times healing was an art, and early medicine was dominated by magic, alchemy, and mysticism. Because its practitioners had only a rudimentary knowledge of the body and disease, many of their treatments, from today's perspective, seem positively barbaric.

> It makes one recoil to think of applying animal excrement or boiling oil to open wounds and blowing septic materials down throats or other orifices. Practices that could not possibly correct an anatomic or physiological abnormality — cupping, bleeding, purg-

ing and inducing vomiting — could only have weakened a person who was already sick. But the remarkable thing is that these treatments were not perceived as harmful by either patient or physician or society. People flocked to receive these treatments.[10]

These ancient healers held a respected position in society, just as physicians do today. They maintained their authority by taking credit for any "cures" they managed to effect, while dismissing their failures as due to forces beyond their control, "the will of the gods."

It's obvious that most medical successes from this pre-scientific era were not a function of competence in biology. Nonetheless, physicians were frequently able to help people in spite of their lack of scientific skill. To understand why, we need to appreciate three factors in the healing process which are as indispensable to the modern doctor as they were to the ancient healer.

1. Most Illness is Self-Limiting   Any physician today will tell you that when you get sick, most of the time the condition you have will clear up on its own, given enough time. All it takes to cure most illnesses is patience, rest, and the willingness to trust in the body's own remarkable defense system. For instance, when we recover from a cold or some other minor viral illness, the cure is due to our own immune system.

And yet, if we visit a physician for that viral infection and receive a totally useless prescription for an antibiotic, who gets the credit? In the same way, the ancient healers plying their potions invariably claimed responsibility for any recovery subsequent to the treatment.

2. The High Variability of Chronic Illnesses   People with chronic illness notice that their condition bothers them more at some times than at others. Usually it's when their symptoms are at their most severe that they seek medical advice. This high variability of some diseases contributes to a false impression that therapies received during an acute stage of suffering are responsible for the subsequent improvement. The fact that such improvements correspond to the natural pattern of the illness is often ignored by patients and physicians alike. For example, people who suffer from mild arthritis usually book a doctor's appointment when their pain gets worse. If, following this consultation, they get a prescription for medication, they will credit any abatement in pain to the treatment rather than to the natural variability of arthritis.

According to estimates, 80% of all people who go to see physicians have nothing wrong with them that wouldn't clear up with a vacation, a salary raise, or relief from everyday stress.[11] Only 10% require drugs or surgery to get well, and the remainder have conditions for which there is no cure. This built-in 80% success rate helps to perpetuate the myth that physicians, both modern and ancient, have special healing powers.

3. The Placebo Effect   It's been found that when people really believe a treatment is going to help, they will react positively to that treatment. A patient given a sugar pill, thinking that it's a strong sedative, will often fall asleep, but it's his *faith*, not the tranquilizing power of sugar, that causes this reaction.

> The placebo effect is as old as therapy itself. Patients with chest pain due to heart disease (angina), will consistently report a decreased amount and severity of the pain when given any therapy that they think is effective. This does not mean that placebos work as well as drugs that go directly to the source of pain, but it does show that pain can be reduced when the patient believes the treatment is working.[12]

Historically, medicine has been duped into embracing a number of totally useless therapies because doctors inadvertently mistook the placebo effect for a cure. Underestimating the power of placebos can play havoc when it comes to evaluating the effectiveness of treatment. In most cases, one can expect that about one-third of patients will improve on the basis of the placebo effect alone.[13] When the therapy is offered by an enthusiastic and trusted physician, the placebo response rate can increase to around 70%.[14]

Drs. Gordon Guyatt, David Feeney, and Peter Tugwell of McMaster University[15] refer to two modern studies which dramatically illustrate how misleading the placebo effect can be. In each case, a type of heart surgery called internal mammary artery ligation was being investigated. Patients involved in these studies were randomly divided into two groups: the treatment group, which actually received the surgery, and the control group, which had only a sham operation. Patients in both groups had no way of knowing whether or not they were going to get the real surgery — there was a 50-50 chance either way. Surprisingly, 75% of patients in *both* groups reported symptom relief. Control and treatment groups alike said they felt less pain, were able to reduce their use of medication, and could withstand more exercise. Electrocardiogram readings taken while they exercised confirmed their assertions!

One way of understanding the strength of the placebo effect is as a function of patient expectations. The doctor/patient relationship is founded on trust: the doctor agrees to base medical decisions on what would be in the patient's best interests; the patient trusts that the physician is competent and knowledgeable enough to do that well. This psychological investment has a great influence on the placebo effect. The ancient healers had the trust and confidence of their patients, if little else. Sometimes it was enough.

For as long as physicians have practiced medicine, they have been prone to an error in deductive reasoning called *post hoc, ergo propter hoc*, a Latin phrase meaning, "After this, therefore because of this." Here's how it works: A doctor tries out a new remedy. If the patient gets better, the doctor concludes it's because of the therapy. This is an error, because it fails to take into account other factors that might have been responsible for the change. As we've just pointed out, the explanation for the improvement might as easily be found in the disease's natural variation, or the patient's psychology.

But in medicine, *post hoc, ergo propter hoc* is usually a one-way street. If the patient fails to improve, or gets worse following treatment, the modern physician (just like the ancient one) is unlikely to dismiss the therapy as useless or harmful. Instead, he'll probably attribute any failures to forces beyond his control (just as the ancient healers did), concluding "the patient's disease was too advanced to be amenable to treatment," or "his attitude was poor; he didn't really want to get well." Ironically, the very factors that were blithely overlooked in assessing those patients who improved, are hauled out as excuses for those who didn't. *Post hoc, ergo propter hoc* continues to be the foundation for modern clinical judgment. The physician makes decisions about how to treat new patients based on the results he got when treating ones who came to him earlier. Doctors, rather than seek out information about the thousands of cases which comprise all of medical knowledge, tend to operate from the narrow perspective of their own clinical experience.

Science and Medicine

One of the first people to reproach medicine for its neglect of science was Abraham Flexner, an educator rather than a doctor, who was asked by the Carnegie Institute to conduct a review of North American medical schools back in 1908. In his report, published two years later,[16] he harshly criticized many of the training institutions of the day for their inadequate laboratory facilities, unqualified instructors, and low entrance requirements. His findings carried a lot of weight with those who funded medical education, and consolidated the growing opinion that doctors needed a thorough grounding in the basic sciences if they were to practice good medicine. Five years after Flexner's review, 35% of North America's medical schools had closed.[17] The message was clear: no longer would such "unscientific" disciplines as homeopathy and hygienics — which until then had been equally respected branches of medicine — qualify for funding.* Only those schools willing to adjust their curriculums to correspond to the model Flexner most admired — the German university system — would be encouraged to flourish. So a mastery of physics, chemistry, and biology became an essential prerequisite for a medical degree.

It wasn't enough. Medicine still remains unimpressed with the scientific method. In medical schools today, "knowledge is

---

*The American Medical Association at that time was the professional organization for physicians who practiced allopathy, a sect of medicine characterized by large-dose drug therapy and, in the early 1800s, bleeding. The AMA was eager to establish its type of practice as the only legitimate medical sect, and to that end, had conducted its own review of medical education in 1906. They knew, however, that their findings would be considered biased and so approached the Carnegie Foundation to undertake an "independent" review — which culminated in the Flexner Report.

imparted by pronouncement, first because the student is deluged with so much biological information to memorize he cannot stop to question what he is told, and second because the medical subculture uses *ex cathedra* statements as a matter of course.''[18] The mere addition of scientific "facts" to the medical curriculum has done nothing to teach students about "the techniques of information gathering, the rules of evidence and inference from data, the need for controlled studies and epidemiological studies for assessing the real effects of therapies or the fundamental fact that human responses to therapies can be predicted at best only as probabilities.''[19]

These failings of medical education have had little effect on the public's perception of medicine. Science promises a world of continuous progress, and people have the proof of it in the changes they have seen for themselves. As for medicine, the public believes more than ever that practitioners have special healing powers. As medicine adopted the new trappings of science — the laboratory, the shiny new instruments, the jargon, the ubiquitous white lab coat — the distinction between medicine and science blurred, and doctors became indistinguishable from scientists. No one seems to notice that medicine has only the look, not the substance, of science, that it has never whole-heartedly adopted the scientific method. In medicine, science is only skin-deep.

The rapid growth of technology in this century has both helped and compromised medicine. Antibiotics to treat bacterial diseases, insulin to control diabetes, and hip replacement surgery to treat joints destroyed by arthritis, are just a few examples of therapies which have more than lived up to their original promise. But other therapies, initially embraced with equal enthusiasm, have turned out to be totally worthless or even harmful. Doctors used to recommend the routine removal of tonsils to prevent recurring throat infections — it didn't work. Neither did freezing the stomach to treat ulcers, or intestinal bypass operations to cure obesity. For years, unmonitored oxygen therapy was used on premature babies to help their breathing. It turned out to be the major cause of blindness in young infants.[20] It used to be standard practice in hospitals to bathe newborns in Phisohex to prevent staph infections. But then it was discovered that hexachlorophene — the active ingredient in the disinfectant — could be absorbed through the skin and cause brain damage.[21]

All of these therapies were widely used before they'd ever been tested for safety or effectiveness. Many times, the clinical trials needed to evaluate therapies are strongly resisted by the medical profession. By their reasoning, it's unethical to withhold a potentially helpful treatment merely because it hasn't been rigorously evaluated. But isn't it even *more* unethical to use a potentially useless or harmful treatment before its safety and effectiveness have been proven? Nothing more clearly demonstrates how *unscientific* medicine remains.

Doctors have known for a long time that even useful medical interventions can cause injury to patients. Complications such as strokes, heart attacks, kidney failure, loss of limbs, and almost all forms of physical and emotional impairment can be caused by modern diagnostic and treatment technologies. There's even a term for illness caused by medicine: *iatrogenesis*, a Greek word meaning "originating with the physician."[22] The patient who suffers an adverse reaction to a prescription drug, or develops an infection from a diagnostic test, or dies undergoing surgery, is a victim of iatrogenesis. Because varying degrees of risk are associated with every diagnostic and treatment option, some iatrogenesis is impossible to avoid. As long as the medical intervention was "indicated" (meaning appropriate), and competently executed, any negative outcome is unfortunate rather than criminal. But what's the excuse if someone is harmed as a result of a needless procedure? Who's to blame if a therapy which has never been evaluated ends up permanently injuring the unsuspecting patient?

In their eagerness to do everything possible to help their patients, doctors often succumb to the terrible pressure to take action. And so they jump the gun in advance of any good evidence to show their intervention will help, and wind up doing more harm than good, or wasting their time. This flagrant neglect of science only increases the danger of medical mistakes, and widens the gap between what medicine promises and what it delivers.

There is a growing awareness among the public about the frequency of medical error. This is starting to interfere with the relationship between patients and their physicians. Litigation, while still not nearly as frequent in Canada as in the United States, is on the rise,* and doctors are feeling more and more defensive. In the absence of scientific standards and guidelines that would give direction to medical decisions, they must somehow determine what's best for the patient. Should they do everything possible, regardless of the chances for success? That option risks harming the patient. Should they do as little as possible in order to avoid exposing the patient to unnecessary risks? That might lead them to miss a potentially useful therapy.

If physicians lack scientific judgment when it comes to treating illness, the same holds true when it comes to investigating it . . . .

Overinvestigation

The Age of Technology has provided doctors with a vast armoury of sophisticated diagnostic innovations, and new ones are emerging at an astonishing rate. Costs associated with testing have risen dramatically in the past decade, even though their contribution to the diagnosis is relatively small in most cases. The CMA task force report on the allocation of health resources quoted one doctor as saying, "Physicians are becoming more reliant on the expensive laboratory test as opposed to their five senses."[23] No doctor, it seems, is willing to base his diagnosis on a careful history and physical examination. Yet in the results of one trial, three-quarters of patients were correctly diagnosed on the basis of the history alone. The physical examination contributed as much useful information as all the investigations put together.[24]

Of course, sometimes testing is necessary to improve the accuracy of the diagnosis. But an alarming number of tests are

---

*Although a Canadian physician is 50 times less likely to be named in a malpractice suit than an American one, insurance rates for doctors in this country have risen dramatically in recent years. The higher litigation rates in the United States are a result of two major differences between our legal systems. First, malpractice cases in America are determined by jury trials, and so awards tend to be much more substantial. Second, American lawyers are more likely to accept malpractice cases on a contingency basis. Juries know that between one-third and one-half of any award will go to the lawyer as payment, and so determine the amount accordingly.

ordered on a routine basis, for no particular reason at all. This is especially true in hospitals, where, for example, blood tests are standard procedure. In an editorial entitled "Medical Vampires" published in the *New England Journal of Medicine*, Dr. John Burnam referred to one study which found that the average adult patient in an intensive care unit of a teaching hospital was leeched of nearly two units of blood during his stay.[25] (A few had almost twice that amount removed.) That represents ten percent of an adult's blood supply — enough to produce anemia in a healthy person! Sure enough, it turned out that the main reason patients in intensive care were given transfusions, was to replace all the blood that had been siphoned from them for lab tests.[26]

The huge escalation in the frequency of testing calls into question whether all these investigations were really necessary. Clinical guidelines and a weekly review of medical records were two measures introduced into a medical unit in a teaching hospital in Britain to promote a more discriminating use of laboratory tests. This strategy resulted in an *immediate* 64% reduction in the average weekly number of blood and biochemical tests, with no apparent compromise to patient health.[27]

Patients may fail to appreciate a doctor's conservative attitude toward investigation as a good thing. Often you'll hear, "Oh, my doctor's just wonderful, *so* thorough. Why, he's had me in for tests three times this month." From the patient's perspective, more investigation is a measure of the doctor's concern. There's evidence, however, that more skillful physicians rely less on testing; one study found that doctors with lower scores on their licencing examinations did more diagnostic investigations.[28]

Doctors who use tests to confirm a diagnosis of which they are already certain, or to rule out illnesses that are highly unlikely, are wasting time and money — and may be doing harm to their patients. The only time testing is justified is when the doctor is actually unsure. If he judges, for example, that a patient has a 30 to 70% chance of having a particular illness, then testing can be a real benefit — assuming, of course, there's a cure.

Being able to correctly label a condition isn't particularly helpful if there's no effective treatment for it. Patients sometimes express relief at having a name to call their condition, even if there's no treatment, but physicians are understandably discontent to discover illnesses they cannot treat successfully. When the ophthalmoscope was invented back in the 1850s, it was greeted with little enthusiasm by practitioners because "the ophthalmoscope [disclosed] . . . . morbid conditions which are not for the most part more curable by being seen."[29]

Of course, it's also possible to underinvestigate and cause harm as a result. For example, a study of a neonatal intensive care unit in a Québec hospital concluded that doctors sometimes failed to test fetal age, or establish the maturity of the fetal lungs, prior to inducing labour or performing a Caesarean section.[30] Prematurity is the main cause of neonatal respiratory distress syndrome (RDS). Results showed that 22% of cases of RDS over the nine-month study period could have been avoided had such tests been performed and the births delayed.

Any rational decision to use or forego a particular diagnostic test requires accurate information about the risks. Iatrogenesis as a result of investigation is certainly possible, but little is known about its frequency or extent. In a literature review on the adverse effects of diagnostic testing, the authors concluded, "Sound clinical judgment requires more dependable data than are presently available."[31]

How a Blood Test Can Kill You

Brian K. a 35-year-old steelworker, went to see his doctor complaining of fatigue. He mentioned that he had recently switched to the graveyard shift at work, and that his wife had given birth to a new baby, but his doctor didn't pay too much attention to these changes in his personal life. Intent on making sure there was no "medical" reason to explain these symptoms, he carefully examined Brian and ordered a number of laboratory tests. Among other things, he asked that Brian's blood be measured for SGOT, (serum glutamic oxaloacetic transaminase), an enzyme produced by the liver. When liver cells have been injured or disease is present, more of this enzyme leaches into the bloodstream, where it is detectable. When Brian's test results showed he had elevated levels of SGOT, the doctor ordered the test repeated, and the second test confirmed the first.

As a consequence, even though Brian exhibited no symptoms of liver disease, the doctor recommended an ultrasound examination — a very safe procedure but one that occasionally produces a false-positive result.[32] The ultrasound results were equivocal: a small shadow on the image suggested the possibility of a tumour. To be on the safe side, the doctor then suggested that Brian undergo a liver biopsy, which is generally a safe investigation as well, though it has a measurably small complication rate. This procedure was done in the hospital, under a local anaesthetic, and involved inserting a hollow needle through the abdomen into the liver and withdrawing a small piece of liver tissue, which was then examined in the laboratory. In Brian's case, the results of the biopsy were negative — he didn't have anything wrong with his liver. But unknown to him or those treating him, the needle used to withdraw the liver sample had inadvertently pierced a blood vessel. Later that night, seemingly safe in bed, he quietly bled to death.

Brian's doctor, on the basis of a single abnormal test result, began an escalating series of investigations, looking for disease that wasn't there, and wound up killing his patient. He was deceived into this dangerous course of action because he failed to understand some of the fundamental statistical limitations of testing.

The Limits of Testing

Laboratory tests are standardized so that 95% of healthy people without symptoms will fall within the normal range. That's all well and good, but it means that five percent of perfectly healthy people getting any test will fall outside that range, half with readings too high and the other half with readings too low to be considered "normal." For these people, the test will come back with an "abnormal" result even though they are not ill.

Also, no test is 100% accurate. Each test can produce "false-positive" and "false-negative" readings.* Many physicians

---

*Readers interested in learning more about the technical limitations of testing can turn to the Appendix at the back of the book.

don't understand that if they perform 14 laboratory tests on a healthy patient, the probability is more than 50% that at least one of those tests will come back with an abnormal result. Modern science's concepts of probability are totally alien to most doctors, even though knowledge of them is essential to good professional practice.

Much of medical testing used to be done in the doctors' office, under the physician's supervision and control. With today's expensive and sophisticated testing equipment, however, most private practitioners rely on private laboratories for their lab work. This does not guarantee high quality, however. A study was done where identical blood samples were sent to 5,000 U.S. labs for cholesterol analysis. The results varied widely, with the highest reading being double the lowest.[33] Private labs, of course, are in business to make a profit, and do everything they can to encourage doctors to use their services. Some even rent out office space to doctors at a discount just to attract a neighbour who will bring them business. They make it easy for the doctor to go overboard when ordering tests. Order forms for blood tests, for example, come in handy tear-off sheets, with 50 or more optional investigations there for the asking. All the doctor has to do is check the appropriate box. When doctors get the lab results back, abnormal readings are conveniently highlighted for the physician's perusal. However, there's no information about the false-positive or false-negative rates of the test. Dr. James Isbister, in the *Medical Journal of Australia*, suggests that "clinicians are bombarded with more and more information about their patients which they have not collected themselves and may not fully understand."[34]

Overtreatment

In the same way that it's possible to overdiagnose illness, it's possible to overtreat it. Since over 80% of all medical therapies have never been evaluated, doctors have little scientific information on which to base their treatment decisions.* In their eagerness

---

*Drugs, the most common therapy, are evaluated of course. RCTs are used to determine their safety and usefulness. But as you'll see in Chapter 5, drugs are frequently prescribed to treat conditions other than those for which they have been proven effective.

to help patients, there's a definite tendency for practitioners to overdo it.

When you compare the surgical rates in Canada with those in other countries, you'll come across ominous clues that many common surgeries performed in this country every day may be unnecessary. The Organization for Economic Cooperation and Development (OECD) has recently compiled statistics from its 24 member countries (all of them Western industrialized democracies), regarding the use of health services.[35] The data show large variations in the frequency of common surgical procedures. For example, Canada's rate for tonsillectomies (surgical removal of the tonsils) is twice that of Denmark and four times that of Sweden (though roughly half that of Holland). Canada has the highest rate for cholecystectomy (surgical removal of the gallbladder) of any country in the world — ten times higher than Denmark, the country with the lowest rate, and five times higher than England. There is no reason to believe that frequency of surgery is related to higher rates of illness in these populations. In fact, several studies have shown that the rate of gallstones (the main cause of gallbladder disease) is approximately the same in most Western countries.[36]

Gallstones can cause infection and severe pain, as well as other complications, such as inflammation of the pancreas and gallbladder cancer. (Cancers resulting from untreated gallbladder disease, however, are extremely rare.) At the same time, many people with gallstones have no symptoms at all. Obviously, many Canadian surgeons have decided it's better to operate even on this latter group of patients, to prevent the possibility of future complications. They point out the low risk of death at the time of surgery (less than one percent), and that the body can get by fairly well without a gallbladder. This argument is quite persuasive when offered to someone who has just barely survived an acute gallbladder infection. But what should be done with someone who has gallstones *without* apparent distress — so called "silent gallstones." To clarify the issue, let's look at an example.

Jane B. was a 52-year-old secretary for a large Canadian life insurance company. Although about 30 pounds overweight, she was in generally good health. Jane visited her family doctor for her annual checkup. Her doctor was very thorough and asked Jane several dozen questions about her physical and psychological functioning. Jane admitted to some "heartburn" over Christmas, but attributed this symptom to ritual self-indulgence. Her physician, however, decided to pursue the matter despite a normal physical examination. The doctor knew by her age, weight, and sex that Jane was at high risk for gallstones, so she ordered an ultrasound examination and, sure enough, found what she'd suspected. So she referred Jane to a surgeon, who recommended operating. Although she felt perfectly well, Jane was pleased that her doctor had been so thorough. And she had confidence in the skills of the surgeon, who promised her that removing her gallbladder would be "preventive medicine." Of course she had to take time off work, but that was covered by her accumulated sick time. She was also told that she would be in a lot of pain for a few days, and wouldn't be able to get back to her full activities for four to six weeks. But all of this looked quite acceptable if it would prevent those awful complications — especially cancer. Unfortunately, in the middle of the operation, which had been routine, Jane's heart stopped beating and she died. Her family, even in their grief, appreciated that the doctors had "done everything they could have." But had they perhaps done more than they *should* have?

If Jane had lived in England she would still be alive. In that country surgeons don't remove a gallbladder unless gallstones are causing problems. An English surgeon would not interpret one episode of mild heartburn pain as an indication for surgery. British surgeons think that, on balance, a person is more likely to have problems from the surgery than from the gallstones, if they haven't yet caused any problems. Canadian surgeons think that, on balance, a person with silent gallstones is better off having the gallbladder removed. Who is right?

Probably the most thorough analysis of this issue was done in Cleveland, by researchers at Case Western Reserve University.[37] They used a technique called "decision analysis," in which the known probabilities that various events will occur are used to compare different ways of approaching the same problem. In this case, they calculated whether someone is more likely to die from having surgery for silent gallstones than from just waiting to see if anything untoward occurs. They found that on average, a 30-year-old man would actually lose ten days of life by having surgery. (It would also cost the health care system approximately six times as much money than if he had chosen instead to wait to see what happened.) Because surgical risks increase with age, a 50-year-old would lose over three weeks of life.

Researchers in Manitoba studied over 2,000 patients who had elective gallbladder surgery in 1974, and found that the operation caused more death than gallbladder disease — which is what the surgery attempts to prevent.[38] Without surgery, some of these patients would undoubtedly have suffered periodic bouts of acute pain, and perhaps even required emergency surgery at some point. But the benefit of surgery to those who had never had any symptoms remains doubtful. In the year of the study, seven people died within six weeks of elective surgery. Although this is a low mortality rate, if any of those seven had been symptom-free prior to surgery — was the treatment justifiable?

Now of course all these operations were not for silent gallstones. But Dr. James McSherry, a surgeon at the Beth Israel Medical Center in New York, has found that even gallstone patients *with* symptoms can often safely delay or avoid surgery. He followed 556 patients with gallstones and gallstone-related symptoms for an average of seven years. During that time only 44% required surgery, on average four years after initial diagnosis. There were only two deaths in this group, and both occurred *after* surgery.[39]

Two recent studies show that a person with silent gallstones has about a ten percent risk of developing complications within a five-year period. One of those studies states that there is only an 18% risk of complications within 20 years. In any case, all the complications were simple gallstone pain, and there were no deaths due to gallbladder disease. Which risk would you prefer — three chances in a thousand of dying, as well as the certainty of several days of pain and four to six weeks of reduced activity? Or would you rather live with one chance in five of developing a few days of pain sometime in the next 20 years, with virtually no risk of dying due to gallbladder disease?

It seems a rational person would opt to wait. Yet Canadian surgeons removed more than 50,000 gallbladders in 1983, at a cost to the health care system of roughly $75 to 100 million.[40] When you consider the cost of lost time from work, and the deaths that do occur secondary to surgery, the total bill for gallbladder surgery in Canada is likely over $200 million a year. This is enough money to put up nearly 6,000 homeless people in $100-a-night hotel rooms for the rest of their lives.

To take another example of overtreatment, the Saskatchewan government discovered a 72% jump in the number of hysterectomies between 1964 and 1971, even though over the same period the number of women over 15 increased by only about eight percent. They also picked up large differences in hysterectomy rates among cities in the province. In response to a request from the health minister, the Saskatchewan College of Physicians and Surgeons set up a surveillance committee that not only established criteria which they felt justified a hysterectomy, but actually monitored decision-making in seven hospitals. The number of unjustified hysterectomies dropped from almost 24% at the beginning of the monitoring process to just under eight percent. As an indication of how powerful this surveillance was, the total number of hysterectomies in Saskatchewan between 1970 and 1974 fell by one-third.[41]

The extracranial-intracranial bypass (EC-IC), a type of brain surgery, had once been thought to prevent strokes. In 1985, 17 years after it was first developed, an RCT proved it to be utterly worthless.[42] Of the thousands of patients who had an EC-IC bypass, over three percent either died, or had a major stroke as a result of the operation that left them worse off than if no surgery had been done in the first place.

Carotid endarterectomy, an even more popular type of brain surgery, is also performed in the belief that it prevents strokes. It involves scraping deposits off the inside of the main artery leading to the brain to improve blood flow. This sounds like a good idea, but in the 30 years since it's been in use, no clinical trial has adequately addressed "its benefit or lack of benefit."[43] Like most surgeries, carotid endarterectomy has never been compared scientifically to the non-surgical treatment — one aspirin a day — or to no treatment at all.[44] Last year, an estimated 150,000 patients in Canada and the United States had the procedure, and between five and ten percent died or had a stroke as a result.[45] Mounting doubts about the effectiveness of carotid endarterectomy led the U.S. government to fund a North America-wide evaluation in 1987. Pending the results, the surgery continues to be performed.

We are by no means suggesting that all testing and surgery equals overtreatment. Nor will evaluation eliminate all the risks associated with medical interventions; many risks are unpredictable and unavoidable. But we believe that much iatrogenesis is the result of overdiagnosis and overtreatment, both of which are symptoms of a medical system out of control. Without proper evaluation, we can't begin to measure the extent of doctor-induced illness.

Overall, the case for medicine as a scientific discipline is very weak. One critic, Dr. Thomas Preston, has gone so far as to call it a "pseudo-science";[46] another, Dr. Richard Taylor, suggested that doctors are practicing "science fiction" medicine.[47] Modern clinical practice has never evolved beyond the principles of Descartes, who believed that fundamental ideas gained by intuition are the surest way to understand the world. Medicine's failure to adopt scientific methods dooms it to be judged an "un-science."

Chapter 4

High-Tech Tradeoffs

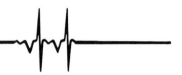

NO DISCUSSION OF WASTE in our health care system would be complete without a word about technology — how it has transformed medicine's practice, and its cost. It wasn't until the 19th century, with the invention of the stethoscope and ophthalmoscope, that physicians began to rely on instruments as well as their own senses when diagnosing disease. But the greatest technological revolution in medicine occurred in the 20th century. Today's medicine encompasses both high- and low-tech strategies; the former is largely associated with advances in computer science, engineering, and nuclear physics, while the latter includes older, more established diagnostic and treatment options like X-rays, drug therapies, and conventional surgeries. The belief that medical technology has been the most important factor in improving our health is a very common one, but many critics are forcing a reevaluation of this assumption. (This is a subject we explore more fully in Chapter 7.)

It's now becoming quite clear that whatever contributions technology made in the past, its influence on improving our health today has dwindled. "We're a long way past the point of diminishing returns," says Ken Fyke, CEO and president of the Greater Victoria Hospital Society.* "We can pour money into

---

*The Greater Victoria Hospital Society (GVHS) is an amalgamation of four hospitals in Victoria.

the high-tech end of the system but at the other end we're not getting our money's worth in terms of results.''

When we commit resources to high-tech solutions, we lose the opportunity to spend them in other areas of social policy which have more influence on health. Our free spending on the sickness sector has brought us well onto the plateau of what Dr. Alain Enthoven calls "flat of the curve" medicine.[1] Like it or not, committing an ever-increasing proportion of resources to the diagnosis and treatment of disease is not improving our health.

At the same time, the rapid growth of medical technology has been a major factor in increasing the cost of hospital care, in terms of both equipment and staff.[2] Getting people to pay attention to the cost impact of technological changes isn't easy, however. That's because proponents of technology (and they're virtually everywhere) always begin their arguments in favour of this new gadget or that new drug with the premise that we need it urgently, that even if we can't afford to fund it, we can't afford not to, either.

It is easy to generate public support for technological solutions. While the claims made for new technologies usually overestimate their benefits, they are nonetheless convincing. The climate of enthusiasm for adopting new-tech solutions is usually strong enough to override the reticence so often associated with the Canadian character. Skepticism in the face of such excitement is a decidedly unpopular stance — one reason why most medical technologies have never been evaluated. Professor David Feeney, who teaches economics at McMaster University, describes the harsh climate for evaluators: "The developers of a new technology spend enormous energy fine-tuning their invention; they not only have the best knowledge about it, they have a personal investment in their own intellectual capital, not to mention a pecuniary one. The guys who pick up on the latest innovation — the early advocates — are no more inclined to be skeptical. Then there are the evaluators, those damned agnostics, viewed from all sides as a disgusting nihilistic bunch. They drive everybody who's lined up 'for' or 'against' the new technology right up the wall.''

Just questioning whether the technology works under scientifically controlled conditions looks like bad manners! Does it make sense to scorn those who question a possibly harmful innovation, to ridicule those who say "this is the kind of evidence I need to decide"?

Surely it's only prudent to be cautious about how technology is adopted into our system. To make rational decisions, it's essential to know how well the new technology works, what conditions and what types of patients it is appropriate for, and whether the benefits *in terms of patient outcome* justify the expenditure. To do anything less compromises both the quality and cost of health care.

One glittering example of high technology is the coronary care unit, or CCU. In 1963, the first report in scientific literature about the usefulness of CCUs to heart attack patients indicated that, overall, survival was no better in these specialized units.[3] Soon after, a number of studies appeared that seemed to contradict these findings. These later studies, however, were of very poor quality; for example, one comparing heart attack patients admitted to CCUs with those treated in general wards during 1968, reported an impressive difference in the death rates: 16% for the CCU group against 27% in the ward group![4] But the groups were not comparable. The ward patients were much older, for example, and therefore more likely to die in any event. Also, because a random process had not been used to establish the groups, there is reason to believe that a doctor, faced with two patients and only one bed in the CCU, might well have assigned the better prospect for survival to the CCU.

Throughout the 1960s, while CCUs were being developed and spreading throughout North America, no randomized controlled trials were performed to evaluate them. The first RCT comparing home with hospital care for patients with uncomplicated heart attacks came from Britain, where the medical establishment had not wholeheartedly embraced CCUs.[5] Their results showed that *patients actually did slightly better at home*, although the difference was not statistically significant.*

This evidence did nothing to slow the proliferation of CCUs

---

*A "statistically significant" finding is one that is unlikely to have occurred by chance.

in North America. They continued to spread like wildfire — every hospital had to have one. Americans and Canadians criticized the British study for looking at a selected group, and claimed that newer techniques, developed since the study was completed, were benefiting new heart attack victims. To answer these critics, another group of British researchers performed a "cadillac" experiment; they sent a hospital-based team to the homes of suspected heart attack victims. Over three-quarters of these patients were randomly allocated, either to a CCU or to home care. *There was no statistically significant difference in survival rates between the two groups of patients.*[6]

What difference has this compelling evidence made to the prevalence of CCUs? None. Are Canadians, following an uncomplicated heart attack, typically released after a few days observation to recover at home? No.

Drs. Eggerton and Berg, who teach family medicine at the University of Washington in Seattle, wrote an editorial in the *Journal of the American Medical Association* in 1984 that summarized the evidence on CCUs. While they admitted the possibility that new drugs and therapies now available in CCUs might benefit some patients, they closed their editorial with a prudent admonition:

> Our current strategy of forcing all patients into the same high-technology expensive care is hardly defensible; it deserves much more critical scrutiny.[7]

Anyone who reads the news is used to seeing quotes from doctors pushing for more money for more of these kinds of intensive care beds. Typically, their arguments explain the need for these technologies in terms of life-or-death consequences. As Bob Evans, an economics professor at the University of British Columbia, says, "Those who stand to benefit financially or professionally make the market offer: 'Your money or your life.' " Unfortunately, the classic rhetoric that's used to promote technology often overstates how important it really is to our health. And in the excitement surrounding its promise more useful, albeit more pedestrian, alternatives are ignored.

Missing the Boat

Let's look at an example of how the glamour of high-cost, sophisticated approaches deflects the medical profession's attention away from more useful interventions. Consider how medicine approaches chlamydia, a sexually transmitted infection that is currently threatening the reproductive health of millions of women.

First a few facts about chlamydia, and the damage it causes:

1. Chlamydia usually resides in the cervix (the outlet of the womb) where it causes few, if any, symptoms. However, in approximately 15 to 20% of women, the organism migrates through the womb into the fallopian tubes and ovaries, causing pelvic inflammatory disease (PID).[8] Chlamydia is fairly easy to diagnose with a swab test (if you're looking for it) and simple to treat. It is, of course, necessary to treat any sexual partners as well, to prevent reinfection;

2. It is now known that 15% of all women under 30 will develop PID, and that the majority of those infected will be under 25 years of age;[9]

3. The scarring caused by PID accounts for almost half of ectopic (tubal) pregnancies, which can be life-threatening;[10] the incidence* of ectopic pregnancies in Canada has increased almost 200% since 1971.[11] In addition, PID causes about one-quarter of all refractory (long-term) infertility;[12]

4. The treatment for infertility caused by PID — either surgery to unblock damaged fallopian tubes, or *in vitro* fertilization (IVF) — is not only very costly, but also largely ineffective. Between 50 and 80% of surgeries fail, despite the use of high-tech laser instruments.[13] The best that can be said for IVF, however "miraculous" it might seem, is that couples in IVF programs have less than one chance in ten of delivering a live baby;[14]

5. In some IVF centres, over three-quarters of the patients have blocked tubes;

---

*The incidence of a disease or condition is the number of new cases in a particular population in a particular time period.

6. The average cost of IVF is approximately $4,000 per treatment, a tab which is currently covered by Ontario's health insurance.*

This scenario suggests there are a number of serious deficiencies in the way young women's reproductive health is being addressed by the medical profession. Chlamydia, the cause of much infertility, is fairly easy to diagnose and very easy to treat. But when was the last time you saw a gynecologist complain about inadequate screening programs for chlamydia? Have you ever heard a doctor complain about the medical profession's woeful ignorance of this preventable epidemic?

Yet not a month goes by without a newspaper or TV story featuring a gynecologist advocating IVF. We have been inundated with pictures of parents proudly displaying their so-called "test tube" babies. Only rarely do we glimpse the other side of the story. In a moving and provocative *Globe and Mail* article, Michele Landsberg describes IVF from the patient's perspective as a "painful, protracted, emotional roller coaster, both traumatic and chancy."[15] One IVF candidate, who like the vast majority failed to conceive, told her, "The process gets us addicted to hope." Usually we're not told of the emotional or financial costs of IVF, or the high failure rate of this intervention. Neither do we hear that a woman might have avoided infertility had the medical profession been as keen on prevention as on high-technology treatment. This is tragic neglect.

Family physicians are often a woman's only source of reproductive advice. But experts like Bonnie Johnson, president of Planned Parenthood of Saskatchewan, say they are often poorly informed: "We've heard stories of women going to four or five doctors trying to get a diaphragm** and none of them [the doctors] knew how to insert one."[16]

It's ironic that it took the rapid spread of AIDS, another sexually transmitted disease, to get doctors to promote condoms. Condoms are a good example of a low-cost technology that's been

---

*In fact, Ontario is one of the few jurisdictions in the world which offers full public coverage for IVF! By way of contrast, the National Health Service in Britain has one public IVF clinic to serve the whole country.

**A diaphragm, used with spermicidal jelly, also protects against chlamydia.

around for centuries. Unfortunately, there's nothing very glamorous about them. Had young women been advised all along to use such barrier methods to protect themselves against disease, millions of cases of infertility could have been prevented, and the billions of dollars that have been spent on expensive and largely ineffective technology would have been saved.

Going Overboard

One way to understand our general bias in favour of technology is by looking at societal attitudes. The public expects progress in medicine — and anticipates it with the certainty of a morning sunrise — and so accepts new medical technology with great enthusiasm and confidence. The backdrop to their expectations is this century's record of medical achievements, which have been considerable. There's no question that the Age of Technology has furnished the medical profession with powerful tools to improve its ability to detect and treat disease. As well, advances in other sciences — electronics, molecular biology, nuclear physics, computer science — have accelerated the development of technologies with medical applications. But implicit here is the misconception that any change in medical practice is *always* for the better, that whatever's new is automatically an improvement over long-established alternatives.

Dr. John Burnam of Tuscaloosa, Alabama, recently criticized the medical profession for being slaves to fashion.

> Consider the irony: as professed scientists and proponents of Cartesian doubt, we physicians find ourselves like lemmings, episodically and with a blind infectious enthusiasm pushing certain diseases and treatments primarily because everyone else is doing the same.[17]

The rapid spread of computerized tomography scanning is a good example of how we've gone overboard for technology. The C-T scanner has so captured the imagination of public and professional alike that in Ontario it's available in virtually every hospital with more than 200 beds. Since provincial governments continue to hold the purse strings where capital costs are concerned, hospitals that have been refused public funding for this device typically make direct appeals to the community. In Sault Ste. Marie, at a time when steel industry layoffs were threatening the community's economic security, people nevertheless reached deep into their pockets to purchase one. The people of Owen Sound, Ontario, engaged in a similar fund-raising exercise, so convinced were they of the vital importance of a C-T scanner to their well-being. These examples, and similar ones from around the country, demonstrate how fervently the public believes that without this technology, we're all doomed.

Now for some perspective. To begin with, let's admit that C-T scanners are an improvement over traditional imaging methods, in that they provide a better and safer look at the condition of the patient. But that being said, the important question still remains — how much effect does the wide availability of C-T scanning devices have on our health?

C-T scanners — along with other new and emerging imaging technologies, like positron emission tomography (PET), and nuclear magnetic resonators (NMR) — are very expensive to purchase and costly to operate. C-T scanners cost about a million dollars each, and anywhere from $500,000 to $700,000 yearly to operate. Clearly, expenditures of this magnitude add to the mystique of the technology: "If it costs a lot it must be good." But the high cost also creates a climate for overuse: "If we've got it, and we paid all that money for it, and we've hired all those technicians to run it, we have to use it." Typically, then, there are waiting lists for C-T scanning. But which patients are being selected to use it?

Denise G., a 28-year-old woman, was one. In 1983, Denise was working in a high-pressure environment as the executive assistant to a federal cabinet minister. She went to her doctor complaining of headaches that had become both more frequent and more severe than she had ever experienced before. "My G.P. then referred me to a specialist and he, in turn, recommended that I have a C-T scan done. I had the test, but the results came back negative. They couldn't tell me what was wrong. Eventually, I took a two-week vacation, and the headaches cleared up on their own."

What happened to Denise illustrates how a useful technology can be wasted on trivial purposes. "To be on the safe side," her G.P. referred her to a neurologist; he didn't really suspect she had anything serious, but he didn't want to be criticized for doing anything less than the maximum. The specialist, in turn, "to be on the safe side," recommended a C-T scan; to do anything less might have reflected badly on the G.P.'s decision to refer Denise in the first place. He didn't suspect anything was seriously wrong with her, but failure to order a C-T scan might have looked like dereliction of duty (his fault) or, as we've said, a professional snub (the G.P.'s fault), so he ordered the test.

It's clear that neither physician applied scientific evidence to inform his decision-making with logic. The incidence of new brain cancers in women 20 to 30 years old is only 2 or 3 per 100,000 per year.[18] On the other hand, 25,000 per 100,000 will have headaches. Can we, or should we, test them all? Even if we did, we'd be left with the uncomfortable reality that there is no cure for most malignant brain cancers. The next time your local newspaper features a radiologist complaining about the lack of C-T scanners, write the doctor a letter asking how many C-T scans are being done for young people with simple tension headaches. (He won't know; no province keeps records of who gets scanned.)

Now there's the possibility that C-T scanners may soon become obsolete because of an even newer and more expensive technology — nuclear magnetic resonance imaging, or NMR (also known as MRI in the alphabet soup of diagnostic technology). Proponents of NMR point out its unique ability to distinguish grey matter from white in the brain stem, and that it uses no radiation at all, and is therefore *presumably* safer. On the other hand, careful evaluation of the effects of NMR technology, which involves subjecting the patient to a very powerful magnetic field, has never been done.

At present there are approximately 700 of these machines in the United States, where technology diffuses more rapidly.[19] In Canada, there were 11 NMRs in use or earmarked as of June 1987.[20] Right now there's tremendous pressure to acquire this technology, much of it coming from a wonder-struck profession that knows how to grab media attention. Ken Fyke refers to the "shroud-waving emotionalism" found in press stories. One article, for example, covering the 1987 Canadian Congress of Neurological Sciences, quoted Dr. Charles Tator of Toronto Western Hospital as saying he believes patients have died for lack of the device: "Patients are being misdiagnosed or undiagnosed by the traditional diagnostic techniques — patients who could be saved or patients who could be treated much more accurately if we had proper access."[21]

Dr. Peter Seland, in the same news story, outlined the advantage of NMR, citing its "unequalled ability to diagnose diseases of the brain and spinal cord, such as tumours, multiple sclerosis, [and] Alzheimer's disease, in a way that could never be achieved before." The article failed, however, to note the dismal prognosis for these conditions — that most of them are, in fact, untreatable. "Remember that to a radiologist, a better picture is a better outcome," says David Feeney. But a better picture doesn't mean better health. Often it just gives you a better look at untreatable disease. Ken Fyke agrees: "It could be argued, with some justification, that all a C-T scanner does is tell a patient a month earlier that he has untreatable brain cancer; he'll still die on the same day, but he gets an extra month to worry about it." He could have said the same for NMR imaging.

Even so, competition among hospitals to acquire NMR is very intense. Feeney notes: "Every teaching hospital in the province except McMaster and Queen's has one of these things.And McMaster certainly wants one. They say what they always say: 'This is the best thing since sliced bread. It will provide tremendous opportunities for research. We can stop shipping people to London to have it.' And yet there's no clearly defined program for evaluating NMR, nor any well-developed proposals as to how it could be used for research."

Although he makes it clear that he is neither a biologist nor a physicist, Feeney admits to "lurking doubts" about NMR's safety. "It doesn't make sense to me that you can put people in a strong electromagnetic field — one capable of making surgical clamps fly around the room — and not end up doing something harmful to them." Under such an intense magnetic field, metals can pass right through the body.[22] Already, patients with metal plates in their skulls or shrapnel fragments are contraindicated for this procedure. What happens then to the unconscious patient who arrives at a hospital unable to supply this information? And what about a welder who took a flying metal fragment in the eye 20 years earlier and has long since forgotten all about it? At least C-T scanning is pretty safe. NMR has the potential to do harm.

The Development of Medical Technology

Private firms engaged in the development of new medical technologies combine "scientific knowledge and applied research to produce technological innovations which are embodied in the products they hope to sell."[23] Often, development costs are supported by public funding as well, through granting agencies and the scientific community.

While still in the development phase, innovations undergo a process of continual modification and refinement. Researchers, when dealing with a product with a very specific use, will try to find ways to broaden its application. In their recent book, *Health Care Technology: Effectiveness, Efficiency and Public Policy*, authors Feeney, Guyatt, and Tugwell note that new technology is seldom developed in a single, major step.[24] Consider the development of X-rays:

It happened quite by accident. Following up on work done by Wilhelm Roentgen, Henri Becquerel — a colleague of Pierre and Marie Curie — had thrown a sample of radioactive ore into his desk drawer before leaving his office. When he returned the next day, he looked into his desk to retrieve the rock and by chance noticed something else in the drawer — a photographic plate. Pulling it out, he saw a strange image on the plate — it had definitely been exposed to something — but what? This is only one of the classic tales surrounding the discovery of X-rays.

But transforming that discovery into a useful medical technology, one that could detect broken bones or tubercular lungs, took decades. And even more refinements were made after X-ray technology became commonplace. Modern radiographic equipment not only looks different from its earliest ancestors, it's also safer and more accurate.

"There are an enormous number of steps going from some good new idea, device, or drug into something that's useful and practical," says David Feeney. "The 'Eureka' model — which supports the myth that all of a sudden a brilliant idea grips you and you run naked from the bathtub into the streets crying 'I've figured it out!' — is not the way it works in real life." Insights happen, but their development into workable technology involves a great deal of refinement. He adds: "Tinkering, fiddling, polishing, sanding — what really accounts for technological advances is a long series of minor modifications, which taken singly are small and insignificant, but cumulatively, very important.''

A peculiarity of health care technologies is that most of the time, they are only evaluated long after they have become well established in the marketplace.[25] Usually, they are subjected to uncontrolled trials, which tend to overstate a new device's effectiveness. Estimates suggest that about 80% of medical technology has not yet been proven by rigorous scientific investigation. In the meantime, crude research, based on the belief that it helped at least one person or didn't appear to harm anybody, seems to satisfy.

This lack of information about the merits of medical technologies means we don't know which are important and which are not, or for what types of illness, or what kinds of patient. As things stand now, we simply don't have enough to go on.

But lack of evidence proving efficacy hasn't tempered the speed at which we adopt innovations. The process of adoption typically has seven stages:[26]

1. a promising report
2. professional and organizational adoption
3. public acceptance and state (third-party) endorsement
4. standard procedure and observational reports
5. randomized controlled trial (RCT)
6. professional denunciation
7. erosion and discreditation

First the doctors get excited, then the media, then the public. Once the medical community has whole-heartedly accepted a new type of surgery or diagnostic technique, and the press hails it as a ''breakthrough,'' and the public clamours for access to it, the climate for objective evaluation gets decidedly chilly. Doctors who are busy using these technologies are hardly likely to seek critical appraisals of them; their own experience — coloured no doubt with optimism for the technology's usefulness — is enough to satisfy them at first. It should come as no surprise that often their initial enthusiasm peters out. Later, their accumulated experience frequently leads to disenchantment, which in turn fuels a desire for reassessment.

It's astonishing how often the careful evaluation of a medical technology shows that the device is much less effective than was first thought. "The results of the RCT are usually less favourable to the innovation than were the uncontrolled studies case reports."[27] Is this because evaluations are conducted only when doubts about efficacy reach some critical mass? Probably, yes. Does this discourage future research efforts? That's likely too. All in all, the burden of proof during the honeymoon stage rests on the skeptics; most of the time, the desire to believe claims about a technology's usefulness is strong enough to override any protest from the unbelievers.

In any case, during the period immediately following the announcement of any innovation, a small number of clinicians will be "early takers." They form the hub of a network of advocates, who then proselytize the technology. Thereafter, widespread adoption can occur quite rapidly, without benefit of scientific research (although new technologies tend to diffuse much more rapidly in the United States than here in Canada). Possibly useless or even harmful procedures quickly become the accepted "standards of care" in the community. Quality becomes compromised.

Whether a new technology has been evaluated or not, doctors know that deviating from what has come to be considered standard practice places them in a difficult moral and legal position. This is, of course, the price professionals must pay for their claims of expertise: if doctors do it, it must be right; if every doctor but you does it, you must be wrong. In the absence of evidence, what is customary becomes correct. That's why careful and early evaluation is so essential.

Appropriate Use of Technology

When Marilyn B. entered the hospital to give birth to her first baby, she was looking forward to the experience. She was young, healthy, and well-prepared for labour and delivery; she also had lots of confidence in the hospital, which was so well-equipped. When the electrodes from the fetal monitor were attached she felt even more secure.

Two hours later, Marilyn's doctor informed her that the baby was showing some signs of distress and needed to be born quickly. Because she was worried about her child, Marilyn accepted the decision for a Caesarean section delivery without question. She realized from her prenatal classes that this was always a possibility, and was just glad that they could do something to save her baby. Of course, she had to stay in hospital longer, and her abdomen was pretty sore for quite a while after, but her baby was fine, and she was happy with the care she received.

Was she right to be?

During contractions, it's sometimes impossible to hear the fetal heartbeats properly with a stethoscope. So when electronic fetal monitors (EFM) were first developed over 20 years ago, they represented a breakthrough for women with high-risk pregnancies. Here was an instrument which could provide continuous monitoring and detect, with greater accuracy than the traditional stethoscope, heart rate abnormalities in the fetus. Because physicians using EFM have more information about the condition of the unborn child, *theoretically* they can make better decisions about the alternative courses of action.

Since its development, EFM has spread to the point where in many hospitals it has become the "standard of care" for all women in labour. This is reflected in its availability. For example, in Toronto, there is almost one EFM for every labour bed, the implication being that all women in labour require monitoring. At first glance, this might seem like a good idea — what's good for the few must be good for the many. But that's not how it works.

One signal that EFM might not be appropriate for everyone is that, concurrent with its growing acceptance as a standard practice, we've seen a disturbingly rapid increase in the rate of Caesarean section deliveries.* Canada's current rate for surgical deliveries is 20% — four times higher than it was in 1970, when EFM was less widely available.[28] It is also four times higher than in the Netherlands,[29] whose five percent rate is the lowest in the developed world.** This information alone is not

---

*Part of the high C-section rate is associated with births to mothers who have previously had surgical deliveries. The myth, "once a C-section, always a C-section" is currently being challenged, but even so, the rate of increase in surgical births cannot be explained from this source alone.

**The Netherlands, where midwives typically attend childbirth, also has a lower infant-mortality rate than Canada (OECD, *Measuring Health Care*, Paris, 1987).

sufficient to dispute the widespread use of fetal monitoring. After all, we could justify this increased rate for Caesareans if, as a result of monitoring, "true" fetal distress were being more accurately diagnosed and treated. The evidence would show better outcomes for mothers and babies.

But recent research now indicates that the indiscriminate use of fetal monitors does *not* improve these outcomes. In fact, we now know that using EFM for mothers who are not at risk, far from representing the best health care, actually leads to unnecessary C-sections. A major study published in the *New England Journal of Medicine* offers compelling evidence that this is so.[30] Over a three-year period, 35,000 births were examined with respect to the impact of fetal monitoring. During the even months of each year, enough EFMs were made available for every woman in labour; during the odd months, the number of monitors "on site" were reduced by two-thirds, so that doctors had to be more selective in order to ensure their availability for high-risk mothers. In the even months, almost 80% of the women were monitored, in the odd months, only about one-third. The rate of Caesarean sections was 20% higher in the even months (21% versus 17%).* *There was no difference in outcomes for the babies.* If anything, babies in the selectively monitored group did better than those who were routinely monitored, although this finding was not statistically significant. The researchers reported that:

> Abnormalities in fetal heart rate were identified almost three times more frequently during the universal monitoring months. Although universal fetal monitoring was associated with a two-fold increase in Caesarean sections performed because of fetal distress, the measures of infant outcome were not significantly different from those observed during selective monitoring.[31]

Clearly, there are risks when technology spreads unchecked to groups for which it was never intended. This in no way undermines the position that fetal monitoring is appropriate for those at high risk. But it does highlight the importance of determining who stands to benefit.

---

*In a large Canadian hospital, this could mean 100 unnecessary Caesarean sections every year.

How are we addressing such evidence in Canada? An organization of obstetricians and gynecologists has recently promulgated a list of indications for C-sections.[32] Will this alone be sufficient to change practice patterns? We doubt it.

Asking the Right Questions

It's important, when evaluating a health care technology, to determine the right questions to ask about its effectiveness. Typically, we want to know how well the innovation works, and for what kinds of cases. This in turn needs to be judged in terms of how it affects outcomes. But which outcomes should we be looking at? Surely among the most important must be the health of the patient, but here we face a number of obstacles. The traditional measure of health status — mortality — is not always appropriate. A "zero" mortality rate associated with a new technology for arthritis may well be an important measure of its safety, but it tells us nothing about its effectiveness in relieving symptoms, or whether it alters the course of the disease.

There are good arguments for expanding the definition of health, so that it embraces more than the mere absence of disease. Consider the case of chorionic villi sampling (CVS), a procedure now being advocated as a better way of testing for chromosomal abnormalities in the fetus than amniocentesis.

Research to date suggests that CVS is less safe, more expensive, and no more accurate than amniocentesis.[33] The only advantage CVS has over amniocentesis has to do with timeliness — CVS can be done within the first three months of pregnancy, so that if a woman decides on the basis of abnormal results to have an abortion, it can be performed at an earlier and therefore safer stage of her pregnancy.* What's more, she can make her decision while the pregnancy is still a private matter.

A further argument favouring CVS over amniocentesis is that many women having the latter procedure will probably begin to detect fetal movement while they wait for the results. This may affect a mother's attitude toward her pregnancy, by reinforcing

---

*CVS can be done from the tenth week of pregnancy, and its results are available in one to two weeks. Amniocentesis cannot be performed until the fifteenth week of pregnancy, and getting its results can take up to four weeks.

her awareness that she's carrying a live being. The assumption is that an abnormal test result at this later stage of pregnancy would make her decision about whether or not to have an abortion a more stressful and difficult one.

All of these arguments sound convincing until we add another fact: during the first three months of pregnancy, women over 35 have a one-in-five chance of miscarrying.[34] There's good reason to believe that many times this is nature's way of disposing of its mistakes. This implies that if we give nature enough time, the body will take care of the problem itself. So, when we introduce a test that reveals an abnormality in the fetus within those first twelve weeks, we force a woman to make a choice she might never have had to make. Often the decision to have an abortion causes much psychological distress. The fact that a woman might have miscarried anyway, and been absolved of any guilt she might feel, puts CVS in a new perspective.[35]

So a terribly important question when comparing CVS with amniocentesis is, "How does it affect quality of life?" Several countries around the world, including Canada, are now conducting trials on the safety and accuracy of CVS. But only researchers at the Chedoke-McMaster Medical Centre and Toronto General Hospital are looking at these quality-of-life issues — and they had a hard time convincing funders of their importance. Admittedly, techniques to measure quality of life are very "soft" when set against the indisputable kind, like counting the dead. But they are improving. At any rate, it's time to admit that this is often the kind of information we need in order to make rational decisions about technology.

Better How? And For Whom?

Dr. Norm Finlayson, executive director of the British Columbia Medical Association, is an enthusiastic supporter of neonatal intensive care (NIC). "Because of the decreasing neonatal death rates there are 500 babies alive this year in British Columbia who would have died in 1972," he says. "It's the health care system, and especially neonatal intensive care units, which deserve the credit."

NIC units offer a range of treatments for high-risk newborns, and provide special equipment and personnel. Clearly, NIC units are expensive to establish and run, but this hasn't hindered their dissemination throughout North America. We aren't saying this is a bad thing, since studies have proven their overall effectiveness in reducing mortality. Still, there is some question about how many we need.

Most of the candidates for NIC are infants weighing less than 2,500 grams, known as low-birthweight babies. The tiniest of these infants often have a wide range of difficult medical problems, including trouble breathing and digesting, and other conditions related to their immature development. And many who survive go on to experience illness and disability for the rest of their lives.[36]

How well a baby does in NIC depends a lot on how much it weighs. In one study, only 18% of babies under 700 grams survived, compared to 62% of those weighing over 700 grams.[37] Still, NIC has been a factor in the survival of even the tiniest infants. Research from McMaster University showed that babies weighing less than 700 grams are two times more likely to survive now than they were before NIC became available. But this study also looked at issues related to *quality* of life, not just mortality and illness. Some parents considered the serious chronic long-term disabilities among their "saved" children to be worse than death.[38]

We're also finding that NIC interventions can sometimes cause iatrogenic illness. Earlier we mentioned a type of blindness (retrolental fibroplasia) caused by exposing premature infants to too much oxygen. There is evidence that this problem from the past continues to be a common complication in NICs; an American study suggests that the number of cases of blindness among premature babies is "close to the estimated number of cases that occurred during the 'epidemic' years of 1943-1953."[39]

With or without NIC, weight is a crucial determinant of infant survival. An article in the *New England Journal of Medicine* cited four critical factors that influence a baby's birthweight: smoking, infections, nutrition, and adequacy of prenatal care.[40] This leads to questions about what society in general, and medicine in particular, are doing to reduce the incidence of low-birthweight babies.

Dr. Gerry Bonham, medical officer of health for Calgary, is concerned that some doctors are even contributing to the problem of low birthweights by warning their obstetrical patients not to gain more than 20 pounds during pregnancy. "This guideline is simply too low to ensure healthy babies," he says. Given society's preoccupation with leanness, Dr. Bonham thinks doctors should be trying to counter this mindset by encouraging healthier and more realistic weight gains. Patients need to be told about the risks of low-birthweight babies, and how this risk is much higher among women who don't gain enough weight during pregnancy. "We see a typical pattern of quite large weight gain by pregnant immigrant women, who rarely give birth to underweight babies." He sees the cultural influences in North American society as much less forgiving: "Suggest to a typical Canadian woman that it's okay if she gains up to 40 pounds with her pregnancy, and she's horrified!" Small weight gains during pregnancy can lead to low-birthweight babies destined for the NIC unit. The real question is not whether NIC can help these children; it's how to reduce the number who need it, through prevention.

Biting the Bullet on Costs

While new technologies are not the only reason health care costs have risen, they are a major source of higher hospital costs.[41] And hospitals, of course, consume the biggest share of health care dollars. Not all of the costs associated with technology are due to high-priced items like C-T scanners and CCUs. Even "small ticket" items can add significantly to costs if they're used very widely. For example, a recent study assessing the usefulness of skull X-rays for patients with head injuries concluded that X-rays were of no benefit to low-risk patients. A simple history and physical examination was enough to rule out serious injury for about 70% of patients with head injury, so there was no need for X-ray investigation.[42] The same study suggested a more rational approach for these patients, and concluded that "use of the management strategy is safe [and] would result in a large decrease in the use of skull radiography, with concomitant reductions in unnecessary exposure to radiation and savings of millions of dollars annually."

Unless governments, the medical profession, and the scientific community start including consideration of costs in their evaluation of technology, there's no way to determine how to use scarce resources wisely. The prevailing attitude among both providers and public seems to be, "If it exists then we've got to have it." Because the acquisition of new technology is under direct provincial control, and separate from the global operating budgets of hospitals, health ministers and hospitals often find themselves on opposite sides of the table on this question.

The prudent *use* of technology is also a major "quality" issue. But government is reluctant to address quality, deferring instead to the profession to answer such questions. Currently Ontario is being pressured into committing funds for 20 additional NMRs. A new NMR costs approximately $2 million, and the equivalent of one-quarter of one NMR would be ample funding for a good evaluation. But none is planned. A common attitude among the provinces is that research is a "public good," that once done it can be used by anybody, so why should we pay for it? Why should British Columbia pay for research that will benefit Ontario?

Funding for research at the national level is also limited. The National Health Research and Development Program is chronically short of funds. Its mandate is really too broad — encompassing issues of public health, native health, and economics, as well as the utilization of health care services. Somehow it has to find a way to do all that with an annual budget of only about $25 million. Meanwhile, the Medical Research Council restricts the types of research it will fund. It favours basic laboratory investigations into the biomolecular nature of disease over evaluative research of programs and technologies.

So governments are leaving "quality" up to doctors and hospitals. And how well are they doing? Well, as we've already discussed, they are hardly likely to be critical of new technologies. And public pressure, heightened by media stories about the "miracles of modern medicine," gives added momentum to the technological imperative. Competition among hospitals to offer the best facilities available generates unnecessary duplication. Waste is one inevitable result; questionable quality, another.

Imagine the benefits to health, *and* the savings, if technology were used appropriately: if fetal monitoring were used only for

high-risk patients; if coronary care units were used only for complicated cases; if the availability of C-T scanners were determined
by need rather than popularity; if prevention programs for low-
birthweight babies and chlamydia were as universally available
as Caesarean sections. How long will it take to learn that there
is no inherent incompatibility between efficiency and quality?

Chapter 5

The Drug Industry, or How to Make Money and Influence Doctors

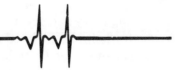

IT'S 1975. Just before dawn on a warm June morning Laura J. was rushed, unconscious with a drug overdose, to St. Joseph's Hospital in Hamilton.* By the time she arrived at the emergency department her pulse had stopped. All attempts to resuscitate her failed. Three years earlier, Laura had gone to her doctor complaining of insomnia, irritability, and loss of appetite. He listened sympathetically as she described how three lively youngsters, an alcoholic and sometimes violent husband, and financial worries were making her miserable. She was particularly distressed about how these tensions were affecting her children — she found herself snapping at them for no reason at all. Laura left the doctors' office that day with a prescription for Valium, which she was to take at night to help her sleep. It worked so well that she soon began using it during the day, whenever she felt jumpy. Her dependence on Valium increased over the next three years. On the last night of her life, terribly depressed after a violent argument with her husband, Laura choked down about 30 of the pills with a large glassful of straight vodka and wound up dead. In 1975, diazepam, the generic name for Valium, was Canada's most widely prescribed drug.[1]

---

*The following three cases of adverse drug reactions are composites created from clinical reports of such adverse drug reactions.

It's 1980. Bill B., a 74-year-old retired postal clerk, went to his doctor complaining of heartburn. His doctor thought he probably had gastritis and prescribed the new drug Tagamet. Only the day before, a detail man had pointed out to him that other doctors were using Tagamet for minor stomach complaints, with good results. So Bill's doctor decided to give it a try, prescribing the usual adult dose. He didn't realize that because of Bill's age, his reduced kidney function might make this dosage too high for him. He also didn't know that Bill's heart medication, propranalol, can interact dangerously with cimetidine.* Shortly after beginning his regimen on Tagamet, Bill woke up one morning feeling dizzy and short of breath. Before he could even telephone for help, he suffered a massive heart attack and died. In 1980, Tagamet was Canada's most widely prescribed drug.[2].

It's 1985. Margorie G., an 80-year-old widow, was admitted to hospital with a severe stomach perforation. For years, Marjorie had been troubled by mild yet painful arthritis in her hands. In deciding how to relieve the pain and reduce the inflammation in her swollen knuckles, her doctor might have weighed the risks of drug therapy against its benefits, and recommended physiotherapy or hot packs for her relatively minor condition. Instead, he decided to use medication, opting for Naprosyn, a drug that had been widely advertised as much easier on the stomach than aspirin. In spite of its claims, Naprosyn *did* irritate Marjorie's stomach — enough to cause a serious bleeding problem. Shortly after she arrived at the emergency department, but before doctors could operate, she hemorrhaged and bled to death. In 1985, naproxen** was Canada's most widely prescribed antiarthritic drug.[3]

These three examples of poor prescribing are more than just additional case studies of iatrogenic disaster. They are also evidence of the extraordinary influence the drug industry exerts over doctors' prescribing decisions — decisions which too often jeopardize their patients' health.

---

*The generic name for Tagamet.

**The generic name for Naprosyn.

Each year Canadians spend hundreds of millions of dollars for drugs they don't need. Even worse, some of these unnecessary drugs can be harmful. Of course, most adverse drug reactions are not life-threatening, but even relatively minor ones like skin rash, headache, nausea, diarrhea, chills, and stomach cramps can be troublesome enough to need treatment with yet more medication. And more serious adverse reactions are certainly not rare; every year they account for between four and ten percent of all hospitalizations, most of which could have been prevented by appropriate prescribing.[4]

Canadian governments now pay for almost half of all prescription drugs, through a variety of provincial benefit programs that cost taxpayers over $1.2 billion a year.[5] But these same governments spend almost nothing to ensure that these products are used wisely. Is it going too far to suggest that governments are paying to poison their populations for the fun and profit of the drug industry?

Drug Research: Quest for Discovery or Profits?

Most people envision drug companies as engaging in rather noble competition with each other in their efforts to find cures for the diseases afflicting modern society. They fully expect that one day the pharmaceutical industry will discover chemical solutions for health threats like cancer, AIDS, and Alzheimer's disease.

To understand why this is unlikely, you need some background about the drug industry. To start with, most of the major pharmaceutical breakthroughs of the past — like penicillin, insulin, and vaccines against infectious diseases — weren't achieved by drug companies, but by researchers working in universities or teaching hospitals. As well, much of the research done by drug companies in Canada today is undertaken by necessity, to satisfy the various legal requirements for testing, without which new products cannot be marketed in this country. Very little of the work done by the industry is likely to turn up any "cures."

The little research money that *is* spent in Canada goes to three basic areas: 70% is used for clinical research, which consists of testing potential drugs on animals and humans; 15% goes to basic research, which seeks to discover totally new drug products, or new ways to use old ones; and 15% is applied to product development, which includes areas such as developing new dosage schedules or different forms of the drug — pills, tablets, creams, solutions, and so on.[6]

Next point: the Canadian pharmaceutical industry is dominated by multinational firms headquartered in the United States or Europe. A firm's research activities tend to be centralized in its home country, and don't get farmed out to branch-plant subsidiaries. But even the research efforts done on "home ground" are not directed at finding "cures." Pharmaceutical companies are in business to make a profit, and know that the best way to do it is to develop slightly different versions of products which *already exist and are successful.* As long as the number of people with a particular condition is large enough to ensure a good market it's much more efficient to develop a "me-too" drug and try to beat out the competition. For example, drug company "research" has brought us scores of competing medications for treating high blood pressure. Because hypertension is so common, the potential market for "new" products to treat it is huge. These drugs may differ by as little as one tiny portion of the molecular structure in the active ingredient.

Since look-alike drugs usually have little therapeutic advantage over other, previously established products, their success in the marketplace depends almost entirely on skillful promotion. Me-too drugs succeed not because they work better, but because their marketing is better. Choosing an appealing name, one that physicians will remember easily, is critical. Placing full-page ads in all the medical journals — a very important source of revenue to these publications — is another essential step in establishing product recognition. Detail men, well-versed in their pitch, dole out free samples to doctors. No effort is spared in launching the latest "discovery."

Overselling Therapeutic Advances

Of course, if the new product turns out *in any way* to be better than its predecessors, the company can announce it as a therapeutic advance. That's how Valium, Tagamet, and Naprosyn rose to prominence. But the clever marketing used to highlight the advantages of these three "new" drugs also tended to minimize their risks. The result has been a lot of overprescribing by physicians.

Roche Canada introduced Valium to this country in 1962. Within a decade it became the most widely prescribed drug on this continent.[7] It owed its remarkable success to a promotion strategy which claimed that here, at last, was a safe pill you could take to relieve the stresses and tensions of everyday life! While it's quite true that diazepam was a better and safer drug than any barbiturate,* Valium was marketed as a treatment for a much wider range of problems than its more dangerous competitor. In the heady enthusiasm that followed its entry into the market, questions about its safety came far too late.

In the 1970s, new information about Valium, citing its addictiveness, the hazards of combining it with alcohol, and its disturbing side effects such as "rage reactions," began to appear in the medical literature.[8] Researchers found that some patients taking Valium developed a tolerance to it, and required larger and larger doses to achieve the desired effect.[9] At the same time, evidence was accumulating that withdrawal from diazepam could cause a host of adverse reactions — even convulsions. Studies conducted in Canadian emergency rooms[10] indicated that between 1973 and 1980, one-third to one-half of patients with drug overdoses were victims of a benzodiazepine.** Ultimately, research results even began to cast doubt on the drug's long-term effectiveness in calming anxiety. Studies comparing a group taking Valium with a control group taking a placebo showed that the therapeutic effect of the drug dwindled after only a few weeks.[11] In one study, prisoners at Millhaven Penitentiary taking benzodiazepines were found to be more aggressive and violent than those who were not.[12]

Yet despite this evidence, the industry continued to promote Valium as a safe product. As late as 1976 the *Canadian Family Physician*, a widely circulated journal, carried an ad for Valium

---

*Barbiturates are far more lethal as overdoses and the withdrawal reaction is frequently fatal.

**Benzodiazepine refers to sedatives and hypnotics of a particular chemical class, including Valium, Librium, and Xanax.

that featured the assurance, "characterized by its safety." Even today, although Valium no longer dominates the benzodiazepine market (having been overtaken by shorter-acting products like Xanax and Halcion), overall use of drugs in its class has not decreased.[13]

Tagamet, the first in its class of drugs, was also sold as a therapeutic advance. Tagamet truly *was* a breakthrough in the treatment of duodenal ulcers, because it was the first effective blocker of a particular histamine receptor in the stomach.* It's rather ironic that Tagamet appeared on the market only just before we had good evidence that large and regular doses of antacids were equally effective in treating duodenal ulcers.[14] This being said, Tagamet still remains a popular treatment choice among physicians, and for good reason: patients find it much more convenient to pop a few pills than to glug down one or two ounces of antacid six to eight times a day.**

The real problem is that Tagamet didn't get to be number one in the drug hit parade by being prescribed for ulcer treatment only. Doctors, impressed by its effectiveness for that indication, began to dole it out for other kinds of stomach ailments, even though no scientific research had been done to prove it was a useful treatment for them. Often Tagamet was prescribed even for minor, self-limiting illnesses, for conditions that clear up easily on their own, especially if antacids are recommended during the acute phase. Also, although few adverse drug reactions are associated with taking Tagamet alone, using it in combination with other common medications can spell trouble. Why risk exposing patients unnecessarily to a potentially toxic drug they don't really need?

One study noted that "the enthusiasm for this drug has led to its use in a number of conditions for which proof of its efficacy and knowledge of the precise dosing regimen required are still lacking." The authors went on to warn that "cimetidine has been

---

*Histamine is a natural substance in the body that triggers the release of stomach acid, and also causes swelling in the lining of the nose in allergy sufferers.

**Nowadays, anti-ulcer drugs are even more convenient to take. A single dose at bedtime taken over three or four weeks is enough to heal most ulcers.

known to 'cure' gastrointestinal symptoms but hide a more serious condition, such as a malignant tumour in the stomach.''[15]

In 1981, Dr. Lilli Kopala from Powell River, British Columbia, did a survey at her local hospital and found that cimetidine was being prescribed inappropriately 80 to 90% of the time. In ten percent of these prescriptions, she could not discover any reason at all why the drug had been ordered.[16]

The promotion of Tagamet as a proven treatment for duodenal ulcers and a small number of other conditions was accurate. Yet doctors clearly were so impressed with the drug's performance for these indications, they overlooked the scientific literature about its limitations. So impressed that they tended to underestimate the risks of combining it with other drug products. So impressed that they commonly used it to treat people with nothing worse than a bellyache. It's a perfect example of how physicians often fail to seek out unbiased sources of information about drugs.

Our third example of poor prescribing was Naprosyn. This antiarthritic drug was widely promoted as being much easier on the stomach than aspirin. In fact, stomach upset *is* more common with aspirin than with Naprosyn. For example, one study found a nine percent rate of severe side effects among patients taking aspirin, but only a three percent rate among those taking Naprosyn.[17] So Naprosyn could be described as having 67% fewer side effects. However, the vast majority of patients have no problem with either drug; the only difference they can tell is in their drug bills — Naprosyn is more than five times as expensive as aspirin.* That's why experienced rheumatologists recommend that doctors start patients on aspirin — especially coated aspirin. In one study comparing the two drugs the authors stated, "The results . . . show naproxen to be a potentially useful drug for the treatment of OA [osteoarthritis]. It should therefore be added to the list of drugs which deserve a trial *if response to aspirin is less than adequate.*"[18] But the advertising for Naprosyn has led doctors to overestimate its advantages over aspirin, and encouraged them to prescribe the costlier drug first.

---

* A one-month supply of Naprosyn (250 mg, 100 tablets) sells for about $47.00; the same amount of 10-grain coated aspirin costs about $8.50.

Drug Safety

Medicine has known for a long time that high cholesterol is a risk factor in cardiovascular disease. The body manufactures most of this sticky blood component on its own, but other factors can contribute to higher levels: smoking, a sedentary lifestyle, not enough fibre, and the typically rich North American diet. In the 1950s, when monitoring patients' serum cholesterol became a very common screening procedure, it was found that many people had elevated levels.

The market for drugs that can reduce cholesterol is hugely attractive to the pharmaceutical industry. In 1960, Richardson Merrell introduced a new product, MER/29 (generic name, triparonal), as the first therapeutic agent for lowering serum cholesterol. Two years later, after hundreds of people had developed cataracts from using the drug, MER/29 was taken off the market.[19]

Shortly after, a new cholesterol-lowering drug called clofibrate was introduced. During the 1960s and 1970s, most doctors advised patients with high cholesterol to modify their diets; if new eating habits failed to lower cholesterol, drug therapy was then tried.[20] Throughout the entire period that clofibrate was being prescribed, no proper evaluation of its safety was conducted.

Then came the shocking results of the first randomized controlled trial on clofibrate.[21] This study on healthy middle-aged men (people with no symptoms of circulatory disease, just high cholesterol levels) confirmed that the drug did indeed lower cholesterol levels by ten percent, and that it reduced both the incidence of heart attacks and the mortality from them. *But the overall death rate was 17% higher among the treatment group than among those taking placebos!* These deaths were largely due to gallbladder and intestinal disease. What's worse, this excess mortality continued for four years following withdrawal of the drug. In the United States, it's estimated that clofibrate treatment led to over 5,000 deaths among people who'd had no symptoms of circulatory disease at the outset.[22]

Another cholesterol-lowering drug is gemfibrozil. This is an expensive product: in Ontario, a year's supply runs about $450 for the drug alone.[23] Pharmacy dispensing fees raise this base figure to about $500. If you calculated the costs of essential laboratory and medical monitoring, yearly costs per patient could easily reach $700 to $800.

Tremendous publicity accompanied the results of the Helsinki Heart Study, an RCT that evaluated gemfibrozil. The media enthusiastically reported that the overall incidence of heart disease among the treatment group in this trial was 34% lower than among the control group, and that deaths from heart disease were 28% lower.[24]

But the press failed to mention that the overall death rate in the Helsinki study was slightly higher (though not statistically significant) in the treatment group! This excess mortality wasn't caused by heart attacks; these people were dying from other causes.

For example, those taking gemfibrozil were five times more likely to have brain hemorrhages. And there was another curious and disturbing finding that no one seemed to take seriously: the rates for accidents and violence were two-and-a-half times greater among those being treated with gemfibrozil. Even though the authors of the research study mentioned that *excess deaths due to violence had been observed in other trials of lipid-lowering agents*, they dismissed this phenomenon as a chance finding![25]

If we followed the Helsinki Heart Study guidelines and so singled out for drug treatment the 300,000 Canadian men between the ages of 40 and 65 with high cholesterol levels, we'd be looking at a yearly cost approaching $300 million.[26] If we added high-risk women and everyone over 65 to the target group, the price tag would climb to over half a billion dollars — for a treatment that, according to the best evidence, does *not* reduce overall mortality.

Victims of Overprescribing: Women

Doctors have often been unwitting partners in drug industry efforts to target products to certain groups within society. An example of this complicity can be seen in the extent to which women have been victims of overprescribing, particularly when it comes to mood-altering drugs.

Much has been written about how pharmaceutical companies

have managed to redefine normal life experiences as illnesses that ought to be treated with drugs. Events like a death in the family, losing a job, or marital breakdown often lead to symptoms of depression or anxiety. Doctors in modern family practice frequently encounter patients who are terribly unhappy, and they know that the source of this anguish is often beyond the scope of medicine to treat. The advent of sedatives like Valium offered sympathetic physicians a way to give patients relief — even if only symptomatic relief — from lives that had become intolerable. But while the drug industry was claiming that "unhappiness" was an appropriate indication for sedation, it failed at first to give doctors sufficient warning about the dangers of using "minor tranquilizers" as a long-term treatment.

There's plenty of evidence showing that women have been particularly at risk of having their problems "medicalized" this way. An analysis of nine separate studies on the use of mood-altering drugs in Canada — all of which were conducted between 1971 and 1979 — found that women were two to three times more likely to receive prescriptions for these drugs.[27]

Certainly the industry aimed its advertising for benzodiazepines toward women: ads featured photographs of weary housewives, anxious college coeds, and ambitious career women striving to achieve, the implication being they were all potential candidates for sedation. Judging by their prescribing habits, physicians seem to have agreed. "Between March 1977 and March 1978, almost 2.25 million prescriptions were written in Canada for all the various brands of diazepam."[28] A study from the family practice units at Toronto General Hospital showed that nearly one-quarter of the patients seen there had taken a benzodiazepine in the previous year, and that one in eight had taken one in the previous two weeks. Over six percent of users admitted they had tried to take an overdose at some point in the past.[29]

Feminists in particular have been vocal in criticizing physicians — and the drug industry — for sedating women whose life situations are intolerable. They point out that the numbing relief such drugs offer may also blunt perception, and in that way discourage people from dealing head-on with the root causes of their problems. The chairman of a 1977 symposium on Valium held in Chicago attempted to point out its usefulness by saying, "We hear much about the adverse effects of the drugs and their costs, while we hear little in terms of *how many divorces Valium may prevent*" (our italics).[30] So an important function of these drugs is to "sustain strained social systems."[31]

Staff from transition houses for battered women indicate that women who use sedatives take longer to leave violent home situations. According to Shirley Small, a Toronto social worker, this is a common social side effect of the drug. "I've been working in the area of battered women for years," she says, "and it's very clear to me that when a woman has been beaten and goes to a doctor, she's more often than not given a tranquilizer, which tends in fact to make her problem worse." She concludes that physicians who prescribe sedatives as a long-term therapy for social problems, and the drug industry, which promotes such usage, are actually encouraging women to remain in high-risk situations. Both are responsible for the consequences of making the unbearable, bearable.

Victims of Overprescribing: Seniors

More and more, however, the drug companies are aiming their promotion in another direction: now elderly people are today's most frequent victims of overprescribing. Dr. Cyril Gryfe, medical director at Toronto's Baycrest Centre for Geriatric Care, says that a lot of drug advertising is promotional rather than strictly informative. He also suggests that the training doctors receive encourages them to overrely on drug therapies. The result is that elderly people are showered with drugs.[32]

Many people over 60 have at least one chronic illness requiring monitoring, and so visit the doctor's office on a regular basis. This gives them the opportunity to inform doctors of other complaints. As a result, they receive more prescriptions for virtually all drugs than any other segment of the population. And since women live longer than men, elderly women are most at risk. According to Dr. Eric Hurowitz, a Toronto specialist in geriatric medicine, the average elderly woman takes 5.7 prescription drugs every day, not to mention 3.2 over-the-counter preparations. "It is faster to prescribe a pill to treat the side effects than to find the source of the problem," he says. "We end up chasing our tails." Overprescribing is so endemic that doctors often can't tell whether a disoriented patient is suffering from dementia or from the side effects of prescribed drugs.[33]

Other factors contribute to medication problems among the elderly. One concerns the dosages they're told to take. Generally, the pharmaceutical companies determine the correct adult dose by testing their products on young, healthy, adult males. The recommended adult dose however, may well be too high for many elderly people; for example, people over 60 often have reduced kidney function, and as a result are less able to flush drugs out of their systems. For them, a normal adult dose could be a relative overdose. In addition to that, elderly people are more likely to be taking a combination of drugs, so a doctor's faulty knowledge about possible adverse interactions can spell disaster for the patient. Too often a doctor responds to a poor medical result from one prescription by increasing the dosage, or prescribing yet another drug.[34]

In 1987, when 170 consecutive admissions to the Geriatric Assessment Unit of the University Hospital in Saskatoon were examined, 19.4% were found to be due to adverse reactions to medication. The researchers concluded that "the results of this study clearly indicate an increasing use of drugs in the elderly, with little or no knowledge of geriatric pharmacology by the prescribing physician, further worsened by inadequate supervision of long-term medication. There is a tendency to treat symptoms of aging rather than the pathology."[35]

Professor Lamy, the director of the University of Maryland's Centre for the Study of Pharmacy and Therapeutics for the Elderly, also lays the blame for these deplorable statistics squarely on the prescribing physician. "We did not teach the doctors, pharmacists, and nurses now in practice about the elderly and their particular needs," he says. "He goes on to criticize physicians for their poor assessment of elderly patients, their overenthusiastic prescribing, and their inadequate patient monitoring.[36]

Victims of Overprescribing: Patients in Hospital

While the risk of being overprescribed is higher if you happen to be female or elderly, it's also significant if you're hospitalized. In 1982, there were 3.5 million hospital admissions in

Canada.[37] Each admission resulted in exposure to an average of eight drugs, for a total of 28 million exposures.[38] Since the more drugs a person is exposed to, the greater the risk of adverse reactions, patients in hospital are in particular jeopardy. (See footnote 4.) In one Ontario hospital the results of 100 autopsies indicated that adverse drug reactions contributed to 36 of the deaths.[39]

Of course, you aren't likely to find many adverse drug reactions unless you really set out to look for them. Symptoms can be easily overlooked, or ascribed to other causes. For example, a *Canadian Family Physician* article reported finding very few adverse drug reactions when family doctors were merely asked to report them. (They found only 314 adverse reactions among a total practice population estimated at 300,000 people.)[40]

On the other hand, a study done in St. Joseph's Hospital in London, Ontario, had nurses carefully monitor patients for signs of adverse reaction. The nurses also accompanied physicians on rounds and reviewed all charts. This study showed that one out of every twelve drug exposures resulted in an adverse reaction. "Among 936 patients monitored, adverse reactions occurred 535 times out of a total of 6,565 drug exposures."[41] These adverse reactions involved commonly used drugs such as digitalis (a medication to improve heart action), heparin (a blood thinner), and antibiotics. Since hospital patients receive, on average, six to ten drugs during their stay, their chances of having an adverse drug reaction while hospitalized are more than 50%.[42]

In an article on hospital drug use, authors Stephen Soumerai and Jerry Avorn list the kinds of errors which can lead to preventable adverse drug reactions: "The use of a potentially toxic drug when one with less risk of toxicity would work as well; use of the wrong drug for a given indication; concurrent administration of an excessive number of drugs, increasing the possibility of interaction effect; excessive doses, especially for elderly patients; continued use of a drug after evidence becomes available concerning major toxic or even lethal side effects."[43] In the same article, they refer to previous research suggesting that "as many as one-seventh of all hospital days are devoted to the care of drug toxicity and . . . that about 70% of adverse effects are predictable and preventable through logical application of existing information."

Doctors and Drugs

Since you can't get a prescription from anyone other than a physician, the responsibility for all this overprescribing falls directly on the medical profession. "Certain drug prescribing patterns are — or should be — an embarrassment to the profession," says Dr. David Naylor, an internist and clinical epidemiologist. He's particularly concerned about the prescribing of antibiotics by doctors in family practice. "Up to one-third of all visits to family physicians in Canada have to do with upper respiratory infections of various kinds — colds, sore throats, and so forth. Only a small fraction of these conditions are caused by bacteria — the majority are due to viruses, for which antibiotics do not constitute effective treatment." All the same, antibiotics are often prescribed for conditions of this type. "The results," Dr. Naylor says, "are allergic reactions, which may lead to hospitalization and are occasionally fatal; bacterial resistance, which makes antibiotics less effective when [they are] really needed; and wasted money. Doctors should first establish that the infection is bacterial in origin, before assuming sore throats require antibiotics."

In 1987 Dr. Joel Lexchin, author of *The Real Pushers*, a well-documented analysis of Canada's drug industry, reviewed ten surveys on antibiotic prescribing in Canadian hospitals. Although he found that prescribing habits did seem to be better in teaching hospitals than in non-teaching ones, he also found that overall only 55% of antibiotic prescriptions were rational, while 35% were irrational, and 10% couldn't be assessed either way.[44]

The raison d'être of medicine is to treat illness, apparently even when no effective therapy is available, and one of the most expedient forms of treatment is the prescription drug. Some doctors transfer responsibility for overprescribing onto their patients, arguing that they *expect* a prescription upon leaving the office. After all, it justifies their visit by assuring them they were "sick enough" to require medication. "I'm not so sure that's valid," says Dr. Lexchin, who works as an emergency-room physician at Toronto Western Hospital. "I think if doctors took the time to explain why a drug isn't needed, most patients would be receptive." Instead, a few scribbles on the pad usually function as the "time's up" signal, ending the consultation neatly and succinctly. Notes Dr. Lial Kofoed, of the Department of Psychiatry at Dartmouth Medical School in Hanover, New Hampshire, "It takes a lot less time to prescribe a drug than to explain to a patient why you won't."[45]

Victims of Underprescribing

But there are also instances where the profession can be criticized for *under*prescribing. A young doctor explains: "Last winter, I broke my ankle and because there were complications, I required surgery to pin the fracture. At four p.m., I arrived at the hospital in agony, 24 hours after the accident. This type of injury is terribly painful and requires a strong narcotic every four hours. Nurses, of course, are not permitted to order drugs, but I didn't get to see a physician until five hours later! All that time, I would have been writhing in pain except that being a doctor, I decided to medicate myself, using painkillers which had been prescribed at the time of the injury.

"Later, after the surgery, I was recovering in a ward and the patient in the opposite bed turned out to be a man I had seen previously with cancer of the prostate. His disease had spread to the bones, making them vulnerable to injury, and he had been admitted with a broken hip. I discovered he'd been prescribed codeine by injection for his pain. I was disturbed because I knew that codeine is relatively ineffective when administered by injection, particularly at the dosage prescribed. Sure enough, in the middle of the night I was awakened by this man screaming in pain. The nurses on duty absolutely refused to summon the doctor on call to alter the prescription until finally, only 36 hours post-op myself, I had to limp out to the desk and threaten all sorts of people to get a doctor to change the order."

This is by no means an uncommon scenario. Although we have drugs that are extremely effective against pain, physicians often fail to use them correctly. Because many illnesses, particularly chronic ones, are characterized by pain, its relief should be a major priority among doctors. But too often that's not the case. When doctors deal inadequately with their patients' pain, they may be reflecting a common medical bias: that merely relieving pain is not therapeutic, that it does nothing to alter the course of disease. Some physicians, in short, tend to underrate the significance of pain relief to the patient's quality of life.

The Information Gap

Since poor prescribing habits are common, we have little choice but to conclude that in general physicians' knowledge about pharmacology is sadly lacking. There are several likely reasons for this. One is that surprisingly little attention is paid to the subject in medical school. Another is that continuing medical education is not usually required of doctors; once licenced, they're free to practice for life, no matter how out-of-date their knowledge may be.* Studies conducted in both the United States and Canada to test physicians' knowledge of pharmaceuticals all indicate a deplorable ignorance.[46]

Although there are better, unbiased sources of information on drugs, like the *Medical Letter on Drugs and Therapeutics***, most physicians seem willing to trust less disinterested sources. Doctors get most of their information about drugs through the promotional activities of the companies that make them. One widely used source, for example, is the *Compendium of Pharmaceuticals and Specialties* (CPS), published by the Canadian Pharmaceutical Association. The CPS lists over 3,000 products available in Canada, giving information on their ingredients, possible side effects, and suggested dosages, as well as the indications and contraindications for their use. All of the information listed in this compendium comes from the manufacturers. The Canadian Medical Association, in its journal, has recommended that doctors use the CPS "to check up on the products they prescribe."[47] In a survey of 75 general practitioners, 91% rated the CPS as their primary source of drug information on overdoses.[48]

But the CPS doesn't appear to be a very reliable source of information: in a study published in 1983, the authors drew a random sample of 230 entries from the 1977 CPS edition and found

---

*Ontario is an exception. As of 1988, the Ontario College of Physicians and Surgeons had monitored all family doctors, internists, and psychiatrists over the age of 70 who were still in independent practice and recommended remedial education as a condition of licencing for those whose skills and knowledge were deemed inadequate. Now, the college anticipates expanding this program to include other specialties.

** This is a U.S. publication for the medical profession, originally started by the American Consumers Union.

that 46.3% of the drugs listed were "probably useless," "obsolete," or "irrational mixtures."[49] In more than half the entries, uses were suggested for which there was no generally accepted clinical, theoretical, or experimental support. In addition, for over 60% of the drugs, well-known risks, dangers, or adverse effects were not mentioned. Dr. Lexchin reports that there have been improvements in the CPS since this study. Nevertheless, it remains suspect as a biased source of information.

Pharmaceutical Marketing: The Secret of Success

The drug industry, like no other industry of its size, has an enormous marketing edge: to sell $2.5 billion worth of products, it only needs to reach a small, readily identifiable group of consumers — the 55,000 physicians practicing in Canada today. (Even the market for luxury cars is larger than that!) And it knows how to exploit that edge: pharmaceutical corporations in Canada have a high advertising-to-sales ratio — in 1983, they spent almost 17% of their sales revenues on promotion.[50]

A drug company's success hinges on its establishing and maintaining a good relationship with the medical profession. Since their profits depend on the prescribing habits of physicians, most of their promotional strategies are aimed at influencing doctors' decision-making.* Above all, they look for ways to inspire doctors' confidence in their products, and to get them to identify strongly with the manufacturer. And companies don't waste any time making connections with prescribers of the future. Dr. Martin Shapiro, in *Getting Doctored*, describes how at the end of first year, medical students in his class were offered free medical bags, each of which contained a stethoscope, a reflex hammer, and a tuning fork. The "gift" came from Eli Lilly, one of the world's largest pharmaceutical manufacturers. Although some in his class spurned the offer, viewing it as an "attempted bribe,"

---

*Drug companies have recently begun to promote prescription drugs to the public at large. TV ads are telling balding men that a new and effective drug treatment is available through their doctors, although the name of the product (Rogaine) is not mentioned. Another example: ads singling out people who want to stop smoking say that pharmacological help (gum containing nicotine) is available through physicians.

most accepted the company's assurance that it amounted to nothing more than good will. "The next year," he writes, "almost all were sporting Lilly equipment when they arrived on the hospital wards."[51]

Probably the most successful technique for promoting drugs is the use of "detail men" — industry jargon for pharmaceutical sales representatives. In Canada, there are over 4,000 detail men visiting physicians in their offices, bringing little gifts like pens, coffee mugs, and flashlights, sharing information about their latest products, and showering free samples "for distribution to your poorer patients." Detail men are well prepared to overcome doctors' resistance to drugs. They arrive with a memorized script, carefully developed to dispel doubts, and concentrate on establishing a trusting relationship. A few detail men have degrees in pharmacy, but according to T. Donald Rucker, a health economist and a professor of pharmacy administration at the University of Illinois at Chicago, most have no scientific background in pharmacology at all. "When hiring a salesman," he says, "some companies figure they're better off with an English or music major than with a pharmacist. If you are trying to bamboozle a physician into thinking a certain drug is the greatest thing since sliced bread, it helps if you don't know anything about the product beyond what your boss has told you."[52]

As an indication of industry confidence in the detailing, drug companies spend almost half their promotional budgets on this strategy alone. Every physician receives, on average, 200 visits a year from detail men — that's almost one for every working day.[53] Of course, the industry concentrates most of its efforts on the high-prescribing physicians, those most likely susceptible to the sales pitch.

Naturally, it's important for the industry to find out who the high-prescribing physicians are. One technique companies use is to pump pharmacists for information about the prescribing habits of doctors in their area. There's no direct financial relationship between physicians and the pharmaceutical companies, because doctors are not the actual purchasers of drugs. But that isn't the case with pharmacists, who can be given price breaks on products in return for such information.

Canadians may remember Bill Crothers as one of the best

middle-distance runners of all time, the winner of the silver medal in the 800 metres at the Tokyo Olympics of 1964. Today Crothers is a pharmacist in Markham, Ontario. He points out that a number of provinces, including Ontario, have tried to stop such practices with legislation, but that it's a difficult area to control. Instead of price breaks, many drug companies offer perks, like free trips and major appliances, in return for high-volume purchasing.* Mr. Crothers says one or two detail men visit his drugstore every day. Do they try to pump him for information about high prescribers? "Sure, it's only natural. They're interested and so are their sales managers."

Dr. Lexchin suggests that the Canadian Medical Directory might be another possible source of information about high prescribers. On the form sent to physicians asking for names, addresses, and so forth, doctors are also asked how many prescriptions they write a day, both in private practice and in hospital.

Print advertising — either through direct mail or in medical journals — is another important promotional technique. In 1983, one Ontario doctor reported receiving "200 pieces of direct mail advertising and about 140 free copies of controlled circulation journals, whose main reason for existence is to be a conduit for pharmaceutical advertising."[54]

Advertising in journals is an especially common strategy. Since nearly all physicians read at least some of the medical literature, it's a sure way to reach the target population. Most journals survive not because their quality attracts many subscribers,** but through the income they earn from drug advertising. Needless to say, journals in this category are less likely to publish articles critical of the drugs advertised on their pages. Even prestigious journals can fall prey to pressure from this powerful industry. At a drug symposium held at McGill University in 1975, Dr. Martin Rizack, a consulting editor to the *Medical Letter*, reported

---

*For example, Crothers told us that Smith, Kline & French offered home computers to pharmacists who ordered a certain volume of Tagamet.

**Only a small number of the hundreds of journals published are responsible for most of the scientifically important articles.

that when the *New England Journal of Medicine* experimented by positioning a *Medical Letter* review of a particular drug alongside an ad* for the same drug, "the drug companies ganged up, threatened a withdrawal of all advertisements, and the objective drug evaluations were eliminated."[55]

Dr. Alan Klass of Winnipeg is the author of *There's Gold in Them Thar Pills*. He notes that the presence of drug advertising in scientific publications lends authority to company claims.[56] Apparently even the advertising director for Smith, Kline & French, a major drug manufacturing company, agreed. "The journal advertising takes on a certain psychological aura of authority by running cheek and jowl with the scientific and expert editorial matter."[57]

Drug companies also rely heavily on "focus groups." This marketing strategy — it's widely employed in other industries as well — involves assembling a group of consumers to learn what motivates their purchasing decisions. A drug company typically brings together a group of doctors, introduces them to a new drug, and then solicits their opinions. The purpose is to find out how they think and why. In particular, the company wants to know about any major concerns the doctors have that might lead them away from prescribing the drug. The company then uses this information as the basis for planning marketing strategies. For example, when thalidomide came out it was advertised as being non-addictive and safe during pregnancy. "These claims were made not on the basis of careful scientific study, but from careful market analysis," says Dr. Lexchin.[58] That's how it happens that unsubstantiated assertions based on flimsy, anecdotal findings end up being pitched to doctors by the detail men, whose main purpose, after all, is to sell the product, not educate the physician. "Rather than coming as a surprise, the predominance of non-scientific rather than scientific sources of drug information is consistent with what would be predicted from communications theory and marketing research data."[59]

Because physician confidence in the product is key to sales, testimonials from prominent doctors used to be especially impor-

---

*Since 1981, Canadian subscribers have received the international edition of the *New England Journal of Medicine*, which contains no advertising.

tant to the industry. Endorsements were sought using a variety of enticements, most commonly "research funding" — often with no strings attached. There are numerous examples of drugs that have risen to prominence this way despite there being little scientific evidence to recommend them. Ads for Zomax, a painkiller that turned out to be no more effective than aspirin, but so dangerous it was removed from the market in 1983, were accompanied by strong endorsements from three prominent Canadian physicians in the 1982 issues of the *Medical Post*.[60]

Because there's so much money at stake, some drug companies haven't been above engaging in dirty tricks to maintain dominance in particular therapeutic fields. For example, between 1970 and 1974, Roche gave away 174 million units of Valium worth an estimated $5 million in an attempt to head off competition from rival firms, and to establish its product in hospitals.[61] The Supreme Court of Ontario later convicted Roche of violating a section of the Combines Investigation Act, and fined the company $50,000.

The fact that the multinational drug industry continues to disparage generic drugs is another example of questionable ethics. Despite widespread agreement among pharmacologists (doctors who specialize in the use of drugs) and government health officials that generic drugs are equally effective, and differ from brand-name products only in being far cheaper, multinationals consistently cast doubt on their bioequivalence.[62] The CMA, and prominent members of council from provincial medical associations, have allied themselves with the multinationals by telling their members that brand names offer "the best guarantee in drug products."

Gerry Rotenberg coordinates the Ontario Medical Association's adverse-drug-reaction reporting program and is the secretary for the OMA's committee on drugs and pharmacotherapy. In the *Medical Post*, he cites the case of an elderly woman who was successfully taking a brand-name drug to control high blood pressure.[63] When she was switched to a generic product, her high blood pressure returned and she reported chest pains and shortness of breath.

Using this kind of example as evidence to deny the safety or bioequivalence of generics is unfair: an individual can react badly to any drug, brand-name *or* generic. Differences in the ingredients used to bind the active agents in the preparation, or in the additives such as those used for buffering, may indeed cause undesirable side effects. While most physicians would agree that it's unwise to switch drugs on a patient whose condition is stable, there's no reason not to start with generic drugs first. After all, for treating high blood pressure, there's more than one generic antihypertensive on the market. The odds are in favour of finding one that would work just as effectively as any brand-name product — and at a much lower cost.

According to figures provided by the Pharmaceutical Manufacturers Association of Canada (PMAC), drug companies spent $240 million on advertising and promotion in 1984 — an average expenditure of about $4,500 per physician.[64] And this amount doesn't include additional funds the industry spent sponsoring medical seminars and providing free hospitality at medical events. Although drug companies insist such sponsorship does not constitute "advertising," their financial support for continuing medical education (CME) is extensive enough to warrant the opposite conclusion. Frank Round, manager of professional relations at Syntex Inc., said that in 1984 his company put on 93 seminars, which often began with a cocktail party and ended with a dinner. "If you give them a couple of drinks, it softens things up," he says. These seminars are a popular way for doctors to accumulate the credits they need to maintain membership in the College of Family Physicians.* However, Mr. Round noted that some doctors do tend to "doze off during the seminars."[65]

Dr. Philip Berger, a Toronto physician, describes one drug-company-sponsored conference he attended at which jellybeans were handed out to promote tranquilizers. Another doctor tells how a detail man mistakenly left behind a sales manual outlining strategies to promote drugs — among them, cookies in the shape of drug capsules, and pizzas with the drug initials "picked out in pepperoni." Though doctors consistently deny that they're influenced by all this, the drug industry simply wouldn't spend upwards of 15% of its revenue on promotion if it didn't work.[66]

---

*Certain specialty societies, like the College of Family Physicians, make CME a condition of membership. Such membership, however, is voluntary and doctors are *not* required to participate in CME to maintain their licence to practice.

Accuracy in Drug Promotion

Since physicians get most of their information about pharmaceuticals from the companies that manufacture them, the accuracy of claims made to promote drugs is vitally important. How valid are industry claims? Judge for yourself:

- In 1947, the first synthetic antibiotic, chloramphenicol, was developed. Marketed by Parke, Davis, as Chloromycetin, evidence linking its use to serious blood disorders began to appear as early as 1949. Yet in 1952, detail men were warned not to mention toxicity unless the physician brought it up.

- In 1962, MER/29, a lipid-lowering drug made by Richardson Merrell, was removed from the market because its use was linked to cataracts. In subsequent investigations it was discovered that one of Merrell's researchers had been ordered to falsify data — data which might have established the drug's toxicity before it was ever brought to market.

- Clindamycin, a broad-spectrum antibiotic known to be associated with a potentially fatal type of colon inflammation, was marketed by Upjohn as Dalacin C. Complying with federal law, Upjohn sent warning letters to Canadian physicians in 1974 and 1975 about this possible side effect. For the first two years a drug is on the market, the Health Protection Branch of Health and Welfare Canada requires that all ads for it contain full prescribing information. After that, "reminder" ads with just the drug's name and a picture are allowed, provided the ad makes no therapeutic claims. So in 1976, Upjohn was running full-page "reminder" ads that simply listed the name of the product, *without* warnings.

- Ads for the antibiotic, Sigamycin, featured the names of doctors who approved of the drug, along with their cities of residence. It was later discovered that those doctors did not exist.

- In the mid-1960s in the U.S., the Food and Drug Administration (FDA) investigated 4,000 drug products. Of the approximately 16,000 claims made about their effectiveness, 66% could not be scientifically substantiated.

- Between 1977 and 1983, FDA investigators in the U.S. found that 24 scientists involved in new-drug trials had misrepresented or falsified their data. In a routine audit of nearly 1,000 investigations, 11.5% were found to have serious deficiencies in their research.[67]

All but the last of these examples are drawn from Dr. Joel Lexchin's excellent and comprehensive analysis of Canada's drug industry, *The Real Pushers*. Dr. Lexchin is regarded as a radical by many physicians, but no one has ever seriously questioned his facts. Indeed, one senior provincial civil servant told us Dr. Lexchin's book was "the best ever written on the drug industry."

Even when a drug's promotion is strictly accurate, the emphasis is almost always on persuading physicians to prescribe it. Ads use very small print to list details about contraindications and potential adverse reactions, and feature a drug's so-called advantages in large type. Often the detailed information appears several pages later in the journal, far from the full-page, full-colour ad to which it pertains. A detail man, if asked, will usually come clean with negative information about his products. But if he's not asked, he's unlikely to volunteer such data.

Leaving doctors at the mercy of such biased information is irresponsible, yet that's what our governments and colleges of physicians and surgeons are doing. In January 1988, Dr. George Carruthers created a furor when he resigned as head of the Drug Quality and Therapeutics Committee, the official advisory body of the Ontario Drug Benefit Plan (ODB).* Dr. Carruthers, a physician and chairman of pharmacology at University Hospital in London, Ontario, accused the provincial government of paying for drugs that were toxic, ineffective, and excessively expensive while ignoring warnings from its own advisory committee. Dr. Carruthers said Ontario's Ministry of Health lacked the political will to stop wasting millions in taxpayers' money.

---

*The ODB pays for drugs prescribed to senior citizens and people on social assistance.

Ontario opposition leader Bob Rae interpreted Carruthers' statements to mean that government is paying for a serious drug problem. But the health minister, Elinor Caplan, neatly ducked the issue by saying it wasn't her role to tell the medical profession how to prescribe, or how to practice medicine.[68] Given the evidence about how little doctors know about drugs, and the lack of action from organized medicine, whose responsibility is it?

Control over Prescription Drugs

There are thousands of drugs currently available on the prescription market, but the World Health Organization identifies only about 230 as being actually "indispensible for health care."[69] Nevertheless, the industry continues to pump out dozens of new preparations every year, so the list of "choice" continues to grow. Health officials and pharmacologists agree that only five or six of each year's "crop" of new drugs really represent a major improvement over what's already available. They note that knowledge about these few products spreads quickly, through contacts with other physicians and articles in the medical literature. As for the rest, the vast majority are either totally useless, or "me-too" drugs — slightly different versions of products already on the market.

How well are Canadians protected from unsafe and ineffective drugs? There are about 3,500 prescription drugs available in Canada.[70] Some 1,500 of these were on the market prior to 1963, and consequently have never been tested using modern methods. New drugs today must be tested before they can be sold, but most of this testing is done by the pharmaceutical companies themselves — and they're hardly unbiased investigators.

Dr. Lexchin points out that when it comes to determining drug safety, Canada depends heavily on testing done in the United States. Nevertheless, our government has no regulations requiring that adverse drug reactions *discovered outside Canada* be reported to Canadian officials. This means that some products which have been removed from the market in the United States remain on sale in Canada. Canada *does* have laws that permit the banning of products determined to be dangerous, but the process requires nothing less than a ministerial order.

On top of that, while our Food and Drug Act forbids false

advertising, the Health Protection Branch has neither the staff nor the budget to ensure good enforcement. In fact, most screening of advertising is done by the Pharmaceutical Advertising Advisory Board, to which the Health Protection Branch merely sends an advisor.

Drug Pricing

With such a proliferation of products on the market, many of them similar to one another, you might expect competition to result in lower prices. But that isn't the case, because of the high level of concentration within therapeutic markets.* "In 1982," Dr. Lexchin states, "in 28 out of 38 major therapeutic markets, two companies accounted for more than 50 percent of sales. For example, two companies had 100 percent of the respiratory stimulant market; two had 66 percent of the diuretic ("water pill") market; and two had 60 percent of the anticonvulsant market."[71] For the majority of products, then, there is no price competition in Canada; competition exists purely on the level of promotion. "This form of competition among patent-holding firms does not result in much lower prices; instead, firms incur heavy promotion costs to promote their brand."[72]

In the 1960s, Canadian drug prices were among the highest in the world. For that reason, the government altered the Patent Act so that other companies could produce copies of import-patented drugs, provided they paid a four percent royalty to the "inventing" company. This "compulsory licencing" brought a small measure of competition to a field dominated by multinational firms.

A small but rapidly growing number of Canadian-owned drug firms benefited enormously from the leg-up this legislation provided. Naturally, companies applied for licences to produce "best-selling" drugs, and as a result, prices for the original, brand-name versions of those products did indeed begin to fall. The multinationals, through their own lobby, the PMAC, fought bitterly against this new competition, which they considered unfair. But how much did compulsory licencing really hurt them?

---

*All the drugs used to treat a particular disease or condition such as high blood pressure or arthritis constitute a therapeutic market.

Not much, according to the Canadian Drug Manufacturers Association (CDMA), which represents Canadian-owned companies producing generics. Between 1969 and the reestablishment of patent protection in 1987, only 70 compulsory licences were issued. And of these, only about 30 drugs actually reached the Canadian market.* The resulting sales represented only three percent of the total sales of all pharmaceutical products in Canada. The Eastman Commission reviewed the impact of compulsory licencing and concluded that it "has not had a discernible negative impact on the profitability and rate of growth of the pharmaceutical industry in Canada as a whole," and that, indeed, "the profits of the industry are substantially higher than those for total manufacturing and for most industries."[73]

Nevertheless, in 1987, the federal government passed Bill C-22, which gives producers of newly patented drugs ten years' freedom from competition with generic drug manufacturers. In return, the drug industry promised to double its investment in Canadian research, thereby protecting existing jobs and creating new ones. Such promises, however, never found their way into the legislation. Consumer organizations, certain that the end of compulsory licencing would mean the start of higher drug prices, pleaded with Ottawa not to fix something that wasn't broken. But the government turned a deaf ear, claiming that the provisions in Bill C-22 for the creation of a Patented Medicine Prices Review Board would control medication costs effectively. The government also ignored the advice of its own Eastman Commission — advice which, had it been followed, would have limited patent protection to only four years, and provided adjustable royalties (from 4 to 14%) so that companies that did more research would receive more compensation. The Senate tried hard to amend the bill in line with this advice, but didn't succeed.

It seems reasonably clear now that the federal government's refusal to consider such reasonable compromises was linked to promises Canada made to the United States in its efforts to get a free-trade deal. Surely it's no coincidence that Edmund Pratt,

---

* The executive director of the CDMA, Mr. Leluk, says there's also quite a backlog of applications for licences waiting for approval by the Health Protection Branch. The CDMA is attempting to negotiate a policy with the HPB to rescue these from limbo.

Jr., the president of Pfizer — a major drug multinational — also chairs both the United States Trade Representatives' Advisory Committee for Trade Negotiations, and the Emergency Committee for American Exports, a group of 60 U.S. multinationals seeking freer trade.[74]

The drug-pricing issue is becoming increasingly important, not just to consumers but to provincial governments as well. Every province has some form of reimbursement scheme for the cost of prescription drugs. Some, like British Columbia and Manitoba, offer universal coverage; others limit benefits to those who are on social assistance or to those over 65 years of age. The costs of such programs have been rising dramatically. For example, in Ontario, which provides free medication for seniors and welfare recipients, costs of the Drug Benefit Plan jumped by 360% between 1978 and 1986.[75]

Friendly Relations

Meanwhile, neither the provincial medical associations nor the colleges of physicians and surgeons seem prepared to criticize the behaviour of the drug industry. On the contrary, the medical establishment has historically favoured the industry's aims and practices over the public's best interests. In 1969, the Canadian Medical Association opposed the legislation that established compulsory licencing; in 1987 it supported Bill C-22, which severely restricts it.

There have long been a number of formal and informal links between the medical profession and the drug industry. Indeed, the first president of the PMAC was Dr. William Wigle, who happened to be a past president of the CMA. "Even today, people who were targets of Dr. Wigle's efforts [to block the original legislation that established compulsory licencing] shake their heads and mutter that it was one of the strongest and most boorish lobbies ever mounted on Parliament Hill . . . ."[76]

In the *Canadian Medical Association Journal* in 1978 the president of the CMA, Dr. Ken Wylie, declared his support for a drug-industry training program for detail men.[77] In this endorsement he asserted that he made a policy of seeing them in his office. This, even though medical specialists in pharmacology urge physicians to get their drug information from non-biased sources.[78]

Could the financial links between medicine and the drug industry be influencing this support? The *CMAJ* took in over half a million dollars in revenue in 1984, most of it from drug company advertising.[79] Is it any wonder this journal almost never publishes articles critical of the industry? The cozy relationship between organized medicine and the drug industry makes it hard not to conclude, along with Dr. Norman Eade of the Montreal Children's Hospital, that they are indeed "in bed together."[80]

The Bitter Pill

The real losers, of course are Canadian consumers. They're the ones who, either directly or through their taxes, wind up paying top dollar for drugs they often don't need.

Doctors remain woefully ignorant about drugs. They've been hoodwinked into relying on the promotional materials prepared by the drug industry — materials designed to sell drugs, not to educate doctors. The result is that prescribing mistakes are common, accounting for a major proportion of iatrogenic illness, particularly among women and the elderly. Meanwhile, governments and provincial colleges have done little to promote good prescribing habits. High industry profits are one indication of just how successful drug companies have been in promoting sales at the expense of health.

Dr. Jerry Avorn of Harvard University has done extensive research on physician prescribing habits. "Nobody's minding the store in academic medicine to systematically inform doctors about drugs," he says. The drug industry, meanwhile, manages to reach just about every doctor in the country with its commercial message. "It's the doctor's fault," says Dr. Avorn, "if that's the only message he listens to, and it is the patient, and society, who is hurt."[81]

Chapter 6

Supply and Demand

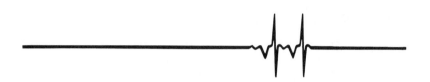

SO FAR, WE'VE DOCUMENTED an appalling level of waste within our health care system, and raised serious questions about quality. There's much less science in medicine than most people would ever guess, and virtually no planning. Finding out that drugs and diagnostic tests are frequently ordered without scientific justification has no doubt alarmed you. That surgical rates for certain procedures are much higher in Canada than in other developed countries must strike you as downright ominous.

Meanwhile, every day specialists see patients who could be handled by family doctors, and family doctors see patients who could be handled by nurses and other non-physician personnel. Indeed, health care providers of all types regularly see people who don't need to contact the health care system at all.

At the same time, many people now in hospitals and nursing homes don't belong in them. Some of these patients could and should be cared for in the community; others are receiving unnecessary treatment, or being kept in the hospital longer than required according to the evidence. This misuse of beds is a major reason why occupancy levels in our institutions are so high. And of course, this overcrowding increases the chance that a patient who does urgently require care will be unable to get a bed.

Who's responsible for this mismanagement, this compromise to quality? Should we blame consumers (patients) for demanding inappropriate services, or the suppliers (mainly doctors) for providing them?

User Fees: Dead and Buried? Or Rising from the Grave?

Many providers — especially doctors — claim that patients are the culprits, and believe we should reintroduce user fees to encourage people to be more selective in their use of health care services. This attitude reflects the belief that a health care system works best when it operates as a free market. It assumes that if patients were at liberty to decide what they wanted *and* were required to pay at least some of the cost, everything would be just fine. In 1982/83, York University researchers conducted a survey of more than 2,000 Canadian doctors and found that about two-thirds approved of user fees as a means to control growth in the volume of medical services, and as a source of additional funding for the system.[1] The Canadian Medical Association took the same position in its 1986 policy statement on health care financing:

> Patient participation has been part of Medicare since its inception and has ensured an additional source of funds as well as consumer and provider responsibility for health care expenditure.[2]

The term "participation" is, of course, a euphemism for "user fees" — a policy Canadians overwhelmingly rejected with the passage of the Canada Health Act in 1984.* Most of us believe that sick people should not have to pay for services at the time they're ill. Still, you may be wondering whether user fees might

---

*The Canada Health Act penalized any province that allowed "extra-billing" or "balanced billing" by physicians. Both terms refer to a physician's practice of charging more for a service than the negotiated fee-schedule allows, and passing on this extra cost to the patient. However, user fees are still being levied in some provinces for some types of services; for example, Ontario residents must pay a portion of their long-term care costs while in a chronic care hospital or nursing home. People in acute care hospitals, who have been designated as "long-term care" patients by their doctors, must begin paying a portion of the cost after 60 days. As a further example of legal user fees, some physicians in Ontario now impose "administrative" charges for services like filling out insurance forms.

not be a good idea. Could they introduce some control over the demand for health services? Could the monies they generated add substantially to the health budget?

Let's begin by admitting that if patients were required to pay more for health care, some people *would* decrease their use of services. The question is, would this decrease only involve "inappropriate" services, or would some people be deterred from seeking *necessary* medical attention because they couldn't afford to pay for it?

A world-famous study on the effects of user charges comes from a natural experiment that occurred in Saskatchewan. In 1968, Premier Ross Thatcher's Liberal government introduced a series of user charges for physician and hospital services; in 1971, Allan Blakeney's NDP government abolished those charges. Two Canadian economists, Professors Glen Beck and John Horne, analysed how 40,000 Saskatchewan families utilized health services before these charges were introduced, while they were in place, and after they were abolished.[3] The main conclusions were:

1. Total provincial health costs remained about the same. There was a small decrease in the use of physician services (about six percent).

2. The elderly, the poor, and those with large families decreased their use of services. For example, use of services by the poor fell by 18%. At the same time, there were more physician-initiated visits, like annual physical examinations, for middle-class patients.

3. There was no change in the use of hospitals — the biggest item in the province's health budget.

From these results, it's clear that user charges are *not* an effective way to control health costs. All they do is discourage people on more limited budgets from visiting the doctor. And if doctors have extra time in their schedules because fewer poor people are making appointments, they bring back their wealthier patients for checkups. As well, we find no effect on hospital use, because it's the physicians who decide who needs to be hospitalized, and people are unlikely to forego what they perceive to be a necessary hospitalization because of cost. So the bottom line on user charges is this: they simply prevent the poor and elderly from entering our system.

Despite the evidence from the Saskatchewan study and other research, the ideology promoting user fees is stubbornly resilient. Many physicians and some politicians continue to favour their reintroduction, with the idea that "patient participation" would cut down on the more trivial use of services. Indeed, the doctors in the York University survey ranked "improved access afforded by Medicare" and "patient visits for minor illness" as the two most important factors in the increased volume of health care services per capita.[4] This implies, of course, that demand for health care comes entirely from the patients. It also implies that inappropriate demands are the patients' fault. How accurate are these assumptions?

The Case for Supplier-Induced Demand

The key to understanding the waste within our system is this: the market for health care isn't like the markets for other commodities. In any normal market, the demand for goods and services is generated mainly by the consumer; when it comes to health care, there's formidable evidence showing that suppliers can generate significant demand on their own. This excessive and inappropriate demand has had major effects on our health system. It's led us into training too many health care personnel — especially physicians — and into building too many facilities — especially hospitals. Indeed, it's skewed planning for the system as a whole by focussing on providers' needs instead of consumers' needs.

The term *supplier-induced demand* may sound academic, but almost everyone has experienced it. Let's consider a health care example: how modern Canadian medicine deals with the common cold.

To begin, we need to explain that the "common cold" is actually caused by any one of several hundred viruses; in fact, over 95% of respiratory infections are viral rather than bacterial in origin. Viruses are the smallest form of life — much smaller than bacteria. But unlike bacteria, viruses can't be killed by antibiotics like penicillin or tetracycline. Apart from vitamin C, which can reduce the duration of cold symptoms (although not the number of colds you catch), there is really no better treatment than rest and plenty of fluids — including granny's chicken soup.

All of this means that antibiotics are a totally worthless cold remedy. Yet many doctors routinely prescribe them for colds.[5] Dr. Howard Seiden, in one of his weekly medical columns in the *Toronto Star*, noted that this inappropriate prescribing habit can lead to a number of complications.[6] Antibiotics are not merely useless against viral infections — they can also be dangerous, in that they can lead to potentially serious side effects among patients taking them. For example, a 1967 study showed that out of 288 patients with potentially fatal aplastic anemia* caused by the antibiotic chloramphenicol, 12% had been prescribed the drug for the common cold.[7] On top of that, the overuse of antibiotics has led to the rise of new strains of bacteria that are much more resistant to treatment. This means that for many bacterial illnesses, higher and higher doses of medication are required, which increases the risk of side effects.

To any readers getting ready to flush their "cold" prescriptions down the toilet, we must point out that *some illnesses that can look very much like a bad cold are indeed caused by bacteria, and do require antibiotic treatment*; strep throat and bacterial pneumonia are just two examples. Fortunately, it's fairly easy to describe those respiratory symptoms that require a visit to the doctor. Listed below are virtually all the cold-like symptoms that really do need medical attention:

- An oral temperature of over 37.7 degrees centigrade (100 degrees Fahrenheit) for more than three days.

- A cough that produces more than a tablespoon per day of yellow, green, brown, or bloody phlegm.

- A nose running with yellow, green, or brown mucus for the whole day, accompanied by facial pain.

---

*In patients with aplastic anemia, the bone marrow fails to produce red or white blood cells.

- An earache.

- Wheezing.

- Any symptoms that are causing the deterioration of someone with a serious chronic illness (heart disease, diabetes,
  cancer, or the like).

So what happens when people catch cold? We all know some
stoics who bravely ignore their symptoms and continue to work,
and others who put themselves to bed and catch up on some reading or daytime television. Some people go to the doctor, others
don't. The average Canadian gets five colds a year. If each of
us went to the doctor every time we caught cold, it would cost
the system about $2.5 billion annually — enough money to build
40,000 subsidized housing units every year.*

In general, most doctors don't discourage patients from seeing
them about minor respiratory complaints. On the contrary, one
study in Saskatchewan found that family physicians there spent
almost ten percent of their time treating patients for cold or flu
symptoms.[8] Other researchers have estimated that as much as
one-third of a family physician's day is devoted to trivial illnesses
like these.[9] One doctor, who works part-time for a Toronto
housecall service, confirms that most of the patients she goes out
to see have colds. Patients who call this service are not screened
in any way, or offered any advice over the phone; instead, the
receptionist merely takes down their name and address and relays
the information to one of the doctors on call. Margaret Wood-
ward, the administrator for a Vancouver walk-in clinic, freely
admits that many people come to her clinic with "sore throats,
flu, and colds."[10] Even hospital emergency departments see
many patients with minor respiratory illnesses for which no effective medical therapy exists.

So whose fault is it when people head for the doctor at the
first sign of sniffles? Should we blame the patient or the doctor?

Before starting a new career in a family planning clinic, Dr.
Debby Copes had a private family practice in Toronto. At the

---

*The calculation is as follows: 25 million Canadians x 5 colds per year = 125
million visits at $20 average cost = $2.5 billion.

end of each day, she used to spend about an hour on the phone talking to patients, most of whom had colds.* She would carefully explain which symptoms required her attention and which did not. Over time, her efforts at health education paid off; her patients learned that they could handle most of their minor respiratory infections on their own. Some colleagues pointed out to Dr. Copes that she could have increased her annual take-home pay by about $20,000 merely by seeing an extra four patients with colds every day. But she felt this would both inconvenience her patients and waste money the health care system could be spending more usefully elsewhere.

Simple patient education has been shown to work in other settings as well. One Seattle, Washington, health maintenance organization, where doctors are paid on salary, found that educating patients about minor respiratory illness reduced the number of calls about flu symptoms by 20%, and cold prescriptions by 18%.[11]

But most patients throughout North America are kept in the dark when it comes to how they might use health care services more appropriately. What's more, many primary care doctors often prescribe useless antibiotics to treat colds. This behaviour reinforces the patient's belief that the visit was justified. If doctors don't tell patients how to distinguish serious symptoms from trivial ones, is it logical to blame patients for seeing a doctor every time they catch cold?

The Agent Is the Expert

This is the key point about supplier-induced demand: lay people — even well-educated lay people — don't know how to practice medicine. As consumers, we simply don't have the expertise to doctor ourselves. If we did, we wouldn't need statutory protection against quackery, we wouldn't need to put colleges of physicians and surgeons in charge of medical licencing; we could judge the quality of practitioners ourselves. But of course none of that is the case. We admit that, by and large, doctors are the

---

*Dr. Copes was not compensated for the time she spent on the phone with patients; doctors cannot bill provincial insurance plans for advice dispensed over the phone.

best ones to judge the competence of other doctors, and that *we have to depend on physicians to advise us about which medical services we should consume.*

We like to think that doctors act as agents on our behalf in a completely impartial way. We want to believe that when they make decisions for us, they do so without bias, combining our preferences for treatment with their expertise about alternative medical interventions. Economists call this "perfect agency" — but how realistic is it?

The physician's interests *may* coincide with the patient's, but we can't assume they *always* do. The professional and economic incentives built into our system exert their own influence over physician behaviour, and can sometimes interfere with what's best for the patient. Can we really blame doctors if, for example, they fail to teach us how to distinguish serious respiratory symptoms from trivial ones? When a doctor on fee-for-service can earn an extra $20,000 a year by seeing four people a day with colds, where's the incentive for spending a lot of uncompensated time educating patients about self-care?

Even if perfect agency were possible, we could still prove that physician-induced demand exists. Once we admit that doctors act as agents for their patients, we're really saying that they're the gatekeepers to our system, that they're the ones who, by and large, determine which services are necessary for a particular episode of illness.

Decisions, Decisions

As you now know, medical decisions are far from clear-cut. The same illness might be diagnosed in a doctor's office with a history and physical examination, or with expensive laboratory tests or a C-T scan. And that illness, once diagnosed, might be treated with a special diet, drugs, physiotherapy, surgery, or even acupuncture. Alternatives abound, and the treatment choices an individual practitioner makes are open to a number of influences: medical education, drug company promotion, other doctors (especially key community specialists), the method of payment for the service, and, of course, the doctor's cumulative clinical experience. This last, while unscientific, nevertheless exerts a powerful influence over physicians' decision-making.

If all these influences served to improve the overall quality of medical decisions there would be no problem. But the extreme variations found in physician behaviour, lead to the opposite conclusion. In fact, there's considerable evidence linking supplier-induced demand with unnecessary treatment.

Health researchers have documented vast differences in physicians' treatment decisions between countries, between provinces, and even between smaller geographical areas, like counties.[12] Of course, physicians claim that these variations occur because the frequency of a given illness varies from place to place, and that higher rates in some areas for a given procedure merely reflect these differences. But research into the prevalence of illness doesn't support this contention. For example, Western countries all report about the same proportion of people with gallstones, yet Canada has by far the highest rate of gallbladder surgery.[13] The same amounts of "illness" are treated in vastly different ways.

- A study of surgery rates in Ontario conducted in the 1970s showed a five-fold difference between counties for hysterectomies, a seven-fold difference for colectomies,* and an eight-fold difference for tonsillectomies.[14]

- There's a 70% difference in the rate of coronary bypass surgery between the area of Ontario with the lowest rate and that with the highest.[15]

- One city in Maine has such high rates of hysterectomy that 70% of women will lose their uterus by the time they're 75. Yet in a city barely 20 miles away, only 25% of 75-year-old women will have undergone a hysterectomy.[16]

- The average length of stay in a Canadian hospital following a normal delivery is about five days. Mothers in most parts of the United States are discharged after only two days.

- Hospital stays are longer on the east coast of the United States than they are on the west coast.

---

*A colectomy is the surgical removal of the large intestine.

Professor Harold Luft, a health economist at the University of California at San Francisco, explains the last point. "A doctor moving from Boston to California will soon discover his colleagues are releasing patients earlier than he was used to back home. The newcomer adjusts to the local standard, once he learns his patients do just as well."*

From the above examples, it's clear that physicians have failed to get together as a group about how to diagnose and treat illness. University of Vermont researcher Dr. John Wennberg concludes that in the absence of authoritative standards, the individual doctor's perception of illness, and choice of treatment strategies, appear to be responsible for the large variations that result.[17] According to Robert Evans, 20 years ago providers of care could ignore or dismiss these differences in their behaviour: "Implicitly, clinical behaviour was its own justification: if the doctor did it, it must have been right." Now he contends that "if physicians cannot find ways either to justify or to correct these variations, others will intervene."[18] And of course, when provincial governments in Canada — or private insurers in the United States — finally accept the challenge of establishing "appropriate rates," they're going to pick the lowest ones possible.

Against All Evidence

Earlier, we documented how evidence from research frequently fails to influence doctors' behaviour. One of the most shocking examples of this can be seen in how Canadian doctors treat lung cancer; it turns out that many recommend a course of therapy which, according to scientific evidence, doesn't work. Even worse, there's some evidence that doctors employ treatments *they themselves would refuse if they were the patient in question*. Here's the background.

Lung cancer is a major killer in Canada. It took more than 10,000 lives in 1983, a toll equal to six percent of all deaths. While there are several different types of lung cancer, over half are "non-

---

*Dr. Luft adds, parenthetically, that new arrivals to California adapt to a different dress standard, as well, and soon dispense with the formality of pin-stripe suits for a more casual "West coast" look.

small cell cancers'' (NSCC). Unfortunately, the survival rate for patients with NSCC is as grim now as it was 30 years ago.[19] Surgery can cure only five to ten percent of patients with NSCC, and over two-thirds of those operated on will actually be worse off for the surgery. Meanwhile, despite dozens of clinical trials in the past three decades, *no regime of chemotherapy has been found useful for these patients.* Yet many Canadian patients with NSCC are subjected to the needless misery caused by this aggressive yet ineffective drug therapy. The question is, why?

- An editorial in the prestigious *British Medical Journal* cautioned against chemotherapy for this type of cancer.[20]

- Dr. Ian Tannock, an oncologist (cancer specialist) at Toronto's Princess Margaret Hospital, says doctors should consider abandoning toxic chemotherapy for NSCC patients because it doesn't work, and because of the sickness it can cause.[21]

- Dr. David Stinson, a specialist in internal medicine in Antigonish, Nova Scotia, goes even further, accusing doctors of causing needless disease and suffering for incurable cancer patients.[22]

- Dr. William Mackillop, a radiation oncologist at Kingston Regional Cancer Centre, surveyed 120 Ontario doctors who treat lung cancers.[23] He found that if they themselves had NSCC that wasn't amenable to surgical treatment, only ten percent would opt for the aggressive therapies currently recommended in standard textbooks.

The Failure to Communicate

Dr. Mackillop and Wendy Stewart also studied cancer patients' attitudes toward and knowledge about their own conditions.[24] Half the incurable patients they surveyed thought they might be cured by therapy. And among those who expressed such hope, half thought their chances for a cure were better than 50%. The investigators also discovered that, although most doctors had informed these patients of their prospects for recovery, they had done this using language that wasn't understandable to lay people.

For example, a doctor may interpret a shrinking of the tumour as a "response to treatment," — a form of clinical success — even though that response may only lengthen a patient's life by a month, and two-thirds of that time may be utterly spoiled by the noxious side effects of chemotherapy. And many times a doctor will refer to a "remission" whenever there's no evidence of tumour — to the physician this is almost the same as a cure. This slides over that fact that many cancers, after going into remission once or twice, will eventually recur and kill the patient.

Dr. Mackillop believes that this kind of misunderstanding prevents patients from making informed choices. "I think most patients with an advanced tumour, who understand that there is a 15% chance of response to chemotherapy, no possibility of remission, and a 100% chance of having nausea, vomiting, and hair loss, would refuse treatment."

Dr. John Evans, chairman of the board of the Rockefeller Foundation (as well as a past dean of medicine at McMaster University, and former president of the University of Toronto), echoes these sentiments. He believes that cancer patients are not offered choices about their treatment in an even-handed fashion. Doctors, he says, have difficulty holding back even when there's no prospect of the patient benefiting. Most provincial medical associations claim that doctors provide the services patients demand. But when it comes to terminal cancer, Dr. Evans disagrees. "We don't have patients calling the shots," he says. "Patients are like the shuttles in a badminton game."

How Fee-for-Service Can Affect Physician Behaviour

Few people would deny that financial incentives affect human behaviour. We're more likely to buy something if it's reduced in price. We'll change jobs if we can improve our income. If we're paid on the basis of how much we produce, we tend to be more productive. But when it comes to health care, we like to think that financial considerations play no part in the care we receive. We tend to forget that physicians and other health care providers are also human beings, that they aren't immune to financial incentives when making medical decisions. Over 90% of Canada's doctors are paid on fee-for-service — the rest work for salaries or on some other fee-for-time mechanism — and it's important to understand how that can affect physician behaviour. Let's begin with an example.

Dr. Ken G. is a fee-for-service family doctor in Winnipeg. He's had a fairly busy solo practice since first opening his office in 1971. In the meantime, however, the number of family doctors per capita in Winnipeg has increased by almost 70%.[25] In addition, that city now has 37 walk-in clinics, most of which have opened in the past five years. As a result, Dr. G. doesn't have as many patients as he used to, and even his regular patients occasionally go to the walk-in clinics because of their extended hours. Dr. G. has been considering expanding his office hours to bring those patients back, but hasn't done so yet.

His first patient today is Jim B., a 27-year-old welder who's usually very healthy. But he injured his back playing with his young son a few days before and is still in pain now. Dr. G. assures him that the injury is not serious, and prescribes one week off work. Dr. G. looks over his patient's chart and notices that Jim hasn't seen him in 15 months. Because he knows he has time available next week, he suggests that Jim come back for a checkup — "just to make sure everything is alright." Is there anything wrong with this? Jim is happy to comply — from his perspective this is proof of his doctor's thoroughness. Dr. G. is happy, too, in that he has filled a hole in his schedule. Of course, there's no real medical need for the visit, but is anybody hurt by it?*

This is one example of how the financial incentives under fee-for-service can affect the delivery of health care. We aren't suggesting that doctors set out in a premeditated fashion to increase their incomes at the expense of the public purse. Except for a few well-publicized individuals, physicians as a group are honest

---

*A prestigious Canadian committee examined the need for regular checkups by family doctors in the 1970s and reported their findings to the conference of Canadian deputy ministers of health in 1979. The committee recommended no routine annual checkups for men between 20 and 50. There are some preventive procedures that should be performed on men in this age group — blood pressure readings, for example — but they can be done while the man is in the office for other reasons. (The Periodic Health Examination, *Canadian Medical Association Journal*, 1979, 121:1193-1254)

and hard-working. But it's only natural that a doctor who has the time, and the capability (like an available hospital bed), will want to treat patients. From the physician's perspective, doing more for a patient is a good thing, and the financial rewards that result from these "good works" are a secondary consideration. But even if income is far from the doctor's mind when those treatment decisions are made, there's evidence that fee-for-service can influence physician behaviour.

Some details about fee-for-service might help you to understand this. Each provincial government negotiates the fee schedule with its provincial medical association — this establishes the overall *level* of the increase. But then it's up to the doctors themselves to apportion this increase across all specialties and for all procedures. This is typically done in a "bear pit" session, in which representatives from the various specialties fight it out among themselves. Theoretically, the fee for a particular service is related to the complexity of the procedure, and to the skill and knowledge required to perform it.

But general practitioners in BC and Ontario complain that specialists have been increasing their fees at the expense of doctors in family practice. Other critics, like Dr. Benson Roe, a medical professor at UCLA, have questioned the fee-setting process. In a *New England Journal of Medicine* editorial, he pointed out that when coronary bypass surgery was first developed in the late 1960s, the surgeon had to direct the preoperation work-up, and a typical bypass took all day.[26] With today's more refined techniques, a surgeon can now do two or three procedures a day; he also has expert support prior to, during, and after the operation. Dr. Roe notes that even so, the fee for this surgery in the United States has not gone down relative to other procedures.

It hasn't dropped in Ontario, either. Between 1986 and 1987, the fee for a double bypass went up nearly nine percent while the fee for a general practitioner's complete examination increased by only five percent.

- In March 1988, the fee for a minor office visit in Ontario was $14.90; a complete physical examination paid $44.60; and a double coronary artery bypass operation paid $1,071.90.

- Ontario's fee schedule provides no payment at all for dispensing telephone advice or discussing cases with a public health nurse, or for the time a doctor might have to spend reading up about a difficult case.

- Doctors on fee-for-service are paid exactly the same amount for a service regardless of how much time it takes to perform. The obstetrician who attends a mother's labour for several hours receives no more than the one who arrives on the scene only minutes before delivery.

- Doctors can't bill Medicare for services provided by nurses,* despite the proven safety and effectiveness of having nurses provide up to 50% of the health care traditionally carried out by physicians.[27]

To see how these characteristics of fee-for-service might influence a physician's practice style, put yourself in a family doctor's shoes for a few minutes. Your first patient this morning is Sally W., a 23-year-old graduate student you've been treating for ten years. Sally is intermittently bothered by tension headaches, which aren't dangerous in any way, but do interfere with her personal life and studies. You know that stress is often the underlying cause of such headaches, but remind yourself that Sally has responded well in the past to treatment with diazepam (the generic form of Valium).

Today, Sally tells you the same old story of school deadlines and problems with her disabled mother. You know she feels guilty about spending time on her schoolwork instead of with her mother. Should you get her to talk about this? The last time Sally came in you referred her mother to a local community centre. Should you follow up on this and ask how things are going?

You hesitate, because the last time you explored Sally's relationship with her mother, she went to pieces, cried for an hour, and left you way behind schedule. Though you were able to bill the Ontario Health Insurance Plan (OHIP) for $84.80 for that

---

*There are a few exceptions to this rule. For example, doctors can bill Ontario's health plan for allergy shots administered by nurses.

counselling, normally you would have seen seven patients in the hour it took to see Sally that day. Since your average billing is $25 for each patient, or over $175 per hour, that visit put you out of pocket by almost $100. You could call Sally back for half an hour of psychotherapy next week, but that would still only pay $42.40. You could be making over twice that in the same half-hour by seeing patients with regular medical problems. You search her face and conclude that Sally doesn't really expect to talk. She's waiting for the prescription. You reach for the pad and start writing.

How Alternative Payment Methods Affect Physician Behaviour

While most doctors in Canada are paid on fee-for-service, some work in alternative practice settings and receive salaries. In Canada, doctors paid on salary are likely to be in group practices, where their behaviour is either formally or informally monitored by the other physicians in the group. Under a salaried-payment system,* doctors have no financial incentive to provide more and more services. Proponents of fee-for-service sometimes argue that salaried doctors might end up offering *less* care than their patients actually require. But a number of studies comparing fee-for-service with fee-for-time refute this criticism.

In 1978, University of Montreal researcher Marc Renaud and his colleagues trained four university students to simulate patients with muscle tension headaches and then randomly sent them either to doctors paid on fee-for-service or to doctors paid on salary.[28] The students were instructed to say that their previous physician had prescribed diazepam the year before, and that they'd continued using the medication. As a reason for the visit, they were told to say they'd moved and that their new pharmacist would not dispense more diazepam without a new prescription. This study found marked differences in physician behaviour according to how they were paid:

---

*Sometimes called a fee-for-time or sessional payments system.

- Fee-for-service doctors spent, on average, only eight minutes with each simulated patient. Visits to the salaried doctors averaged over 21 minutes.

- At the same time, 40% of fee-for-service doctors were rated poor or fair in their investigation of these headaches, compared to 14% of the salaried doctors.

- When it came to taking the medical history, 46% of the fee-for-service doctors were rated poor or fair, compared to 28% of the salaried doctors.

- Even though the same proportion of physicians from each practice setting prescribed medication, there were major differences in the duration of the prescriptions, the warnings issued, and the suggestions about non-drug therapy:

	Salaried Doctors	Fee-for-Service
Prescription—More than three months	14%	50%
Explicit warnings re: medication	64%	30%
Explicit advice re: non-drug therapy*	54%	23%

Overall, the researchers rated 50% of the encounters with salaried doctors as adequate. *Only 17% of the encounters with fee-for-service physicians met this standard.*

The payment system can also affect the delivery of preventive health care services. Under fee-for-service, immunization, well-baby care, annual cancer detection visits for women, and the like, typically pay much less on a money-per-time basis than other fee-for-service procedures.

---

*Examples of non-drug therapy for tension headaches include physical activity, relaxation techniques, or psychotherapy.

- Two studies showed that salaried doctors in Québec were more likely to follow approved protocols for cancer detection than doctors paid by fee-for-service.[29]

- Another Québec study showed that fee-for-service doctors were less likely to vaccinate young children according to the proper schedule than salaried personnel at public "well-baby" clinics. By the time 90% of the children attending the public clinics had received all their first five immunizations, only 65% of those attending private doctors had completed their first series.[30]

- In 1967, researchers examined the use of health care services by steelworkers and their families living in Sault Ste. Marie, Ontario. Some of these people were attended by fee-for-service doctors; others, by salaried physicians at the Sault Ste. Marie Group Health Centre. The study groups were very similar except in their source of medical care. The results showed that the salaried doctors provided more preventive services and were much less likely to hospitalize their patients. In fact, patients at the centre used 24% fewer hospital days per capita than the patients cared for by fee-for-service doctors.[31] While much has changed in medicine since 1967, the 42,000 patients who go to the Group Health Centre still use 25 to 30% fewer hospital days per capita than the rest of the population of Algoma District.[32]

- Health maintenance organizations (HMOs) in the United States charge their patients a fixed premium and then accept responsibility for providing and paying for all their health care, both in the doctors' office and in hospital.* These groups have a dramatic effect on health care utilization. Most HMO doctors are paid on salary, work in groups, and are subject to peer review. A summary of the evidence published in 1981 concluded that HMO patients cost approximately 25% less to treat than patients attended by fee-for-service doctors, and that HMO patients spent about 40% fewer days in hospital.[33] Subsequent research has confirmed these findings.

---

*Health maintenance organizations will be discussed more fully in Chapter 9.

To summarize: The evidence that supplier-induced demand exists is based on the fact that the market for health care is like no other. Patients are the "consumers" of medical service, but must rely on doctors to tell them what types of care they need. Whether you call this supplier-induced demand or the "trust me, I'm a doctor" syndrome, the result is the same: doctors decide what services we consume and then patients — individually and collectively — pay for them.

If medicine offered only one way to diagnose and one way to treat any particular episode of illness, then doctors could justifiably claim that their decisions were totally objective. But as you now know, medicine is full of choices, and the way doctors make those choices is often not very scientific at all. At least 80% of therapies have never been rigorously evaluated, and there's even less scientific evidence about the appropriate use of diagnostic tests. The result is that "appropriate care" is defined differently by different doctors, different hospitals, and different communities.

Meanwhile, our suspicion grows that there's a strong link between supplier-induced demand and the provision of unnecessary services. We see wide variations in health-service consumption between different geographical areas that are not explained by differences in illness rates. At the same time, we find that physicians' behaviour can vary greatly according to the payment system they're under, and whether or not their work is being monitored.

The ability of physicians to generate demand for their services has seriously affected our ideas about how many health care personnel and hospital beds we need. Let's look first at how this has led us into training too many physicians.

Finding the Magic Number: Doctors

Canada presently has 55,000 active physicians — one for every 465 people.* We don't know how many of them are in full-time practice, which presents a problem when it comes to interpret-

---

*Health and Welfare Canada considers a physician "active" if the doctor has billed a provincial Medicare plan at least once in each of the preceding four quarters (Health and Welfare Canada, 1987).

ing these figures. What can be said is that most health care researchers agree we have too many doctors now, and are producing too many for the future. Here's why:

- Since 1975, Canada's supply of doctors has been growing at an average rate of 3.4% a year. Canada's population has been increasing at a much slower pace — only 1.1% a year over the same period.[34]

- Each year about 1,800 doctors graduate from Canadian medical schools and enter our health care system; another 300 to 400 immigrant doctors are licenced every year. Meanwhile, we lose only about 950 doctors a year to retirement, death, or career changes.[35] Just to maintain the current doctor-to-population ratio, which most experts agree is too high, we would have to reduce our yearly output of physicians by at least 500 immediately.

Right now there are over 5,000 medical students in Canada who will enter the pool of active physicians in the next few years. Even ten years ago some health policy experts were saying we had too many doctors, which suggests we're facing a crisis now. If nothing is done, we may achieve what some cynics call the ultimate ratio for family doctors: every family will have one — all to itself!

Governments, of course, are becoming concerned about the cost implications of this explosion in the number of physicians. They're beginning to listen to the university academics, who have been warning for over a decade that controlling the supply of physicians is essential to controlling health-care spending. Professor Richard Plain, a health economist at the University of Alberta, is proud to be a fourth-generation Albertan and a lifelong Tory. But his political allegiance hasn't stopped him from fighting for equal access to health services. He's been a consultant to the Consumers' Association of Canada and other pro-Medicare groups. Plain says that the main problem facing health care financing in Alberta is that the province is oversupplied with doctors. It's a problem Alberta shares with the rest of Canada.[36] Robert Evans echoed this view in October 1987 when he told delegates at a health conference in Winnipeg, "I think it would be better for the country as a whole to stop producing so many physicians."[37]

A curious feature of this problem is that no one has taken a close look at how many physicians we actually need. In 1964 there was one practicing doctor in Canada for every 800 people. By 1975 the ratio had dropped to one for every 580; by 1987, to one for every 465. How do we determine the most appropriate ratio?

Before beginning to answer this question, we have to deal with the fact that physicians are not a homogeneous group. General practitioners, family physicians, and some pediatricians, gynecologists, and internists work in primary care — patients refer *themselves* to such doctors for treatment. In other specialties, patients arrive mainly through referral from other doctors — radiologists, psychiatrists, various types of surgeons, and many internists fall into this category. All of this means that while the overall ratio of physicians may be adequate or even too high, some specialists in medicine — like geriatricians and oncologists — could be *under*represented in terms of actual patient needs.

Also, the distribution of doctors in Canada is uneven. Most choose to practice in large urban centres; smaller communities often report difficulty attracting doctors. Those living in the far north, in particular, often complain about the shortage of physicians. But research into the use of medical services by rural people — in Manitoba, for example — has shown that they don't differ significantly from their urban counterparts in the amount of health care they consume.[38] In any case, merely increasing the pool of doctors does nothing to ensure a more equitable geographic distribution.

Establishing the ideal doctor-to-population ratio is made still more difficult by the fact that many doctors spend much of their time inappropriately. Specialists and subspecialists have gone through years of additional training to develop particular expertise in treating the very ill. Yet many of these specialists see patients who could easily have their needs met by family physicians, nurses, or other health personnel. Indeed, there is no documented evidence anywhere that a specialist can provide better well-person care than a nurse. So we have to ask, why do so many healthy women get their Pap smears and birth control prescriptions from an obstetrician/gynecologist? And why should perfectly healthy babies need a pediatrician? After practicing in Newfoundland

and New Guinea, Dr. Nancy Harris set up a family practice in Toronto. "I was shocked to discover that most of a Toronto pediatrician's day was spent with well children," she says. (When it comes to getting health care for herself, Dr. Harris goes to a nurse practitioner.) Until we address the important question of who will do what — based on what patients actually require — we can't determine the appropriate physician-to-population ratio or plan for the future supply of doctors. What's more, we have to suspect a serious oversupply right now.

While governments focus on the cost impact resulting from an oversupply of physicians, some doctors are worrying about how an oversupply may be affecting the health of Canadians. Well they might, considering the evidence for unnecessary interventions of all kinds. For example, Dr. Fraser Mustard, former dean of McMaster University's medical school, and now president of the Canadian Institute for Advanced Research, says the biggest menace to an older population is an excess of doctors. "What am I going to do as a doctor who needs an income? I need patients. So there I have you — an older person and your physiology is changing. Now, if I can medicalize that . . . ."

Sure enough, a look at how different age groups use medical services reveals that patients over 65 are a susceptible group. As Bob Evans points out, "The intensity of servicing (the number and cost of interventions) is rising rapidly among the elderly themselves; the age-use profiles are shifting upwards and twisting."[39]

The aging of our population is often cited as the driving force behind the growing use of health services. It's also used as an excuse for increasing our supply of doctors. But like other simple explanations for complicated problems, it's wrong. It's true that elderly people use more services per capita than younger people. It's also true that the proportion of our population which is over 65 is growing now, will grow even more quickly as the "baby boom" generation ages, and will reach about 20% in the year 2020.[40] Now if the rate of service utilization stays the same as it is now for each age group, so that elderly people in the future receive the same level of care that seniors get now, this demographic change presents no cost problem, in and of itself. The overall increase in costs will only amount to about one percent a year — far less than our current annual rate of inflation, and well within the bounds of what our economy can afford.[41]

Professor Morris Barer, from the University of British Columbia, recently shed some light on this poorly understood public policy issue. He points out that the only real problem will be if we continue to increase the level of servicing. "If there is a crisis," he says, "it is the disproportionate growth in the use of health care services by the elderly, not the growth in the number of potential elderly users."[42] Given the nature of supplier-induced demand, if we continue to flood the market with doctors, what are our chances of maintaining current service levels for *any* age group?

How did this happen? How did a well-meaning program intended to improve Canadians' health by increasing their access to doctors turn into a sorcerer's-apprentice nightmare of unnecessary surgery, adverse drug reactions, and wasted social spending?

Mistakes from the Past Return to Haunt Us

Our current oversupply of physicians is mainly the result of some wildly inaccurate forecasting about Canada's population growth, and our failure to plan on the basis of what we know about appropriate patient care.

We started going wrong in 1964, when a medical manpower report for the Royal Commission on Health Services* incorrectly predicted that Canada's population would continue to grow as fast as it had during the baby-boom years.[43] This report estimated that Canada would have 30 million people by 1986. This figure turned out to be badly off — by 1987, Canada's population was only 25.6 million. The report also forecast that by 1986, 44,000 doctors would be needed to serve our population. In fact, by 1987, Canadians were being served by 55,000 doctors.[44] In other words, even though the commission overestimated our population's growth, its forecast called for fewer doctors than we have now. This is because it based its estimate on the assump-

---

*Justice Emmett Hall's *Report on the Royal Commission into Health Services* is nevertheless a landmark document. It paved the way for the federal Medicare legislation and has guided the development of our health-care system for over two decades.

tion that one physician for every 693 people was ideal. Today we have one for every 465 of us.

Where do these ideal figures come from? By what means do provincial governments, medical associations, and university medical schools decide how many doctors we need today? And why do official reports on physician supply usually conclude that we don't have enough doctors?

The planning process is flawed because it assumes and accepts the present pattern of utilization. In other words, it deems all services currently provided by physicians to be necessary and appropriate. This flies in the face of evidence we've already presented about waste in our system. We know conclusively that many medical services offered today are inappropriate, and that some are even dangerous.

Professor Jonathan Lomas is the assistant coordinator of the Centre for Health Economics and Policy Analysis at McMaster University's faculty of medicine. He's been studying physician manpower issues for over ten years, and is appalled that this major flaw in methodology continues to warp today's forecasts. For example, look at how the Macdonald Task Force, a manpower planning exercise conducted in Ontario in the early 1980s, repeated the same error: "A 'demand-based' approach . . . determines physician requirements consistent with the amount of health care that people actually demand and receive. The demand- or utilization-based approach essentially tells you how many physicians will be required in the future *if the present structure and policies of the health care system are maintained.*"[45] (Italics ours.)

According to Lomas, a much better approach would follow the methodology of an American manpower-planning exercise done by the Graduate Medical Education National Advisory Committee (GMENAC). This group didn't assume current utilization patterns were necessarily appropriate. In other words they didn't begin with the providers' side of the equation. Instead, they looked at the population and its needs. GMENAC estimated future needs for health care based on epidemiological data and expert opinion on how much illness would occur in 1990 in the United States. Then they looked at the most effective and efficient ways of diagnosing and treating those illnesses — again according to medical research. Using this information, GMENAC then estimated how many full-time-equivalent physicians would be needed to perform those services.*

It's interesting that GMENAC, the only North American manpower-planning report to use a needs-based approach, was also the only one ever to conclude that there was an impending surplus of physicians. Recently, some experts have suggested that even GMENAC overestimated the need for doctors, by failing to predict the rapid growth of health maintenance organizations. When GMENAC released their report in 1980, just over 9 million Americans were enrolled in HMOs; by June 1988, over 31 million Americans had joined an HMO of some type. HMOs typically use far fewer physicians to serve their populations, because they're offered no financial incentives to overservice, and because they use non-physician personnel more effectively. As a result of this growth in HMOs, one researcher and his colleagues forecast that by the year 1990, America would have 20% too many children's primary care physicians (pediatricians and family doctors), and 50% too many adult primary care physicians (internists and family doctors).[46]

While we in Canada have no HMOs, we do have alternative practice settings that use fewer doctors than the fee-for-service system. For example, Lomas has documented that Ontario's health service organizations (HSOs) — like the Sault Ste. Marie Group Health Centre, where doctors work in groups and are paid on salary — use roughly 25% fewer doctors per capita than the fee-for-service system.[47] In other words, once the economic and professional incentives change, we don't need nearly as many physicians.

When governments back in the 1960s and 1970s believed we were facing an impending doctor shortage, they had little difficulty dealing with the problem — they simply expanded our medical schools. Now they're finding that it's much harder to *decrease* the number of doctors we're producing. As Lomas and his colleagues point out, very little evidence was required to prime

---

*This approach is comparable to what accountants call "zero-based" budgeting. You don't assume the current budget level is appropriate at the outset; instead, you examine your future financial requirements in terms of predicted needs.

the pump, but rigorous evidence is being demanded by doctors and medical faculties alike, now that governments are trying to stop the flow.[48]

Finding the Magic Number: Other Health Personnel

As the GMENAC planning exercise recognized, health services needn't always be supplied by physicians. Deducing the future demand for services says nothing about who should be providing those services. If we factored in the appropriate use of non-physician personnel, our estimate about how many doctors we need would drop even further.

Let's look at an example. Mr. and Mrs. D. have a young son with brain damage who sees a neurosurgeon at Toronto's Hospital for Sick Children every six months. They are terribly frustrated because they only get to see the doctor for a short time during these visits, and because he seems to lack much interest in their son's progress. They expect the neurosurgeon to encourage them to continue their hard work. Instead, they find their encounters with him brief and unsatisfying.

On the surface, it's easy to sympathize with the D.s' complaint. But is it really appropriate to expect a neurosurgeon to spend a lot of time with these parents? He isn't trained in patient education, nor is he particularly knowledgeable about available community services. He does know how to operate on people's brains — a very specialized skill. Wouldn't it make much more sense if the parents had frequent access to a nurse or social worker, that is, to someone trained in health education and the use of support services? This contact person could always call in the doctor as the need arose, whenever the parents wished to discuss their son's medical condition.

To determine the appropriate service provider for a patient, you have to begin with a clear understanding of that patient's needs. Often those needs can be met more effectively and more efficiently by non-physician personnel.

For example, many studies have shown that specially trained nurses can safely and effectively provide over 50% of the services generally provided by family doctors. Probably the best-known of these studies was conducted in Burlington, Ontario, in the early 1970s. Patients in a group family practice were randomly assigned to either a doctor or a specially trained nurse practitioner for their basic care. There were no differences in the health outcomes or in the level of consumer satisfaction between the two groups of patients.[49]

Julie A. is a 17-year-old grade twelve student in Toronto. She started having intercourse with her boyfriend three months ago. Before this she had gone to her family doctor for advice about birth control and he started her on the pill. Soon after, Julie found she'd put on five pounds; on top of that, she sometimes forgot to take her pills. When she was two weeks late for her menstrual period she went back to her doctor, who chastised her for not taking her pills properly and warned her that she might be pregnant. Julie began to cry and the doctor, feeling a little over his head and mindful that he had six other patients to see that hour, told her to go to a clinic where she could get an abortion referral. In tears, Julie was advised by her friends to go to the Hassle Free Clinic in downtown Toronto. (Hassle Free started as a crisis centre for street kids in the early 1970s and has evolved to become Toronto's busiest venereal disease and family planning clinic.)

At Hassle Free, Julie was booked with a nurse named Laura for a 45-minute appointment, during which she poured out her story. Laura did a pregnancy test and assured Julie that she was probably not pregnant, and that her missed period was probably due to the pill. But Laura's training enabled her to probe for the likely causes of Julie's forgetfulness. As Laura suspected, Julie wasn't really ready to begin having sex, and had been pressured into going on the pill by her boyfriend. She told Laura she wasn't enjoying sex and felt very guilty about the whole thing. She felt even worse for taking the birth control pill. Like many of her peers, Julie thought it was all right to have sex as long as it wasn't premeditated, that sex wasn't immoral if you were caught up in a grand passion. But taking the pill removed that illusion and made sex a planned act. Laura suggested that Julie take the next week off sex and come back to talk some more.

Let's compare the two visits. Julie's encounter with her doctor accomplished almost nothing and cost the Ontario Health Insurance Plan $15; Julie's visit to Laura changed her life and cost the Ontario government about the same amount.

There are 200,000 nurses working in Canada and without them

our health care system would come to a complete stop.[50] They form the backbone of the hospital work force, not only carrying out physicians' orders but directing the work of nurses' aides, orderlies, and other staff.

Yet everywhere you look there are signs that the nursing profession in this country is in crisis. Today's hospital nurses complain of overwork, too much responsibility, and too little authority. In his book *Hospital*, Martin O'Malley quotes Bev McParland, the nursing manager of the coronary care unit at Toronto General Hospital. "Most doctors would not have survived their medical education without nurses . . . . We've all seen it. We've defibrillated patients and run full resuscitations with a junior doctor limping along behind. When it was over he'd sign the papers and get credit for it. What do you do? You know what you do? You say, 'Oh well, another day in the salt mine'."[51]

O'Malley goes on to quote a *Journal of the American Medical Association* article from 1906: "Every attempt at initiative on the part of nurses . . . should be reproved by the physicians . . . . The professional instruction of nurses should be entrusted exclusively to the physicians who only can judge what is necessary for them to know." Since this bit of turn-of-the-century chauvinism was published, nursing has become a more complicated and sophisticated profession. The rapid introduction of new technologies since the Second World War has meant they've had to specialize more, and attain ever higher levels of skill.

Even so, until very recently nurses were principally seen as handmaidens to physicians. They're still expected to do whatever doctors tell them — and quickly at that. Gail Donner, executive director of the Registered Nurses' Association of Ontario, says she was taught in nursing school to always stand when a physician entered the room. "It got so I stood up no matter who came in — doctors, other nurses, even patients."

The average Canadian doctor earns five times more than the average Canadian worker. These high incomes no doubt reflect the attitude many Canadians hold, that services considered essential to life are worth paying for. But it could be argued that the work of nurses is just as essential, if not more so. Consider that Ontario law prohibits nurses from striking because they're considered an essential work force. No similar prohibition against the right to strike has ever been enacted against Ontario's doctors; indeed, the government allowed a doctor work stoppage to continue for more than three weeks in 1986.*

But however essential nurses are, they haven't nearly the financial security or decision-making authority doctors have. Senior hospital nurses make only a few thousand dollars more than graduates fresh out of nursing school, even though they frequently manage six-figure budgets. Nursing administrators' salaries are minuscule when set against those of their physician colleagues. The same can be said of their clout within the health care system — compared to doctors, they have little or none. We're paying a price for this imbalance.

- As of February 1987, up to 750 nursing positions at Metro Toronto hospitals were unfilled, and, according to health officials, could not be filled.[52]

- Bright, well-trained nurses are likely to leave practice for business, medicine, or law when they find that they're barred from living up to their potential as nurses.

- Hospital wards in some cities — Toronto being a good example — remain in mothballs because there aren't enough nurses to staff them.

- Nurses in Alberta, concerned about pay and working conditions, went on an illegal strike in January 1988. The Manitoba government narrowly averted a nursing strike later that spring over similar issues. Then in October, Saskatchewan's nurses won a settlement following a seven-day walkout.

While Canada's supply of nurses continues to grow at a faster pace than our population, we're opening so many new facilities that the demand for nurses today is outstripping the supply. For example, Ontario announced plans for $850 million in new investment in hospitals in 1986, and Alberta is still opening new acute care beds. Both Gail Donner and Ginette Rodger, who is executive

---

*This "strike" was over Bill 94, legislation which the province of Ontario had passed to ban extra-billing.

director of the Canadian Nurses Association, take this as a sign of poor planning. How, they wonder, can provincial governments voice concern about the nursing shortage in existing facilities, yet announce in the same breath that they're going to open new ones? This leads inevitably to questions about how Canada plans its supply of institutional beds.

Planning for Institutional Beds

Determining the "magic number" for the supply of institutional beds is no different from determining how many doctors we need, in this sense: before we can answer, we have to ask a series of other questions. What types of illness are seen in the community? What types of care do these illnesses require? Is there good evidence showing that an institution is the most appropriate setting for delivering that care? And so on.

Once again, the GMENAC methodology provides the most accurate projections. You start with the amount of illness seen. Then you search the medical literature to ascertain the most effective treatments for those illnesses, and the most appropriate settings for providing those treatments. Finally, using this information, you add up the number of hospital beds required. It sounds simple in theory — but let's look at the confusion we have in practice.

"People are waiting longer and longer for needed surgery and some people are dying before they can have it." John Laplume, executive director of the Manitoba Medical Association, in the *Winnipeg Free Press*. December 28, 1987.

"Equating good health with hospital beds is a myth." Wilson Parasiuk, former Manitoba health minister, in the *Winnipeg Free Press*. December 26, 1987.

"Manitoba doctors are sending elderly patients to hospital who don't need to be there, a research study prepared for a conference on health care costs suggests." *Winnipeg Free Press*. May 6, 1986.

"I don't think health care will suffer at all [from hospital bed cuts]. For example, the hospital performs 400 tubal ligations annually on an inpatient basis, but elsewhere the procedures are being done on a not-for-admission basis." Rod Thorfinnson, president of the Winnipeg Health Services Centre, in the *Winnipeg Free Press*. October 23, 1987.

This is typical of what we hear across the country. Provincial medical associations claim that without more money — and specifically, more institutional beds — our health will be in danger. Only rarely do we get an honest comment from someone like Thorfinnson, who acknowledges the overwhelming evidence that we are using our present resources inefficiently. Meanwhile, government officials and university academics point not only to the waste in our system but also to the evidence that some people are actually *worse off for being in a hospital.*

We've already discussed how, from the 1950s to the mid-1970s, patients with uncomplicated heart attacks were kept in hospital for six weeks. Back then, it was routine for patients to remain in bed for two or three of those weeks. Dr. Fraser Mustard former dean of McMaster University's medical school, is one of the world's leading researchers in blood clotting disorders. He estimates that thousands of Canadians may have died from blood clots to the lung caused by the conventional treatment.

Gradually hospital stays for heart attack patients have shortened to about two weeks, but this is still much longer than it needs to be. Heart attacks occur when clots form in the coronary arteries; heart attack patients are more susceptible to other clotting disorders. If you make heart attack patients rest in bed for several weeks, many will develop blood clots in the veins of their legs and pelvis. A piece from such a clot may break off and travel through the bloodstream and into one of the lungs, where, if it's big enough, it can block blood circulation (a pulmonary embolism) and cause death. Are we still killing some people who've had heart attacks by keeping them in hospital too long? Probably.[53]

Of course, this is only one example of how hospital beds are being misused. Doctors themselves, when surveyed by York University researchers, estimated that 15% of the days patients spent in the hospitals where they worked were unnecessary.[54]

It doesn't take much insight to understand that an oversupply of doctors, who are able to generate their own demand for services, ups the pressure to build more institutional beds — particularly in acute care facilities, where doctors do much of their work. What effect does the supply of hospital beds have on the provision of service? How does bed supply affect physician behaviour?

The classic illustration of what happens when more beds become available comes from Ithaca, New York, in the late 1950s.[55] When the supply of acute care beds increased from 2.8 per 1,000 people to 3.8 per 1,000 in a single year,* hospital occupancy rates fell slightly, but the overall utilization of hospitals beds jumped 20%. This happened *even though there appeared to be no increase in the amount of illness in the community. And there was no improvement in the health status of the county's population in return for the drastic increase in health care expenditures.* Dr. Milton Roemer, then at Cornell University, conducted this famous study, and his name is still used to describe the phenomenon he discovered: Roemer's Law states that "a built bed is a filled bed" — a rule that has been found to hold true wherever there's third-party, fee-for-service payment for physicians and hospital care. In other words, it's also true in Canada.

Other examples of how bed supply can affect physician behaviour come from several studies of intensive care units. These special facilities are home to much of today's highest-of-high-tech medicine; as medical technology mushroomed in the 1960s and 1970s, every hospital of any size or reputation added an ICU. Today, when physicians and hospital administrators complain about hospital underfunding, they often cite how it's endangering the standard of care provided by these elite units. But are all these ICU beds really needed?

- The Strong Memorial Hospital in Rochester, New York, opened a 14-bed ICU in August 1970. Dr. Paul Griner, a specialist in internal medicine, decided to examine the effect the ICU had on patients with acute pulmonary edema.** He looked at patients with this condition who had been admitted to the hospital one year before and one year after the ICU became available. He found that the same proportion of patients died after the unit opened (eight percent) as had died before. But at the same time,

---

*The increase in bed supply came about when a tuberculosis hospital was converted to general use.

**Pulmonary edema, which is sometimes called "fluid on the lung," is a life-threatening condition treated with oxygen, intravenous drugs, and special life-support technology.

the average hospital stay was 2.3 days longer after the ICU
was opened and the costs were 46% higher.[56]

- In the summer of 1981, an acute nursing shortage forced
  Massachusetts General Hospital* to reduce bed capacity
  in one of its ICUs from 18 to 8 beds. Dr. Daniel Singer
  and his colleagues looked at the effect these bed closures
  had on patients admitted to the hospital with chest pain.
  They found that as physicians were faced with fewer available beds, their accuracy in diagnosing heart attacks (a reason for admission to an ICU) increased from 40% to 62%.
  But *the proportion of chest pain patients who died
  remained the same, and overall costs fell.*[57]

In other words, before the bed crunch physicians had tended to
admit patients for observation, if they had any concerns about
their condition. But this monitoring had no effect on patient outcomes. Remember, it wasn't a matter of the patients/consumers
demanding to be in the ICU. It was the physicians/suppliers who
felt it was necessary and recommended the unit. In this case, there
was no financial incentive encouraging doctors to opt for the ICU,
because most were residents in training, and would have been
paid on salary. It was the availability of beds that influenced their
decision-making.

While neither the Singer nor the Griner study was as rigorous
as a randomized controlled trial, both strengthen the arguments
of those who would like better evaluation of specialty units.**

Another recent development in specialty care is the burn unit.
While intuition suggests that these facilities save some patients
who would otherwise die, burn units have never been thoroughly
evaluated. Dr. Bernard Linn, a surgeon at the Veterans' Administration hospital in Miami, Florida, and his colleagues, compared
the outcomes of patients treated at burn units with those of com-

---

*The Massachusetts General Hospital, which is associated with Harvard
University, is arguably the world's most prestigious hospital.

**Readers will remember from Chapter 4 that RCTs were performed to evalu-
ate the need for CCUs for patients with uncomplicated heart attacks. The results
indicated that patients did as well at home as they did in hospital (H.G. Mather,
et al., 1971; J.D. Hill, *et al.*, 1978).

parable patients treated on regular hospital wards, and found no significant difference.[58] But the cost of care in the burn units was 30% higher. Once again, the design of this study was not particularly rigorous, and we're not suggesting that burn patients don't need special treatment. But at the same time, no one should question the authors' call for a thorough prospective evaluation of burn units before more are developed.

All the above examples should raise doubts in your mind the next time you see a headline calling for more ICU, CCU or burn unit beds in your community. A day in an ICU can easily cost $1,000 more than one in an ordinary ward.* By taking two beds away from your local hospital's ICU for one year, you could free up about a million dollars to spend somewhere else. That's enough to give 300 single mothers a year's worth of $300 monthly rent subsidies. Everybody would likely be better off.

Specialty units, like most medical high technology, are appropriate for certain types of patients. But problems arise when they're used by a broader group of patients, by those whose chances of benefiting haven't been established by evidence. ICUs are nasty places for patients. There's too much light and noise to rest. Deaths are quite common. If you don't stand to gain anything from being in a specialty unit, you certainly don't want to be in one.

Finding the Magic Number: Institutional Beds

So what's the magic number for institutional beds? Right now Canada has about 4.4 acute care beds and 2.4 long-term beds for every 1,000 in our population. The average occupancy rate in our institutional facilities is very high — 85.4%.[59]

Health economists often express these measures in another way, by stating that Canada uses 1,200 bed-days a year for every 1,000 in our population. While our doctors continue to clammer for even more beds, health professionals in other countries consider even our present utilization rates to be staggeringly high, and amounting to clear evidence that Canada has a considerable over-supply of hospital facilities. Take, for example, the reaction of

---

*An average day in hospital on an ordinary ward costs between $100 and $700, depending on the hospital and the condition of the patient.

Dr. Richmond Prescott, the assistant medical director for Kaiser-Permanente in northern California, an HMO serving 2.2 million people. Dr. Prescott is an administrator, a practicing internist, and a former lawyer. His tall, distinguished carriage and well-tailored clothes testify to a man not given to hyperbole. Still, when he heard that Canada annually uses 1,200 bed-days per 1,000, his jaw dropped in astonishment and he cried, "That's outrageous!" His HMO gets along very well with a ratio two-thirds lower.

- Research on HMOs in the United States consistently shows they use 40% fewer hospital bed-days than third-party insurance plans.[60]

- Manitoba compared its hospital utilization rates with those of the Group Health Cooperative of Puget Sound, in Seattle, Washington, an HMO. Even when Manitoba excluded the bed-days used by its elderly and obstetrics patients, it still turned out to be using 60% more bed-days per capita than the HMO population.[61]

What about beds in nursing homes and other chronic care facilities? The claim that we don't have enough is a constant theme in news reports. We're forever reading about how elderly people, unable to get a long-term care bed, are taking up space in acute care hospitals, thus preventing people who desperately need to be in hospital from getting admitted. The fact is we have more than enough beds both in short- and long-term institutions. The problem is how they're being used.

Almost ten percent of Canada's over-65 population are in chronic-care hospitals or nursing homes — an appalling world record. In the United States and Australia only about six percent of seniors are housed in institutions, and in Britain, only five percent.[62] How is it possible to believe we don't have enough long-term care beds, when we institutionalize more of our elderly than any other country in the world? An example showing how people end up in nursing homes might help explain this mystery.

Georgina N. of Saskatoon is 82 years old. She was widowed three years ago and since then her health has gradually deteriorated. She has osteoarthritis (a degenerative form of arthritis), adult-onset diabetes (the type of diabetes that comes on with age and usually doesn't require insulin), and mild emphysema. She has a son in Calgary and a daughter in town. She has great difficulty getting out in the winter because of her arthritis.

One day in January she runs out of milk. Because she knows her daughter is unavailable, she sets off on her own to get some. Along the way she slips on a patch of ice and breaks her hip. She has surgery, but after three weeks her doctor thinks she isn't making suitable progress and suggests to the daughter that perhaps her mother should be in a nursing home. The daughter considers taking her mother into her own home, but with three teenagers there just doesn't seem to be room. The daughter and mother reluctantly agree to set the nursing-home admission procedures in motion. Once Mrs. N.'s papers are sent to the provincial agency responsible for nursing homes, the hospital staff back off on her rehabilitation and she spends more time in bed.[63] She becomes withdrawn and eats poorly.

Stories like this one abound in Canada. An elderly person is managing to stay at home with some difficulty. He or she develops an acute illness or suffers an injury and is admitted to hospital. The doctors and family — and often the patient as well — then decide that a nursing home would be best after all. This could hardly be called scientific medicine.

Why aren't other options available for Mrs. N., and for thousands like her? For example, she should have been getting more active rehabilitation while in hospital. Perhaps her condition, instead of deteriorating, might have improved enough that she could have returned home with appropriate supports, like home care. She could even have been brought to a rehabilitation centre daily to continue her treatment.

Patricia Spindel helped to found an effective lobby group advocating better care for senior citizens — the Concerned Friends of Ontario Residents in Care Facilities. She believes that if government funded humane residential services for disabled seniors, a lot of hospital beds would become redundant. But she concludes, like Dr. Roemer, that until hospital resources are managed more appropriately, doctors will find ways of filling available beds.

The 1984 Canadian Medical Association Task Force looked

at the allocation of health care resources, paying particular attention to the plight of senior citizens in institutions. They were adamant about the need to *reduce*, not increase, the number of elderly in institutions. They too called for more alternatives to institutionalization.

For example, Canada could establish social policies like those in Sweden and Japan, where grown children are given financial incentives to care for their parents.* We could dramatically reduce the number of elderly people in nursing homes and acute care hospitals by making adequate home care supports available. We could simplify the assessment process to make it more responsive to each individual's changing needs. Unfortunately, in our system there's no planning of long-term care for the elderly or chronically ill. Neither governments nor the medical profession are acting on the priorities of Canada's senior citizens. Indeed, long-range thinking is absent from all aspects of our health care system. There's almost no attempt to find the most cost-effective methods of delivering care to any age group.

Robbing Peter to Pay Paul?

In looking at Canada's overall supply of institutional beds, we find a curious shift. The number of acute care hospital beds actually fell slightly (by 5.6%) between 1975 and 1986. In the same time period, the supply of long-term care beds ballooned by 59%.** Of course, this means that today we're in a better position than ever to institutionalize elderly and disabled persons.

But it also means that the demand among doctors for acute care beds is reaching fever pitch. This slight drop in the acute-care bed supply must be viewed in the context of the rapid rate at which we are pumping more and more physicians into our system. Individual doctors practicing today are facing greatly reduced access to hospital beds — more so now than ever before. And they're not taking it very well.

---

*We'll look at these and other options in more detail in Chapter 9.

**The actual number of acute care hospital beds in 1975 was 119,077. This had dropped to 112,436 by 1986. Long-term care beds in chronic care hospitals and nursing homes swelled from 37,766 in 1975 to 60,077 in 1986 (Health and Welfare Canada, 1987).

Mass Media Extortion

Most large hospitals have public relations departments. More and more of them employ professional fund-raisers as well. Together with the physicians, they work to convince the media that our health care system doesn't have enough money. In particular, they claim our health is in jeopardy because they don't receive enough funding for institutional beds and high technology. Here are a few examples:

> "People are going to die waiting for surgery if hospital beds continue to be closed," Dr. Barry Gilliland, president of Saskatoon's City Hospital medical staff, told reporters at a press conference called in response to a provincial government decision to cut back on the number of hospital beds in Saskatchewan.[64]
>
> Dr. Thomas MacLachlan, president of the Saskatoon and District Medical Society, said there were 8,500 on the waiting list for surgery in Saskatoon, and that people requiring cataract operations, for example, have to wait a year for the surgery. He wanted the public to become aware of the crisis so they could "perhaps reach their MLAs and change it."[65]
>
> Toronto's Northwestern General Hospital took out an eight-by-ten fund-raising ad in *The Globe and Mail*, headlined, BY THE TIME YOU FINISH READING THIS MESSAGE WE MAY HAVE SAVED SEVERAL LIVES. The ad reads as though the entire community is at risk because the "demand for emergency services outweighs the supply . . . . We desperately need to extend our emergency facilities. Lives depend on it. We need your help . . . because someday, you may need ours."[66]

The public doesn't get balanced reporting when it comes to health care issues. Reporters rely on doctors and hospital officials as their principle source of information, and so are at a distinct disadvantage when it comes to uncovering inefficiencies within our system. After all, these sources are hardly likely to volunteer information about their wasteful use of resources. Also, some reporters may shy away from asking hard-hitting questions because they don't want to risk offending their sources. Many times, though, reporters don't even know what questions to ask — they're as confused as the public is. But by far the biggest threat to balanced health reporting is the editorial process itself.

In the fall of 1987, Chris Wood wrote a long story for

Maclean's about how transplant surgery is revolutionizing medicine. The article was full of first-person accounts of how people's lives had been transformed by new hearts, lungs, kidneys, and livers, and included a glowing biographical sketch of one of Canada's pre-eminent transplant surgeons, Dr. Wilbert Keon.[67] The original article contained a great deal of material questioning whether high technology isn't deflecting scarce resources away from strategies that would do more to improve our health. When it appeared in print, however, this critical commentary was reduced to only two sentences in the entire eight-page story. And one of those sentences was neatly deflected by a quote from Dr. Keon, who said, "No one has the right to start placing price tags on human life."*

Wood admits that he finds it easier to point to the stretchers lined up outside an emergency department than to the inefficiencies of our system. The economic arguments, he feels, are too diffuse and difficult to present.

Keith Watt, a CBC reporter in Edmonton, agrees. He says reporters don't feel comfortable departing from conventional wisdom — which in this case is that the government is underfunding the system and people might die. Watt did a story about health care in Alberta for CBC radio's "Sunday Morning" in the spring of 1987. Originally his program contained comments from two Alberta health economists and an Ontario doctor, all of whom criticized the waste in our system. But their opinions were edited out of the broadcast version, which focussed instead on the moral choices physicians face when they have to ration health care. The piece contrasted a middle-aged woman awaiting elective heart surgery with an 80-year-old man dying in an expensive ICU bed. There was no mention of our system's inefficiency. All the interviews were with doctors. Even the ethicist interviewed was a doctor.

---

*Of course, society places a price on life all the time. We allow homeless people to sleep outside in the winter. We pay single mothers allowances that are substantially below the poverty line, even though it's well-known that poverty endangers the life and health of children. Because of costs, we don't insist that ambulances in remote areas respond as quickly as those in urban areas. Every day governments, through the decisions they make in the health and other ministries, formally or informally place a value on human life.

Bob Carty, at the time a senior producer for "Sunday Morning," says it's hard work to dig beneath the surface to get to the root of these problems. "It's difficult to challenge the status quo." Both Carty and Watt believe that our system's inefficiencies may be too complicated to explain to a lay audience in a short item. And of course, doctors and hospital administrators are quite keen to talk about patients who may die because they lack a particular service. They're hardly likely to volunteer information about patients who have received unnecessary services.

These explanations from journalists are very understandable. But the media's inability to offer a more critical view of our health care system plays right into the hands of hospitals and physicians, who want more of society's resources. When a newspaper, magazine, or TV or radio program does a medical story, it usually concentrates on one of two types of messages. The first is what Robert Evans calls the "your money or your life" message. In this type of story, doctors and hospitals claim that people are dying for lack of funds. The reporters fail to mention the inefficiencies in our system, and its mismanagement, and accept at face value the assertions of provider groups, who have a vested interest in convincing the public they need more money.

Dorothy Lipovenko, a *Globe and Mail* reporter, once wrote an article like this, in which she claimed that because people were older and sicker, our system needed more money.[68] When told that fewer Canadians are dying now in all age groups and that, in fact, we've never been healthier than we are today, she replied, "I don't regret at all reporting that Canadians are sicker than ever." She maintained that every doctor and hospital administrator she spoke with had told her so. When facts based on hard statistical data are dismissed in favour of unsubstantiated opinion, what chance does the public have of understanding the real problems of our health care system?

The second type of message, like the one in the *Maclean's* story described earlier, combines intense human interest with new and emerging breakthroughs in technology. Such stories are particularly insidious in that they inevitably reinforce our faith in the progress of medicine, and in doing so tend to overstate the overall impact of such advances.

For example, Dr. Keon, we're told, does two dozen heart transplants a year, at a total cost for the surgery and aftercare of about

$200,000 per person. The one-year survival rate for his patients is 85%. By contrast, if we convinced ten percent of smokers to quit, we would save 500 to 1,000 people who would otherwise have been lost to heart disease, and 2,000 more who would have died of other smoking-related illnesses. To match this level of "cure" — that is, to save 3,000 lives — we'd have to transplant hearts into 3,600 people at a total cost of nearly three-quarters of a billion dollars! Yet this kind of analysis virtually never appears in the "look what they can do now, Martha" stories.

Both the "people are going to die" messages and the "miraculous discovery" ones are dramatic, interesting, and — in media terms — newsworthy. But they also play on public fears and raise public expectations, and in the long run mislead people about the real issues affecting our health care system. Ann Silversides, the *Globe and Mail*'s health policy reporter, notes that "doctors overwhelmingly induce priority attention and financial support for the existing treatment system and curative medicine." The predominance of such stories dims any chance the public has of viewing our health care system more objectively.

Summary of Supply and Demand

By now you should be convinced that physicians — not patients — determine which health services we consume. But the lack of science in medicine, and its inherent uncertainties, put their decision-making abilities in question. The diagnostic and treatment choices doctors make are frequently influenced by how they are paid, whether they work alone or in groups, and whether there's a hospital bed available — factors that have little or nothing to do with cost-effectiveness. The variations in physician behaviour are so striking that we must conclude that Canadians are getting many unnecessary tests, hospitalizations, surgical operations, and drug prescriptions. At the same time, some consumers are unable to get what they *really* need. They have to wait too long for a hospital bed, too long to see a specialist, too long to get home care supports arranged.

The cost implications of this mismanagement are enormous now and growing worse every day. Every new doctor we add to the system ups the ante, for we not only pay for his or her training, but also for the next 30 or 40 years he or she spends in practice. You can't train physicians at double or triple the rate of population growth and expect to remain unscathed. Once out of school, these doctors will want their share of access to hospital beds, too. But let's be clear who we're building them for — it's to meet doctors' needs, not their patients'. As health budgets strain under the pressure, the shortfall between what doctors and hospitals want, and what governments can afford, is labelled "underfunding."

Meanwhile, the media plays along with this farce, sometimes innocently, sometimes knowingly, as the cry from doctors and hospitals for more money continues unabated. Governments are raked over the coals as unfeeling when they try to hold the lid on costs. And journalists — even good ones — hesitate to buck conventional wisdom. The economic arguments about what's wrong with our system are too subtle, they claim, for a lay audience. It's too complicated, they say, to explain that poverty and illiteracy are far more dangerous health problems than lack of money for high-technology medical solutions. What do you think?

Welcome to one of the greatest mass delusions of the 20th century. With what you now know, you don't have to share in it anymore.

Chapter 7

What Makes Us Healthy?
What Makes Us Sick?

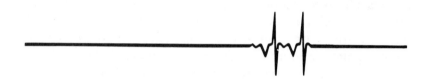

YOU HAVE JUST PATIENTLY waded through a subtle and complex account of the problems pervading virtually every aspect of our health care system: its planning and priorities, its organization and financial incentives, the training and monitoring of its practitioners, and the medical technologies they employ. If our evidence has been convincing, then you're probably beginning to experience what Professor Robert Evans, from the University of British Columbia, calls "the tunnel at the end of the light."

Do not despair — there *are* solutions. But to find them, you need a new perspective about what makes people healthy. After that you can look at what makes us sick, and what to do about it. The conclusions of this chapter should not be surprising: how we live — how we eat, how we work, how we love, and how we take our minds off our troubles — has far more impact on our health than the efforts of hospitals and doctors.

The Role of Medicine

People living today in the developed countries of the West are much healthier than any people at any other time in history. In fact, over the past three centuries, we've added an extra 30 to 40 years to the average life span.[1] Medicine, too, has made some impressive advances in the course of its history, most of them occurring in our own century. The past 60 years have brought a dramatic expansion in our understanding of biological processes, and in our ability to treat certain diseases successfully.

So far, so good. Medicine is better than ever, and we live longer than ever before. But there's a problem. People put these two facts together and wind up assuming a cause-and-effect relationship between them that simply doesn't exist. The fact is that medical advances, however impressive, have *not* been responsible for very much of our improved longevity. The health we enjoy today is *not*, for the most part, a by-product of better treatment for our illnesses. The reason modern medicine can't take the credit is very simple, straightforward, and irrefutable: it's all in the timing.

Dr. Thomas McKeown, a British epidemiologist, began to question the role of medicine in making people healthy when he was a medical student in a London hospital:

> There were two things that struck me almost at once. One was the absence of any real interest among clinical teachers in the origin of disease, apart from its pathological and clinical manifestations;* the other was that whether the prescribed treatment was of any value to the patient was often hardly noticed, particularly in internal medicine . . . . I adopted the practice of asking myself at the bedside whether we were making anyone any wiser or any better, and soon came to the conclusion that most of the time we were not.[2]

These early doubts were confirmed by Dr. McKeown's research. He found, after painstakingly working through hundreds of years

---

*Today's medical students will notice that little has changed. Doctors in training are taught little about the determinants of health. They spend virtually all of their clinical time dealing with sick people rather than healthy ones. (Obstetrics is an obvious exception.) Often, too, their patients are ill with very rare diseases, and clinical professors impress upon the student doctors the awesome responsibility of never missing something that's treatable. The medical school curriculum devotes very little time to epidemiology, economics, or sociology. Students are as familiar with these disciplines as most Americans are with Canada.

of death records, that most of our gains in life expectancy occurred long before medicine had effective treatments for infectious disease. Until the early 20th century, cholera, typhoid, tuberculosis, whooping cough, measles, scarlet fever, diphtheria, and other infectious diseases were the most common causes of death. Infants and small children were particularly vulnerable to these infections; in the 18th century seven out of every ten children didn't survive to reach adulthood.

In his famous book, *The Role of Medicine*, Dr. McKeown demonstrates that we started living much longer lives well before doctors had any real help to offer us! Using European records going back as far as 1751, he reconstructed a pattern which showed that death rates began to decline at the beginning of the 19th century. He found that *almost all of the decline in death rates due to infectious disease occurred long before medicine had any effective treatments for them.** Effective medical means simply arrived too late to justify awarding the glory to physicians. By the time antibiotics and vaccines were available, all that remained was a "mop-up" job. Sulpha drugs didn't appear on the scene until the 1930s. Penicillin wasn't generally available until after the Second World War. Until these major 20th century discoveries, medicine really had nothing useful to offer against infectious disease.

For example, in 1900, tuberculosis was the number-one killer in Ontario, claiming 160 lives for every 100,000 people in the population.[3] There was no effective medical treatment for TB back then. Patients were told to rest in bed, eat nourishing foods, and if possible, move to a "healthy" country environment. Sanatoriums were set up all over Canada for this purpose; in these, patients waited through their disease, with the strongest surviving, and the rest slowly deteriorating until death. It wasn't until 1948, when the antibiotic streptomycin was developed, that medical practitioners had an effective treatment for TB. But by that time, it was no longer a major cause of death. In Ontario, for example, the TB death rate had already dropped by 90%.[4]

---

*Smallpox is an exception to this phenomenon. A crude but effective vaccine was developed against smallpox in the late 18th century by an English physician, Dr. Edward Jenner.

This analysis for TB holds true for most of the other infectious diseases of the 19th and early 20th centuries.

If medicine can't take the credit for this turnaround, what *was* responsible? Dr. McKeown attributed the conquest of infectious disease to better and more food, access to clean drinking water, improved housing conditions, and the sanitary disposal of wastes. Dr. Thomas Reves, in a reanalysis of Dr. McKeown's work, adds family planning to the list, suggesting that smaller families also contributed to improved health status for a number of reasons. Continuous childbearing is hard on a mother's constitution. Also, in large families, children born later in the birth order are more likely to have health problems and less resistance to disease. Smaller families meant less crowded conditions at home and a better chance for parents to provide their children with an adequate level of nutrition.[5] In short, better living conditions made health possible, and created a context in which it could flourish. People were less exposed to infection and had better resistance to it. Prevention, not cure, prevailed. For this success, we owe an enormous debt of gratitude to public health measures, and in particular to the enlightened social policies of the 18th and 19th centuries that gave them priority, and the widespread economic growth that financed them.

Professor John McKnight, from the Department of Urban Studies at Northwestern University in Illinois, summarized Dr. McKeown's work at a conference on prevention held in Waterloo, Ontario, in 1987. In his speech, he nominated clay pipe, improved roadways, and the heating of milk as the three greatest healers of the past two centuries. Clay pipe, because it provided the means by which sewage waste and drinking water could be separated. More roads and better vehicles, because they made it possible to transport more food to growing urban populations. And the chemist Louis Pasteur's discovery that heating milk could eliminate bacterial contamination, because it greatly reduced deaths due to gastrointestinal disease and tuberculosis. None of these innovations came from clinical medicine. Indeed, most of the benefits from public health measures, and improvements in social and economic conditions, had already been realized as early as 1910 — which was just about the time when medicine was beginning to emerge as a "scientific" discipline.

But Dr. McKeown's work offers more than just a new perspective on the overall impact of medicine in the past. It also provides historical evidence about how to reform health policy now. Since Dr. McKeown began publishing his results in the 1960s, most major health policy documents have acknowledged the importance of his contribution. We now have a much better understanding about how living conditions affect health. The implications for modern times are obvious: to improve health in today's world, we need look no further than the past. Sadly, Dr. McKeown's message is realized more often in empty rhetoric than in concrete policies and programs. But this can change.

Today's Killers

Today's most common health threats are different from those of the past. At least among Western developed nations, infectious diseases have largely been routed (although our complacency has been seriously shaken by the emergence of AIDS). Most of our modern "killers" pose a very different challenge. For one thing, unlike infections, which can be traced to a single, biological disease-causing entity (a virus, parasite, or bacterium, for example), most modern illness cannot be attributed to a single cause.* Multiple factors interacting in complex ways lie at the source of the two greatest threats to life today: heart disease and cancer.

Heart Disease: Progress and Puzzlement Cardiovascular disease (disease of the heart and blood vessels) is far and away the greatest life-taker in Canada, as it is in other Western countries, accounting for about half of all deaths.[6] Since 20% of these deaths occur before age 65, and another 20% between age 65 and normal life expectancy, we're looking at a major cause of *premature* death.[7] In 1982, 80,000 Canadians died of cardiovascular disease. Direct hospital costs for treating it have been estimated at $2 billion a year.[8]

Heart disease is the most common form of cardiovascular disease, and the sudden heart attack its most feared consequence. This fear is justified — about one heart attack victim in three

---

*The obvious exception, which we'll discuss later in this chapter, is lung cancer, over 80% of which is caused by tobacco.

dies before ever reaching the hospital.[9] Indeed, many people only find out they have heart disease *after* their first heart attack, and about one-quarter of all new cases of heart disease are only discovered when the victims die suddenly from heart attacks. In 1982, there were over 28,000 deaths from heart attack in Canada.[10]

On a cold evening in January 1978, Carl G., a 58-year-old accountant, was shovelling snow from his driveway when suddenly he was seized by a crushing pain in his chest. Describing the sensation, he recalled, "It felt like an elephant was standing on my chest. The pressure was relentless and unbearable." Ellen, his wife, and Randy, his teenage son, rushed him to the nearest emergency department and got him there within ten minutes. Emergency room staff quickly assessed his condition, confirmed that he'd had a heart attack, and gave him some morphine. Then he was started on an intravenous drip and whisked off to the coronary care unit. Carl remembers his enormous relief at reaching the hospital in time. "I was so damn scared I was going to die before getting there. I can't describe how much relief I felt as soon as I made it through the doors."

A few hours later Dr. Clifford J., the staff cardiologist, explained to Carl and his family that he was fairly confident the heart attack hadn't done any major damage. "But I'm going to keep you here in the coronary care unit for a few days just to be on the safe side."

After three days in the CCU, Carl was still grateful for the care he was receiving, while admitting there were a few drawbacks to being there. "Visiting was limited, for one thing. And of course, it wasn't easy to get much rest — nurses were constantly coming in and out to check on us. And every so often some poor guy's heart would start beating funny and all hell would break loose. People rushing around, yelling orders, trying to bring him around. But overall, I'd have to say I was mighty glad to be there, knowing help was so close to hand."

During rounds on the third day, Dr. J. found that Carl's heart was beating with a steady rhythm and that he was maintaining good blood pressure — two major indications that he hadn't suffered any complications from his heart attack. "You're out of the woods now," the doctor assured him, "so I'm going to transfer you to the internal medicine ward for two or three weeks to rest up. Then you'll be able to go home and get on with your life.''

"I was so grateful I could have cried," Carl recalls. "I felt I'd been given a whole new lease on life." All the same, in the following weeks, Carl developed a few new problems. He had a nasty red swelling on his wrist, right where the IV needle had punctured the skin — a sign of infection. Then he had a bad reaction to the antibiotic used to treat the infection. "I broke out in hives all over — the itching drove me crazy."

Still, 20 days after admission, Carl was discharged and returned home to his family. With the hives gone and the infection healed, he had nothing but praise for the compassionate care he had received at the hospital. "They were there for me when I really needed them," he says. "I owe my life to those guys."

Carl's assessment is a very common one among heart attack patients, who feel they've been "rescued" from imminent death. But how accurate is it?

You now know from earlier chapters that lengthy hospital stays for people with uncomplicated heart attacks are no safer, and may even be more dangerous, than early release. The evidence suggests that after the first 48 hours or so, Carl could have done as well if not better at home. Certainly he would have had more peace there. And he could have avoided both the infection and the hives, both of which were a direct result of his treatment.*
Remember, his long stay in hospital didn't improve his chances of avoiding future heart attacks, nor did it do anything to slow the advance of his disease.

How would Carl have reacted if his doctor had suggested he go home after the first few days? "I think I would have felt he was abandoning me. Neglecting his duty. I was too scared of having another attack. I just felt safer in the hospital."

Carl's attitude is very understandable in human terms: he was frightened. But his confidence in the health care the hospital provided led him to overestimate its real impact on his health. Meanwhile, prior to his attack, he had little understanding of what made him sick in the first place. He had a sedentary job,

---

*Both are examples of iatrogenic illness, which was discussed in more detail in Chapter 3.

a diet high in animal fat and low in fibre, and he smoked. He knew smoking caused cancer, but he didn't realize it could cause heart disease as well.*

The calcified arteries of Egyptian mummies, and medical records down through the centuries, suggest that heart disease has been around since antiquity. Still, it's mainly thought of as a modern illness, because heart disease deaths rose so dramatically during the first half of this century. But what most people don't know is that heart disease mortality has actually been falling by about one percent a year ever since the early 1960s.[11] In Canada, between 1951 and 1982, death rates for heart disease fell by 31% in women and 26% in men; indeed, death rates for all cardiovascular disease have fallen, by one-half among women and about one-third among men.[12] And since 1982 this encouraging trend has continued. The puzzle is, why?

As with infectious disease, there's a strong temptation to ascribe this success to medical advances. The high profile of innovations like heart transplants and coronary bypass operations, the widespread use of medications to control high blood pressure and angina, and new drugs like TPA (tissue plasminogen activator) to treat heart attack patients, all lead us to overestimate the role medicine has played in this improvement. But Dr. Andy Wielgosz, a cardiologist and epidemiologist at the University of Ottawa, points out that the drop in mortality rates from cardiovascular disease began *before most of these modern techniques had been developed.* Sound familiar?

Dr. Sidney Pell has been researching the health of Dupont Corporation employees in the United States for over a quarter of a century.[13] He documented an almost 30% decline in deaths from heart attack among these workers between 1958 and 1983. Using Pell's data, it's possible to conclude that, at most, only 25% of this decline was due to the effectiveness of the health care system.[14] This means that other factors had to be responsible for at least 70 to 80% of the drop in heart attack deaths. What were these factors?

While an exact answer continues to elude researchers, environ-

---

*According to a Gallup poll conducted for the Canadian Cancer Society in 1987, only 29% of adults knew smoking was a risk factor for heart disease.

mental and lifestyle factors are clearly much more important influences than improvements in medical care. Evidence pointing in this direction comes from the markedly different rates of heart disease found in various parts of the world. Research has shown that, generally, industrialized countries with high standards of living are at greatest risk: Scotland and Finland have the highest mortality rates, while Mediterranean countries have the lowest.[15] An exception is Japan, an industrialized country with a high standard of living; the Japanese nevertheless, have among the lowest death rates from heart disease in the world. Even within Canada itself, we find regional differences. Why does western Canada have lower mortality rates from heart disease than eastern Canada?[16]

These variations are far from easy to account for, but do seem related to differences in diet, physical activity, smoking habits, the incidence of high blood pressure, social class, and perhaps social integration. One thing, however, is certain: these differences have nothing to do with racial origin. To illustrate, North Americans have five times more coronary heart disease than the Japanese. But studies have shown that Japanese who have emigrated to the United States and adopted a North American lifestyle soon "acquire" the same risks as the native-born population. According to cardiologist Dr. Gary Fraser, "These trends for both heart disease and stroke are of environmental origin, as there is no evidence of genetic differences or reason to suspect such."[17]

Cancer: The Pretense of Progress   Cancer is the second main cause of death in Canada, accounting for one-quarter of all mortality. One in three Canadians can expect to develop some kind of cancer, other than skin cancer, at some point in their lives.* The booklet *Canadian Cancer Statistics 1987* estimates that this year 94,700 new cases of cancer (other than skin cancer) will be diagnosed in Canada, and that 49,200 Canadians will die from cancer.

In 1986, Adrienne P. was on top of the world. At age 45, she was working as a successful tax lawyer in a prestigious Calgary

---

*We exclude skin cancers for a number of reasons: although they're very common, most are basal cell carcinomas, which never spread, except locally, and which can be completely cured by removal while they are small.

law firm, which had just made her a senior partner. In early March of that year, Ms. P. caught a bad cold, and a month later she was still troubled by a persistent cough. Forced to admit she was feeling awful, and worried about having dropped 15 pounds, she phoned her doctor for an appointment.

He listened as she described her symptoms, did a physical examination, and then ordered a full diagnostic work-up, including a C-T scan and a flexible bronchoscopy.* The results confirmed his worst fears: Adrienne had non-small cell bronchial carcinoma — in other words, lung cancer — and the prognosis was grim. Already there were signs the disease had spread to her liver and lymphatic system; neither surgery nor chemotherapy held any hope for recovery. Six months later, Adrienne was dead.

Like the vast majority of lung cancer victims, Adrienne smoked cigarettes, and there's little doubt they caused her cancer. Lung cancer deaths have increased enormously in this century, but until the late 1960s, most of the victims were men. Of course, until then most smokers were men, too. But not anymore. Studies have shown that it takes about 20 years of smoking before lung cancer occurs. Women started smoking in large numbers after the Second World War, but it took until the 1960s before women's rates for lung cancer began to increase. Over the past 20 years, lung cancer death rates among Canadian women have quadrupled.[18]

We've all heard the slogans, "Beat cancer with a checkup and a cheque," and the hopeful "Cancer can be beaten," but in fact we're not much further along in finding cancer cures today than we were 20 years ago. True, doctors have found a few new and effective treatments, but these discoveries are mainly for some rarer types of cancer, like Hodgkin's disease and childhood leukemia. But apart from these gains medicine can't claim any improvement in prognosis for patients with the most common forms of the disease.[19] There's a widespread belief that we're making progress against cancer. It's an illusion.

For example, since 1950 there's been very little change in the survival rates for breast cancer — the leading cause of cancer death in women — or for cancer of the prostate.[20]

---

*Bronchoscopy is a diagnostic procedure during which a flexible fibreoptic tube is passed through the mouth down the trachea and into the lungs.

Meanwhile, the incidence of most cancers has been rising, not falling, which means we're failing to prevent or control the causes of cancer.* Lifestyle and environmental factors seem to play a pivotal role in the development of cancer, just as they do with heart disease. Evidence suggesting this can be found in the large differences in the rates of certain types of cancer between and within countries.

- We know that colon cancers are rare in countries where people eat a fibre-rich diet, and that breast cancers are associated with a high-fat diet and alcohol consumption. Breast and colon cancers are five times more common in North America than in Japan. The mortality rate in Halifax from colon and rectal cancer is twice that of Regina.[21]

- Cancers of the esophagus and throat are related to the consumption of alcohol. France consumes more alcohol per capita than any other nation; cancers of the esophagus and throat are about three times more common there than in Canada.

- Stomach cancer is five times more common in Japan than in North America. Within Canada, cancer of the stomach is more than twice as common in St. John's than in Calgary. Smoked fish and other smoked foods are staples in the Japanese diet, and very popular in Newfoundland as well. Are differences in diet responsible for this variation in cancer rates?

Exposure to toxins in the workplace and the general environment is also associated with certain types of cancer. Dr. Rick Bedard, medical officer to the Canadian Cancer Society, criticized a Nova Scotia study which, in attempting to explain why cancer rates in Cape Breton are one-and-a-half times higher than in other parts of the country, failed to examine key environmental factors —

---

*Stomach cancer is an exception; mortality rates for stomach cancer have fallen significantly, not because of better medical treatment but because fewer people are getting it in the first place. One possible explanation is that today people don't eat much food cooked over open fires. Carcinogens produced in the charred surface of meats prepared this way are thought to be a major cause of stomach cancer.

Mortality Rates for Selected Cancer Sites   *Figure 7.1*

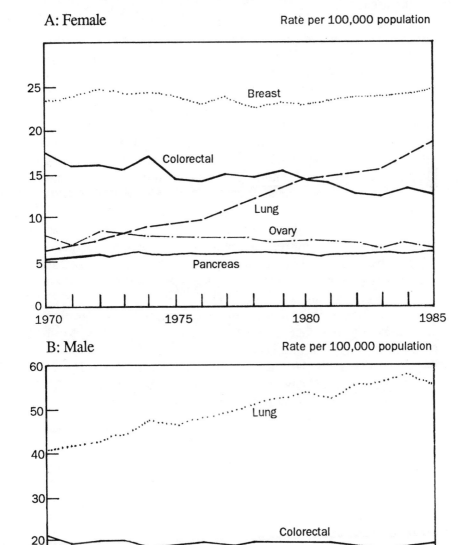

A: Female   Rate per 100,000 population

B: Male   Rate per 100,000 population

(1) Rates are adjusted to the age distribution of the world population
(2) Figures are for Canada, 1970-1985
Source: Vital Statistics and Health Status Section, Health Division, Statistics Canada

particularly those linked to industrial coke and coal tar produced in the area.[22]

Trying to find the key factors that would explain why some people get cancer and some do not, and working out all the variations, should be a major research priority. But instead, most cancer research is devoted to gaining a better understanding of the biomolecular processes of the disease. We're not suggesting this is unimportant, only that this narrow focus on "finding cures" is misleading the public and deflecting resources away from other terribly important research efforts. In 1986, the *New England Journal of Medicine* published an article by John C. Bailar III and Elaine M. Smith that shattered many illusions about medicine's progress against cancer. Bailar is a renowned statistician and a consultant to the *New England Journal of Medicine*. He and Smith concluded that "some 35 years of intense effort focussed largely on improving treatment must be judged a qualified failure . . . . Although no one can be certain about the benefits of preventive efforts, history suggests that savings in both lives and dollars could be great."[23]

No example of this failure is more striking than the alarming increase in the incidence of and mortality from lung cancer. Most cancers arise from multiple causes. Lung cancer is an exception — cigarette smoking accounts for almost all of it. The role that smoking plays in causing this deadly illness is now "widely recognized as a medical, social, and political scandal."[24]

Cigarettes: Public Enemy Number One

Just how bad for our health is tobacco? The answer may shock you: cigarettes are quite simply *the single greatest cause of disease and disability in Canada.*[25] There are many different ways to count the bodies: a liberal estimate might claim that cigarettes cause as many as 50,000 deaths every year, but even a conservative one would attribute at least 30,000 deaths to smoking.* In

---

*Evidence from various other epidemiological studies provides a range of percentages to indicate, for each relevant illness, the proportion caused by smoking. For example, these studies indicate that between 80 and 90% of all lung cancers are due to smoking. The difference between a liberal and a conservative estimate, therefore, depends on whether you apply the higher or lower percentage to the total mortality of each condition.

1986, there were 182,000 deaths in Canada, so depending on which estimate you choose to accept, *cigarettes were responsible for between 15 and 30% of all deaths that year.*

How does tobacco compare with other causes of death? Alcohol doesn't even come close. The figures for heart attacks and cancers caused by poor diet pale in significance. The number of lives lost or ruined in car accidents, while a national tragedy, amounts to a small fraction of those lost to cigarettes. Every workday three Canadians die on the job because of unsafe conditions; it would take almost 50 years of work-related deaths to equal the number caused by tobacco in a single year.[26] Lung cancer is the illness most of us associate with tobacco use; indeed, smoking causes between 80 and 90% of all lung cancers, and was responsible for between 7,000 and 8,500 lung cancer deaths in 1983. But few people realize that in terms of absolute numbers, *cigarettes kill more people by causing heart disease than lung cancer.* For example, in 1983, 48,000 Canadians died of coronary artery disease. As many as 20,000 of these deaths were due to cigarettes. A recent study of over 100,000 nurses in the United States showed that cigarettes caused more than half of all the coronary deaths in that group.[27]

We also know that smoking is linked to other circulatory diseases, including stroke, and to many other cancers besides lung, including those of the bladder, kidney, mouth, esophagus, liver, pancreas, nose, and cervix. Smoking is also a major cause of accidental death: about half of all fires resulting in death are started by cigarettes. Smoking also appears to be a major factor in the development of osteoporosis ("thin bones") and subsequent hip fracture. Finally, 100,000 Canadians are disabled by chronic lung diseases — chronic bronchitis, emphysema, and the like — almost all of which are caused by cigarettes.[28]

What about the tobacco industry's claim that no one has ever proved conclusively that cigarettes cause lung cancer or other diseases? Some of our readers may be familiar with the British television series "Yes, Prime Minister," which satirizes the relationship between politicians and civil servants. In one episode, Sir Humphrey Appleby, the cabinet secretary, pooh-poohs the scientific evidence establishing tobacco as a major health threat.

"Oh, Prime Minister," he scoffs, "you should know that you can prove *anything* with statistics."

"Yes," responds Jim Hacker, the P.M., "*even the truth.*"

In their attempts to deny the "truth," the tobacco industry is playing a game with the scientific definition of cause and effect. They say, and we agree, that the best way to prove causation is by experiment, which in clinical medicine means by an RCT.* But it's pretty obvious that we can't perform an RCT to study the effects of smoking; clearly, it would be neither ethical nor feasible to randomly allocate a group of teenagers to smoke or not smoke cigarettes, and then follow them for 30 or 40 years. But even though an RCT is the best way to determine cause and effect, *it is not the only way.* Over the past three decades remarkable progress has been made in developing other methods of establishing causation. Even the most skeptical epidemiologist would accept these alternatives to an RCT as good evidence. Below are three criteria most scientists would accept instead:[29]

1. Is the association between the effect and the purported cause strong? In 1951, two Oxford professors collected personal data —including information about smoking habits — on almost 35,000 male doctors in Britain. They then followed those doctors for the next 20 years.[30] Less than one-third of one percent of the subjects were lost in the follow-up process. Although the smoking and non-smoking groups weren't established through randomization, all the subjects were male doctors, and in 1951 one could assume a fair degree of homogeneity between groups. Among the subjects, there were 441 deaths from lung cancer. Smokers were over 14 times more likely to die of lung cancer than non-smokers.

2. Is the effect more likely after greater exposure? The Oxford study showed that the more a doctor smoked, the more likely he was to develop lung cancer. Compared to non-smokers, light

---

*Readers will remember from Chapter 3 that an RCT (randomized controlled trial) is an experiment that allocates subjects at random to receive either the active intervention or a placebo.

smokers (less than 15 cigarettes per day) were 8 times more likely to develop lung cancer; moderate smokers (15 to 24 cigarettes per day), 13 times more likely; and heavy smokers (more than 25 cigarettes a day), 25 times more likely. The rates among ex-smokers for lung cancer fell about midway between those for non-smokers and those for current smokers. But if a smoker quit his risk of lung cancer gradually decreased until, over five to ten years, it matched that of non-smokers.

3. Is the effect consistent from study to study?   Dozens of studies show that smokers are more likely to develop lung cancer. In fact, *no study has ever demonstrated a contrary finding.* We consistently find that light smokers have rates of lung cancer 5 to 10 times those of non-smokers, and that heavy smokers have rates 15 to 30 times those of non-smokers. A heavy smoker has about a one-in-six chance of developing lung cancer before age 75.[31]

Naming the Illness: Cigarettes or Cancer or Heart Disease or . . .

So which is really the disease? Is it cigarettes themselves, or the two dozen or so illnesses with which they've been linked? Should we focus on the single underlying common denominator, or use a scattered approach to deal with its various manifestations? Instead of dissipating our energy trying to deal separately with all the diseases smoking causes, wouldn't it be more sensible to label cigarettes the problem and launch a concerted assault against smoking itself?

There are medical precedents that lead us to favour this strategy. For example, syphilis can cause many different clinical syndromes from heart disease to insanity. But until the microbe that causes syphilis was identified about a century ago, each of those different pathological conditions was thought to be a separate disease with a separate cause. Treating the secondary effects of syphilis instead of the disease itself was a wasted effort. Until there was an effective treatment for syphilis itself, the only useful strategy was prevention. Even today, when we have medications for curing syphilis, no one doubts that it's far better to never need treatment in the first place.

We often speak of strategies for treating disease using military terms: we wage war against cancer, we battle against heart disease, we fight infection. Perhaps we ought to carry this parallel even further. A competent field general would try to destroy his enemies before they had a chance to establish themselves on home territory, before they could disperse to start two dozen different fronts of action. Are we losing the war against cancer and other diseases by trying to deal with them individually, and by focussing on treatment instead of prevention?

Who Gets Sick?

Although our health care system is oriented almost entirely toward treating and curing illness, we know instinctively that health is more than just the absence of disease. The World Health Organization (WHO) recognizes this, and defines health very broadly as a state of complete physical, mental, and social well-being.

This view of health acknowledges that *feeling* well is an important component of *being* well, and that our social relationships, physical environment, and economic status directly influence our health.

Canada has been in the forefront of changing how the world looks at health. As we mentioned earlier, the now-famous Lalonde Report, *A New Perspective on the Health of Canadians*, established the concept that factors *other than the health care system* are important determinants of health. Our health status is governed by the kind of work we do, by what we eat, by whether we smoke or drink alcohol, by how much money we make, and so on — in short, by how we *live*. This widely praised report — it was heralded as the most important health document of the postwar era — has had a tremendous influence on health and social policy in Europe. But Canada has been slow to respond to its implications.

Still, in the years since the Lalonde Report came out, the scope of health research has broadened considerably even here. More and more investigators are trying to match social and economic indicators with mortality and illness rates. They want to know how important income, education, and social standing are to our health status. What they're finding out from this work is that the most revealing statistics about health in Canadian society are *not* about what kinds of diseases kill us or make us sick — they're about *who* gets sick in this country.

This research offers chilling evidence that the Canadians most vulnerable to disability, chronic illness, and premature death are those who don't have enough money to afford the living conditions the rest of us take for granted. In other words, poverty is the greatest health threat of all.*

How can this be? Poor people in Canada have the same access to health care — Medicare guarantees it. But as you now know, health care makes very little difference in determining who gets sick. It's irrefutable that poor people get sick more often, and when they do the consequences are more serious. Take, for example, the results of two studies comparing Montreal neighbourhoods: the working-class community of St-Henri and the much more affluent Westmount, only a few kilometres away:

- On average, men living in St-Henri died nine years sooner and had 13 more years of disability than men living in Westmount.[32]

- Men and women living in St-Henri were three times more likely to smoke and twice as likely not to wear seat belts. Women in St-Henri were more than three times as likely to neglect breast self-examination. Births to teenagers were 20 times more in common in St-Henri.[33]

We've known for some time that Canadians of lower socio-economic status (as defined by their level of education) have higher rates of heart disease. But researchers from Health and Welfare Canada have also found that these Canadians are more likely to smoke, and to be overweight and physically inactive. They also have higher cholesterol levels than the rest of us.[34]

---

*The best research detailing the health risks of poverty comes from Britain. Popularly known as "the Black Report," because the chairman of the working group for this study was Sir Douglas Black, *Inequalities in Health* (Penguin, 1982) is a landmark document offering compelling evidence that poverty causes ill health. When the British Ministry of Health, which commissioned the report, tried to bury it, authors Peter Townsend and Nick Davidson decided to go public and publish the results commercially, in order to reach a wider audience.

The links between a low income and ill health are well established. But who exactly are the poor in Canada?

Monica J. is 60 years old. She's been struggling to make ends meet ever since her husband died. "I was doing okay as long as Phil and I were both working. We were making ends meet, if you know what I mean." But Monica's husband Phil died five years ago, just before he was about to retire. He'd been an unskilled factory worker in a small plastics plant, and since his employer didn't offer any pension plan, Monica had always expected to continue working past his retirement. The problem for Monica now is that she simply doesn't earn enough money working as a cashier to support herself. "I never expected to end up this way," she says, "I never dreamed I'd spend my old age in poverty."

Greg T., who's 27 now, is also poor. Greg had a diving accident one summer and wound up a paraplegic when he was 16 years old. "I was never really a very good student before the accident, and afterwards I didn't go back. I keep trying to find work but people are put off by the chair. They don't think I can do anything." Greg depends on a small disability pension that puts him under the poverty line like Monica.

Jennifer S. is 19 years old and the mother of two small children. She married at 17. Her husband, who's a year older, skipped town right after their younger son was born, and now mothers' allowance is her only source of income. She's on a waiting list for subsidized housing but has little hope of getting an apartment for at least a year — maybe two. In the meantime, she's living in a damp basement flat in downtown Ottawa that eats up more than half her welfare cheque. "I hate this life," she says. "I've had three jobs since Jerry left me and got fired from each one because my kids kept getting colds and ear infections. The day-care won't take them when they're sick and this place is just too cold and damp."

According to the National Council on Welfare, almost 15% of us — that's over three-and-a-half million Canadians — live below the poverty line.[35] But this figure is undoubtedly an underestimate, since it excludes key groups that are prone to poverty: people living in the Territories, native peoples, and those living in institutions. Monica, Greg, and Jennifer are representative of the largest groups of poor in Canada — elderly women, disabled people, and single mothers. There are millions like them; in fact, single mothers, together with their children, make up the fastest-growing group of poor in our society — and they're already the largest proportion of those who live in poverty. And there's another group . . . .

Native peoples are among the poorest of all Canadians. They also have lower life expectancies and higher rates of infant mortality and chronic disease than other Canadians. The infectious-disease rates among native peoples are much higher as well, and compare with those found in the Third World.[36] The overwhelming risks to health that poverty imposes on this sector of our population are in no way lessened by access to quality medical care.

Mortality rates on Indian reserves are actually 50 to 100% higher than anywhere else in Canada. They're especially high among those under the age of 40.[37] But disease isn't the only major cause of death on reserves. Deaths from violence are also much higher — three or four times higher — than in the rest of Canada. Between 1977 and 1982, over one in six deaths among males on Indian reserves were from intentional violence — suicide and homicide. "The most significant differences between mortality on Indian reserves and that experienced by Canadians as a whole [are] the much higher mortality rates for accidents, poisonings and violence on reserves."[38]

The continued poor health of our native peoples is an illustration of what happens when you introduce First World health care to people living in Third World conditions. For example:

- About 30 years ago the Navajo Indians of Arizona asked the U.S. Public Health Department and the medical school at Cornell University to organize medical services for them. They did this. After five years the services were found to have had only marginal effects on health status. Maternal deaths and infant mortality did fall somewhat, but the health risks associated with deplorable living conditions remained unchanged.[39]

Michael Mendelson, who has held senior positions in both federal and provincial governments, is now an assistant deputy minister in Ontario's Ministry of Community and Social Services. In his opinion, until the economic climate for native people improves, no amount of medical technology will have much impact on their health.

Not having enough money for the basic necessities of life — food, clothing, and shelter — is bad enough. But to make matters worse, poverty also stigmatizes its victims, which in turn undermines their hope and self-esteem. Despair is a health threat, too. Many more fortunate Canadians contribute to this problem by blaming the poor for their own poverty, by holding them personally accountable for their circumstances. Whether you believe this is fair or not, there's at least *one* group of Canadians suffering from poverty who *can't* be blamed this way — the children of poor parents. In Canada, one child in six is trapped in poverty, and this economic hardship takes its toll on their health as well.

- Children from poor families are twice as likely to die at birth or in infancy as those from wealthier homes. Throughout childhood, they experience higher death rates from respiratory problems, gastrointestinal ailments, and accidental food inhalation. Children living in poverty are also two-and-a-half times more likely to die in an accident or from an infectious disease.[40]

Dr. Chan Shah, a professor from the University of Toronto, who conducted this research, notes that much of this disparity is related to poor living conditions and lack of education.[41] "Not all solutions to health problems are in more doctors and more nurses," he said. "The health model usually ranks diseases as the cause of death. But if you look at what causes disease, poverty is at the top." Comparing the overall effects of poverty on life expectancy with those of cancer, Dr. Shah concluded that poverty is more deadly. "Eliminating the disparities between rich and poor would increase overall life expectancy more than the prevention of all cancer deaths."

In fact, there's substantial evidence that cancer victims who are poor have substantially higher death rates than those who are middle-class. This is true even if the patients are diagnosed at the same stage and given the same treatments.[42]

Too Early, Too Little, Too Late

Poverty is a threat to health even *before* you're born! A host of medical problems are associated with low birthweights from mental retardation to sudden infant death syndrome (SIDS). About three-quarters of all babies who die in their first week of life, die from the effects of prematurity and low birthweight.[43] In fact, birthweight is such a potent predictor of health that many researchers are beginning to add it to other more traditional measures of health status, like life expectancy and mortality. Now they're finding that the risk of having a low birthweight baby is much higher if you happen to be poor.

What's worse, an underweight infant who survives to leave the hospital is at a double disadvantage if his parents are poor, according to Dr. Henry Dunn, professor emeritus of pediatrics at the University of British Columbia. He says these children are much more likely to have learning and behaviour problems than premature babies who leave hospital for better homes. Dr. Dunn also reports that children from the lowest socio-economic class who were low birthweight infants have IQ levels *25 points lower* on average than children, also born small, from the highest socio-economic class.[44]

- Data from 125,000 births over a five-year period in Montreal showed that unwed mothers had more than a 60% chance of being poor, and that more than half were very poor indeed, with incomes 30% or more under the poverty line. Single women with the lowest levels of education were three times more likely to deliver an underweight baby.[45]

We can make this contrast still more concrete. Researcher Russell Wilkins notes that better-educated, married women in Canada deliver low birthweight babies at rates comparable to those found in Sweden, Finland, Norway, and the Netherlands. But among poorly educated, unmarried women, rates for low birthweight are closer to those found in North Africa, Central America, and Mexico. Are we to conclude that Canada's poor comprise a Third World enclave in the midst of affluence?

Thanks to neontology, the survival chances for low birthweight babies have improved dramatically; overall, infant mortality in Canada has fallen by 50% in the past decade. It's easy to get lost in admiration for this accomplishment, and to forget that many of the babies in intensive care nurseries could have been born healthy enough not to need this expensive therapy.

Wilkins stresses that over the five-year period he was studying births in Montreal, there was no significant change in the frequency of low birthweight deliveries. Poor nutrition, smoking, and inadequate prenatal care increase the chances of a mother having a low birthweight baby. All of these risks are more common among the poor. "I'm all for treatment," says Wilkins. "It's really marvellous to see what can be done to improve the survival of these infants, and that even the poorest people can get that service, but wouldn't it be nice if we could eliminate the problem? Neonatal intensive care is expensive and not without risks — prevention could reduce our reliance on it."

Health and Work: Is Your Job Making You Sick?

People have known since ancient times that certain jobs made people sick in certain ways. The hatter went mad because he was poisoned by the mercury he used to treat his hat fabric; asbestos miners were stricken with asbestosis, a lung disease. In Canada in 1986, there were 586,718 work-related injuries that resulted in lost time or a workers' compensation claim, and an estimated 700 to 800 work-related deaths.[46] Internationally, Canada falls in the middle range for work-related fatalities among OECD* countries. Canada's rate of 11 fatal occupational injuries per 100,000 workers in 1977** was much higher than the Netherlands' (2 per 100,000) but much lower than Switzerland's (22 per 100,000). Our record was particularly dismal in the mining industry, where the rate of fatal injuries was 102 per 100,000 employees per year. This compares to 26 for Spain, and 20 for Italy.[47]

Dr. Clyde Hertzman is the director of the occupational health program at the University of British Columbia's faculty of medicine. He says that because jurisdiction over occupational health

---

*Organization for Economic Cooperation and Development.

**The most recent international data.

and safety is held primarily by the provinces, there are no national standards for workplace inspection, and no national policies for establishing preventive clinical services. The result is a patchwork of programs, and wide variations in how much money provinces commit to them. Dr. Hertzman cites the forestry industry as an example of this lack of national coordination. Forestry is a major economic activity in most Canadian provinces and an extraordinarily dangerous one, yet we have no national strategy to address its health and safety issues.

Canadian organizations for workplace safety have far less power than you might imagine. The Canadian Centre for Occupational Health and Safety (CCOHS) in Hamilton has none of the clout of its American counterpart, the National Institute for Occupational Safety and Health (NIOSH). NIOSH inspectors can enter workplaces, suggest standards, and even draft legislation. In contrast, the CCOHS has a much more narrow mandate, one that limits its role to data collection, research, and information dissemination.

Employment patterns in Canada are changing. Job opportunities in manufacturing and resource extraction are drying up, while employment in service industries is expanding rapidly.[48] We're in the midst of a massive industrial labour transfer. For example, the steel and mining industries are using new technologies to produce more with fewer people. Will laid-off miners and steelworkers eventually find themselves working for McDonald's? Will this shift to the service sector make work any healthier?

Dr. Hertzman doesn't believe so. He says that while there may be less chance of dying making a hamburger than setting dynamite in a mine shaft, the overall risk of injury may be the same. Indeed, the risk of injury in service-sector jobs may actually be increasing, as employers introduce technological changes to improve efficiency. As an example, Dr. Hertzman cites the high rate of strains and sprains among check-out cashiers in grocery stores. New technology now requires cashiers in many stores to glide each item over an optical scanner, which "reads" the price. Such repetitive motions can lead to many wrist injuries, says Dr. Hertzman, who also notes that clever management can make the problem even worse. "Grocery-store managers carefully estimate the number of shoppers at each time of day and reduce the number of cashiers accordingly. This means that the cashier is busy all the time. There's no time for sore wrists to rest.'' Musculoskeletal problems may be the most common occupational health problem, but Dr. Hertzman notes that monotonous, hectic work, and workers' increasing lack of control over the pace of work, are also risk factors for cardiovascular disease.

Since 1982, the purchasing value of wages and salaries has fallen.[49] If the net effect of this, and of new employment patterns, is to increase economic disparities in our society, there will be adverse health consequences for many people. As we've already said, poverty kills.

People Needing People: Loneliness Is Bad for Your Health

For thousands of years we've known that recently widowed people are much more likely to die than people of the same age who haven't lost a spouse. It used to be quite common to hear the sad pronouncement, ''She died of a broken heart,'' as a tacit acknowledgment of the importance of being loved to a healthy life.

Such observations can't be dismissed as mere sentimentality. There's now substantial evidence that being part of a social network — what's known today as having ''social support'' — is an important determinant of our health. In other words, everyone needs friends. Dr. Eugene Broadhead, of the Duke University Department of Family Medicine, found that improving people's social support improved health, while decreasing that social support led to decreases in health status.[50]

There's even some biochemical evidence to defend the idea that social support is an important determinant of physical health. Recently, scientists have found that the conscious portions of the brain can have a major impact on the body's involuntary systems. This possibility had been quite controversial: many scientists firmly believed that the conscious mind had little influence over these other systems. But according to Dr. Broadhead, we may soon have even more scientific evidence to support the premise most societies have always accepted on faith: *that being lonely is bad for your health.*

Roslyn Lindheim, of the Department of Architecture at the University of California at Berkeley, agrees with Dr. Broadhead, and adds that when a society ignores basic human needs — and she includes among these basic needs a sense of connectedness to others — it does so to the detriment of that society's health.[51]

Resource Allocation: The Power to Define Health Problems

All societies give special status and special powers to physicians. In Canada a doctor can have a psychiatric patient detained against his or her will. We give enormous powers to medical officers of health, who are always doctors; for example, in an infectious epidemic they have the right to quarantine the sick and restrict transportation in order to limit the outbreak. But perhaps the most significant power we give to physicians is the right to define what is and what is not a health problem. This is important, because as a society we accord the highest priority to those conditions "defined" as health problems. How we allocate our social spending is, to a large degree, based on these definitions.

To illustrate what this means, let's compare the experience of Carl G., the heart attack patient from our earlier example, with that of a battered wife and her children who happened to arrive at the hospital on the same cold January night in 1978.

As you will recall, Mr. G. spent 20 days in hospital with his first heart attack. Unfortunately, over the next ten years his health deteriorated further. Despite warnings from the hospital's dietician and his personal physician, Mr. G. never quite managed to quit smoking, nor did he change his eating habits or his sedentary lifestyle. In 1981 he had another, more serious heart attack, and the following spring, he had coronary artery bypass surgery. This helped a bit for a time, but gradually his arteries clogged up again as he continued his unhealthy habits. By 1984, even walking a few blocks had become impossible for him. In 1986 he had a third heart attack. The doctors tried angioplasty * in early 1988, but it was too late. He had a stroke shortly after the procedure and died in January of the same year. Ten years of health care related to Mr. G's heart disease — including hospitaliza-

---

* Angioplasty involves inserting a catheter into the patient's groin and moving it into his coronary arteries. A balloon at the catheter's tip is inflated to squash the plaque and (hopefully) open the artery.

tion, physicians' fees, and drugs — cost almost $100,000. Over 95% of this expense was paid with tax dollars.

Jane H. was a 23-year-old housewife when she turned up at the hospital in 1978 with her daughter, aged two, and her son, aged five. Her husband had beaten her and she had a lot of back pain as well as a bleeding laceration on her left arm.

Bonnie T., a nurse in the emergency department, played quietly with the kids and tried to help. Jane told her she had no money, but that after five years of escalating violence, she was determined to leave her husband. Bonnie phoned a local women's shelter for her, only to find it was full.* Staff at the shelter indicated there might be a spot in a couple of weeks. So Jane arranged to stay with her sister temporarily and left the emergency department in a taxi paid by the hospital.

Jane, like Carl G. , had a tough time over the next ten years. While she was with her sister she learned that without a permanent address, she couldn't get on social assistance. This was a Catch-22, because without money from social services, she couldn't get a permanent place to live. Meanwhile, her husband found her and, as usual, professed his love for her and the children. If they'd only come back, he promised, he'd never abuse her again. Jane felt trapped. Because it was clear that she had no hope of finding another place to live, she reluctantly returned to her husband — with predictable results. He continued to abuse her and occasionally the children as well. Soon the family began to experience other problems. At age 11, Jane's son was picked up for shoplifting. The following year he began sniffing airplane glue and stopped going to school for weeks at a time.

One day in November 1987, Jane came home early from a shopping expedition and was horrified to find her husband drunk and undressing her daughter in front of two friends. That afternoon Jane went to a newly opened legal-aid clinic and started to make plans for her "escape," with help from a social worker, Fran H. Fran found Jane a place in a hostel and started work on her

---

*There were less than 70 shelters in Canada in 1978. There were over 230 by 1987, but the average shelter still turned away two women for every one they could take in.

legal case to retain sole custody of the children. The next day, while her husband was at work, Jane packed a few essentials and arrived at the shelter with her children. Things began to look up for this family when, three weeks later, they moved into a small apartment. But despite a court order instructing him to stay away, her husband showed up in a drunken rage on New Year's Day and stabbed Jane to death. For the ten-year period between 1978 and 1988, social services and health care related to Jane's circumstances cost $7,000. An additional $3,000 had been spent on her children.

Comparing Carl G.'s case with Jane's makes it clear how confused our society is about what's really important to our health. The fact that we insist on making so much money available for treating "health" problems, and so little for treating "social" problems, reveals a dangerous bias, a kind of discrimination that deserves to be exposed. Because Carl G. had a clear-cut medical problem, his doctors were allowed virtually unlimited draws on the public purse to give him whatever treatment they felt would be of benefit. Even the fact that some of his care was known to be useless and potentially harmful didn't limit their decision-making authority. Carl's doctors didn't have to justify the need for the bypass operation or the angioplasty. They simply ordered whatever treatments they wanted, without having to concern themselves with cost.

Compare this kind of freedom to the maze of restrictions and endless application forms that Jane's social workers had to contend with while arranging for her "therapy." Compare the total amounts spent on her treatment to those available to the heart patient.

Why was there such a discrepancy? Because our society takes the position that Jane had a "social" problem rather than a "health" one. Of course, we were more than willing to pay for any *medical* treatment Jane required for her physical injuries. If she'd needed more costly "health care" — in its narrowest medical definition — her doctors could have ordered it, and it wouldn't have mattered at all that she was poor. But strangely, we failed to respond to her most pressing health needs. Indeed, once we defined her needs as "social," their priority plummeted. Money for surgery? Certainly, no problem. But money for housing? For a decent level of social assistance? For legal aid? For counselling? For treating her violent husband? Resources for these types of services are much more limited.

In 1978 there were hundreds of thousands of Canadian women being abused by their husbands, but fewer than 1,000 beds for them in shelters. Even now, hostels are forced to turn away thousands every year for lack of space. Treatment programs for wife-batterers and their victims are in very short supply. Waiting lists for non-profit and public housing are years long in some communities. Housing agencies have strict clamps on over-spending, and social assistance increases have been held to the rate of inflation for many years in most provinces.

Meanwhile, when Ontario's doctors overspent their projected budget by nearly $200 million in 1987, the province's gentle response was to create a committee of civil servants and physicians "to study the issue." The deficit was covered by taxpayers. There's no strategic plan to deal with the increasing costs of physicians' services. (By the way, $200 million is enough money to build about 3,500 units of assisted housing.)

Medical and Social Problems: The Margins Begin to Blur

The line we draw to separate medical issues from social ones begins to blur when we look at the health consequences of social problems. Consider that in Jane's case the ultimate result of inadequate therapy for a "social" problem was death — the most undesirable "health" outcome imaginable. Unfortunately, such cases are not at all rare.

In 1986, 40% of Canada's 561 homicides were "domestic." Of these, 37% involved women who were killed by their husbands or male lovers.* In most of these cases, a history of earlier phys-

---

*The domestic category includes all of those homicides where the parties were related by blood, common law, or in-law. As mentioned in the text, 37% of these murder victims were wives killed by husbands; 29% were children killed by parents (almost always the father); 10% were parents killed by children (almost always a son); 10% were husbands killed by wives (almost all of these wives had lived in chronically abusive relationships); and 4% involved siblings. Other family relationships, including those that involved grandparents, uncles, aunts, and so on, accounted for 9% of the domestic homicides. (Holly Johnson, "Homicide in Canada," in: *Canadian Social Trends* Statistics Canada, Winter 1987, pp. 2-6.)

ical violence had preceded the murder, and the police were aware of the potential risks to the family. In some cases the courts had ordered the husband to stay away from his estranged wife, but the police failed to enforce the restraining order.[52] The Toronto police used to have a special domestic response team to deal with family violence, but it was discontinued in the fall of 1987. Bob Couchman is executive director of the Metropolitan Toronto Family Services Association, the largest family counselling agency in Toronto. He told the *Toronto Star* in February 1988 that his agency hadn't received a single referral from the police since the team had been abandoned.[53]

But murder is only the most extreme health problem experienced by families living with violence. Records show that in the first six months of 1987, Toronto police investigated 1,764 cases of spousal assault. Most workers in the field believe this is just the "tip of the iceberg," and that many cases go unreported even when police *are* called to intervene. Bob Couchman says that all the paperwork involved in filing such reports often deters police officers from reporting such cases. "We know from talking with senior officers that there are far more incidents of family violence than those statistics would indicate . . . . We know it takes about 20 minutes for an officer to fill out an occurrence sheet, and it's our guess that a lot of these officers are not filling out these forms."

Although Canada's attorneys general have instructed police officers to lay charges when abuse is suspected, it still remains far from common practice. Susan Goodfellow, a counsellor at Interval House in Toronto, says she still sees many cases where a woman is forced to lay charges because the police won't. Inspector John Dennis, head of the Toronto police department's family and youth bureau, explains why the average peace officer is sometimes reluctant to deal more harshly with domestic violence. "Time and time again we'll arrest the guy, get a court order to keep him away from the woman, and then the woman will turn around, let him back in, and try to get the charges dropped. Three months later we'll be called back because he's hitting her again."

It's not easy to estimate the amount of wife assault in Canada with any accuracy, but if we apply the reported figures for Toronto to Canada as a whole, there were about 40,000 cases in 1987. If these represent only one-tenth of the true number —

as many social and legal workers believe — the figure could be as high as half a million. A study from the Canadian Advisory Council on the Status of Women offers an even higher estimate, suggesting there may be as many as a million cases of wife assault every year.[54]

Physical injuries from family violence run the gamut from bruises to cigarette burns to skull fractures. But when adding up the cost to society, we must include with this bodily suffering the host of mental health problems found among women and children subjected to abuse. Although the figures have never been tabulated, the annual costs to our health care system from wife assault must be tens and perhaps hundreds of millions of dollars.

And what about the suffering? Does anyone really believe that a woman who breaks her leg at the hands of her husband suffers less than someone who slips on some ice? Is the ongoing agony of a woman living in an abusive relationship any less than that of someone with another chronic disease like rheumatoid arthritis?

What Makes Us Healthy?

So what keeps us healthy? One experienced doctor says that if you ask patients about their eating, sleeping, and sex life you get a good idea of their health status. A major study from California agrees with this doctor's clinical judgment. Starting in 1965, a group of investigators followed the health of 7,000 residents of Alameda County in California. The subjects for this study were selected as representative of the general adult population of a California urban community.[55] They found a strong correlation between good health (as indicated by low death rates) and regular eating and sleeping habits, regular physical exercise, normal weight, moderate use of alcoholic beverages, and adequate income. We also know that married people live longer than unmarried people, and that death rates are lower among those who have a lot of friends and social contacts.[56]

The way we define health is related to how we measure it. A lot of epidemiological research uses fairly classical measures of health status — rates of mortality and morbidity (illness), and especially life expectancy — all of which are rather narrow and limited in approach. Dr. John Frank, from the Department of Social and Preventive Medicine at the University of Toronto, explains that the field of epidemiology has been led by technical people, who like to base their findings on absolute and undeniable outcomes — like death. The problem is that measures of this type are pertinent to an ever-tinier fraction of the population. "Most people," he says, "don't worry about their kids dying during their first ten years of life. And they're right. Between the ages of one and ten, the chances are astronomically low.* What parents worry about is social failure, social deviance (criminal or other kinds), and mental illness. Those are the bad things they fear [might happen to their children], and they are, in fact, the most common to happen." Hundreds of thousands of Canadian children are affected by these kinds of problems. So if we want to look at improving health, it doesn't make much sense to confine our investigations to mortality rates.

Dr. Dan (David) Offord, with his colleagues at the Child Epidemiology Unit of McMaster University, conducted a massive study in the early 1980s to look at the prevalence of chronic illness and psychological and social problems among Ontario children. The results support Dr. Frank's assertions. Dr. Offord and the other researchers found that 15 to 20% of children had some psychiatric problems. Four percent had a physical disability. All of these conditions were more common in poorer families.[57]

Modern epidemiology, as a science, is less than 30 years old. The diffusion of its techniques to other disciplines such as social work, psychology, and economics has been slow. "I blame epidemiologists who teach and practice" says Dr. Frank, "for being more interested in furthering their technical prowess, producing ever more refined results using the same old data, instead of broadening their approach to include newer areas." But he points out that there's really no commitment to social epidemiology in Canadian medical schools. "Only in Britain is there a strong tradition, where being on the faculty of departments of social and preventive medicine accords high status and respect. In North America, the departments themselves are becoming vanishingly rare, and those who work within them receive little recognition."

---

*For example, a five-year-old child in Ontario has more than 997 chances out of 1,000 of living until the age of 14. (Ontario Vital Statistics, 1985.)

All the research done so far suggests that many factors are involved in creating a context for health. This has forced both governments and students of public policy to relearn an old lesson: our health care system is *not* a major determinant of health. But we're only at the beginning of this research, and meanwhile, our ideas about the other more important influences on health remain very general. For instance, we know that housing can affect health — there's plenty of data to support that conclusion. But *what* exactly about housing is key to improving health? Its cost? Its design? The neighbourhood in which it's located? Its physical size? How much private space it contains? All of the above?[58] The challenge remains: we have to refine our understanding so that we can develop specific strategies to promote health.

We Don't Know How Healthy We Are

It's sad but true that neither governments nor health care personnel really have much incentive to look for the real determinants of health. The Canada Health Survey of 1979 was meant to be the first in a series of studies designed to pinpoint changes in health status over time. But the federal government suddenly dropped its plans for subsequent investigations. Doug Angus, now the executive director for the Institute for Health Care Facilities for the Future, was working with Health and Welfare Canada when the government called a halt to the project. He recalls that his first reaction to the news was "utter disbelief. We'd only been underway a few months when the program was cut. Yet we'd spent six million dollars in start-up costs, developing the questions, the physical measures, and analytical techniques. Now all of a sudden, instead of a continuing program, it was a snapshot. Its potential value was never realized."

Angus is particularly critical of the thoughtless way the survey was cut. "They broke a lot of trust with people," he says. "It takes a lot to bring together a scientific core of such competence, and that group had some of the sharpest minds. When they disbanded, we lost a golden opportunity for quality research."

Still, there are some signs that governments are beginning to change their minds about the potential value of knowing how healthy their populations are. Québec conducted a survey in 1987.

Ontario has recently announced its intention to conduct a regular provincial health survey, and other provinces may well follow suit. It's rather ironic that the best data on Canadians' health status doesn't belong to governments at all. Rather, it's been carefully collected by insurance companies, who for business reasons have to be able to identify health risks. By contrast, governments have traditionally displayed much less interest. In fact, the only time governments really become concerned about the health of their people is when they're at war. Then health becomes strategically important!

Considering the potential payoffs, we believe it's strategically important even in peacetime to find out more about our health and what affects it. There's so much to learn, so many details to fill in. But we can't even get started until we begin asking the right questions.

Health planners could take some advice from Willie Sutton, the famous American bank robber of the 1930s. When asked why he robbed banks, Willie replied, "Because that's where the money is." Putting more money into hospitals and doctors promises fewer and fewer health returns. Instead, we should be investing our money where it will do the most good — that is, on those social and economic interventions which promise the greatest health dividends.

Chapter 8

Don't Get Cured, Stay Healthy

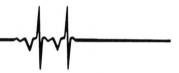

The Case for Prevention

"NO MASS DISORDER OR condition affecting humankind has ever been eliminated or controlled by treating afflicted individuals."

Professor George Albee from the University of Vermont made this statement in May 1987, at a Canadian conference on disease prevention. He repeated this forceful pronouncement twice, stressing, "If that's the only thing you remember from what I have to say, that's enough." The quote — which actually comes from John Gordon, a Harvard professor of epidemiology — remains for Albee the most important piece of health information he ever received. "I make all my students memorize it," he says, "and regurgitate it back to me on exams, because it holds the key to all past, present, and future hopes for improving health — which is, of course, prevention."

One way to understand preventive interventions is to think of them in terms of two categories: those which strengthen our resistance to disease, and those which deflect potential hazards or risks. Along the same lines, specialists in infectious diseases talk about "host" resistance, and the virulence of the disease "agent." Eating correctly increases our resistance to infections, heart disease, cancer, and most other illnesses. So does exercising regularly. Reducing excessive alcohol consumption decreases the potential ill effects from that "agent" of disease.

In this chapter, we'll examine how preventing illness encompasses a very broad spectrum of strategies. At one end is the individual who makes healthy choices, like deciding not to smoke. At the other, is the society which implements healthy public policies, like safe speed limits. Our health care system, or more particularly, preventive medicine, plays a relatively minor, though important, role in keeping people healthy.

Prevention Isn't Sexy

Most people don't give much thought to their health until they fall ill. Illness, not health, is the real attention-grabber. And of course, by the time illness strikes, prevention is beside the point, an irrelevance. We take health for granted as the most natural state in the world. Then when we get sick we run for treatment, which, if successful, strongly reinforces our belief that medical care is the most important factor determining our health. By the same token, when treatment fails or is unavailable, we tend to think the answer lies in more research to find cures. Alan Backley, a former deputy health minister in Ontario, sums it up: "We scream around the fast track of life with carefree abandon until suddenly something goes wrong. Then we pull in to the nearest pit stop and expect a quick fix will be able to patch us up so we can get back in the race."

The way we allocate our health dollars reflects these attitudes. Fear of disease — along with the mistaken idea that health care is totally responsible for our well-being — has fueled the development of a hugely expensive sickness treatment system. When contrasted with the high public profile of curative medicine, prevention seems very low-key and undramatic — it just isn't "sexy." That's why, when it comes to funding, prevention programs lose out to those for sickness treatment time after time. Medical research is a good example. Most research resources are spent looking for cures in the laboratory. This emphasis on germs and genes makes it unlikely that medicine will be able to shed much light on the true underlying causes of illness — the social and environmental context in which diseases flourish. In saying this, we're not dismissing the importance of treatment; we're simply arguing that more emphasis on prevention could obviate the need for treatment in the first place.

Perhaps the most famous event in the history of disease prevention occurred in 1854 in London's Soho district, when the city was in the grip of a raging cholera epidemic. In those days, very little was known about how diseases spread; Pasteur's germ theory of illness wasn't to appear for another ten years. That's why it's so remarkable that a physician named John Snow was able to deduce that cholera was a water-borne disease, and that the source of this particular epidemic was the water from one particular pump.*

Snow was very much a product of the Victorian age, in that he believed science held the answers to all of humanity's problems. Tracking cholera epidemics was one of his passions. In this instance, he documented that most of the cases came from the neighbourhood that drew its water from the Broad Street pump. While he believed this water was the source of the contagion, his data revealed a few discrepancies — a brewery and a public workhouse in the area had mysteriously escaped the epidemic. Why? Snow knew he was on the right track when he discovered that both of these institutions drew their water from other sources. Snow, on the basis of his careful analysis, was now certain the Broad Street pump had to be turned off. Much to the consternation of the local private water company, he went to the local officials and convinced them to remove the pump handle. They did so, and thus halted the cholera outbreak. This is one of the first documented, definitive public health measures arising out of statistical research. And it was a smashing success! It's interesting that public health officials of the time were slow to give John Snow any credit. His extraordinary contribution wasn't recognized in the scientific community until 30 years later, when the German microbiologist, Koch, identified the cholera bacterium.

---

*Although he's now revered as one of the fathers of epidemiology, in his own lifetime, John Snow was better-known as a pioneer of anaesthesia. It was he who administered chloroform to Queen Victoria during the births of two of her children. At that time the use of anaesthetic in childbirth was a hotly debated issue among religious leaders, some of whom claimed that God intended women to bring forth children in "sorrow," which they interpreted as meaning "pain." To the relief of many women of the day, Queen Victoria's use of anaesthesia for childbirth temporarily ended the controversy. In more modern times, it has resurfaced as an issue, but now the question is one of the "medicalization" of childbirth, and the merits of returning to a more "natural" delivery process.

Dr. Brian Holmes, former chairman of the Ontario Council of Health, thinks this typifies the kind of reaction one gets in prevention work. "Curative medicine is much more challenging and interesting," he says. "You can see the results almost right away. With prevention, you might not see any for 25 to 30 years — there's no drama to that. That's why it's difficult to attract people to prevention careers." Besides, successful prevention results in an *absence* of illness, and that's hardly likely to attract much attention: few of us call our doctors to thank them for the vaccination that keeps us free from polio, and public health departments rarely get praise from us for inspecting restaurants. Prevention just doesn't attract the kind of attention it really deserves.

Fluoridation is another more recent example of prevention. During the Second World War, American recruits had to take medical examinations to certify their fitness for service. Army dentists began to notice that draftees from Deaf Smith County in Texas had remarkably healthy teeth.[1] "Every time we saw a man with no cavities and asked where he came from, the answer was the same," reported one dentist. After the war, subsequent investigations showed that the water in that part of Texas contained naturally occurring fluoride. Although fluoride treatments had become common in dentists' offices, the profession — as well as governments — recognized they could extend this protection to a much wider population by adding fluoride to drinking water.

Thus began a heated public debate about whether or not this was desirable. Fluoridation finally won the day. As a result, most communities in Canada today have a fluoridated water supply. This has greatly reduced the incidence of dental cavities in children; for example, between 1971 and 1982, the number of cavity-free 13-year-olds in Toronto jumped by 200%.[2] The dental profession has responded to this dramatic change by placing more emphasis on prevention, by teaching dental self-care, and by treating gum disease at an earlier stage. Orthodontic procedures, once considered " frills," now occupy much of the time dentists used to spend drilling and filling decayed teeth.

In both of these examples of disease prevention, the most striking element is that they didn't depend on personal choices in order to work. When John Snow found out that cholera was caused by water from the Broad Street pump, he closed it down — he didn't start a public information campaign to warn people against drinking from it, or try to convince people to change their habits. Today, when we drink a glass of tap water, few of us give much thought to the fact that we're giving our teeth a fluoride treatment. While it's true that individual behaviour can have an enormous impact on individual health, the most effective preventive measures in history have operated on a societal basis, precluding individual choice. But although success may favour those preventive endeavours which *don't* depend on individual choice, this poses a political problem for societies dedicated to individual freedoms and property rights. Remember the opposition when provinces began to pass legislation requiring automobile passengers to wear seat belts? And it took years of effort after we learned about the toxic effects of asbestos and lead before we started to clean up those industries. In Chapter 10 we discuss these public-policy areas further.

Personal Responsibility and Victim Blaming

We still place much of the responsibility for health on individual behaviour. The voices of health promotion continually admonish us to change our habits: "Don't smoke." "Don't drink too much." "Drive carefully." "Eat less fat, more fibre, less salt." "Stay away from junk food." "Get plenty of rest." "Exercise." All these slogans put the burden on the individual.

There's good evidence to show that some people are listening to this advice and applying it. But there's a disturbing subtext to all these demands to change our ways: a message that reads if we get sick, it's *our fault*. We should have known better and done something about it. Professor Leonard Syme teaches epidemiology at the University of California at Berkeley and has long researched the connection between health and social factors. In his opinion, people often have a limited range of choice available to them. He notes, for example, that many teenagers have to fight a tough battle not to smoke. It's also more difficult for shoppers to choose healthy food when it lies hidden on the bottom shelf and unhealthy food is prominently discounted and stored at eye-level.[3]

Fortunately, most Canadian professionals involved in health

promotion and disease prevention know that victim blaming is unfair precisely because choices are often limited by circumstances beyond the control of the individual. The mother on welfare may well be overweight because she feeds herself and her children on starchy, but filling foods. Sure, she knows that fresh fruits and vegetables would be healthier for her family, but she can't afford them. Similarly, the unemployed worker, who faces being cut off from UIC, knows he shouldn't smoke. But he's under stress, hardly a propitious time to consider quitting.

All the same, some health education efforts targeting people at high risk have proven effective. As a good example, the gay community itself initiated public education about acquired immune deficiency syndrome (AIDS), to warn homosexuals about unsafe sexual practices. Rates among gay men for all sorts of sexually transmitted diseases have fallen dramatically during the 1980s. This is a good indication that the message promoting "safe" sex has been heard and understood.*

At the same time, however, fear of AIDS among the general public often expresses itself in homophobia (fear or hatred of homosexuals) — a classic example of blaming the victim. We hear stories about doctors and other health professionals refusing to treat AIDS patients. Certain religious leaders suggest that AIDS is God's punishment for promiscuity or what they feel is "deviant" sexual behaviour. Some politicians have advocated quarantine for AIDS victims, even though it's well established that AIDS isn't spread by casual contact. These are only some of the ethical and legal issues beginning to emerge around AIDS, but they should be enough to show that blaming victims for their disease is both cruel and useless.

It's important to recognize that the choices we make that affect our health are very much influenced by our society and culture. For example, society's diminishing tolerance for tobacco smoke is often cited by ex-smokers as a major influence on their decision to quit. "I couldn't take the disapproval any more," says

---

*It's generally agreed that the most likely way to pass on the AIDS virus sexually is by engaging in anal intercourse. Between 1982 and 1987, the number of rectal gonorrhea cases seen at the Hassle Free Clinic, Toronto's largest V.D. clinic, dropped from 575 to 52 — more than a 90% decline.

one man. "My kids were always on my case. Then when it started at work and on social occasions, too, I decided I had to give them up."

Sometimes the social context encourages behaviours that are promoted as healthy, but actually have detrimental effects. For example, Dr. Gerry Bonham, the medical officer of health for Calgary, considers society's worship of body leanness to be a major contributor to ill health, especially among women. "First we have to face the unhealthy behaviours women exhibit in their desperate attempts to be thin," he says. Women often use cigarettes as an appetite suppressant. Constant dieting and excessive aerobic exercise are two other frequently used weight-control strategies. But there's a problem: women need more body fat than men — it's essential to their biological functioning. A woman faces a host of health problems, all preventable, when she becomes too lean. For example, when her body fat falls below a certain level, her metabolism of the hormone estrogen changes. This can affect ovulation, and since women who stop ovulating can't get pregnant, a common result of leanness is decreased fertility.

Estrogen also protects women from bone loss due to osteoporosis. This condition is usually found in older women, because after menopause estrogen production is drastically reduced. But when young women are too thin, they fail to produce estrogen as well, and so are at serious risk for premature osteoporosis.* "We're seeing more and more of this," says Dr. Bonham. "Ballet dancers are among the most seriously affected. I examined one young dancer whose bones were so light and hollow, they were like those of an 80-year-old woman."

Self-perceived overweight is a major women's health issue. A recent poll of *Glamour* magazine's readers found that 75% of respondents said they thought they were "too fat."[4] Among those women who felt they were overweight, twice as many said they considered losing weight to be more important than being successful at work. Anorexia nervosa (not eating) and bulimia (binge-eating followed by induced vomiting and/or diarrhea) are especially prevalent among teenage girls. Dr. Bonham says one

---

*The problem is aggravated among women who smoke, because cigarette smoke has anti-estrogenic activity.

high-school survey reported that over 80% of the female students were dieting. Lisa, a Toronto nurse in her mid-twenties, says that when she was in high school, nearly everyone was trying to lose weight. Role models for young women reinforce these unhealthy behaviours. Toronto's Monika Schnarre has been a world-famous model since she was 14. In a *Toronto Star* article, Monika (who was then sixteen) announced that she had recently shed 14 pounds from her already slender frame.[5] "I feel great," she said. "My energy is so high." Even worse, Monika admitted she was still growing. Growth requires additional calories. What happens, then, when young girls are encouraged to emulate a thin, growing 16-year-old model who is dieting? They have to struggle hard against the current in order to stay healthy.

The message here is that social and cultural norms can influence healthy *and* unhealthy behavioural decisions. The challenge is to create a climate that favours healthy behaviours.

The Limits of Preventive Medicine

What effect on health can we expect from preventive medicine — the services delivered by doctors, nurses, and other health professionals? Even though much of the information we get about disease prevention comes from non-medical sources — newspapers, magazines, television, radio, and the like — many people expect their physician to be the best source. Susan L. is a 30-year-old ad executive who suffers from recurrent bladder infections. She gets two or three of these bothersome infections every year, and each time gets a prescription from her physician for ampicillin, an antibiotic. As sometimes happens, a few days after taking this medication, she develops a secondary infection in her vagina. This new infection is caused by yeast organisms, which are normally present in small numbers in the vagina. But thanks to the antibiotic Susan's been taking, the normal vaginal bacteria that keep the yeast in check have been wiped out. The yeast isn't killed by the antibiotic. On the contrary, these little beasts are flourishing and causing discomfort and irritation. She returns to her doctor and leaves with a new prescription, this time for vaginal suppositories whose active ingredient is an antifungal agent. Eventually her problem clears up, only to return a few months later. One afternoon, discussing this problem with a few friends, someone suggests that she try a few preventive measures — like urinating after sex, drinking plenty of cranberry juice, and not sitting around in a wet bathing suit. Simple, benign suggestions — although not validated by scientific evaluation. She asks her doctor about them, but he isn't impressed. Still, she decides to give them a try and is delighted with the results: no more bladder infections.

While these measures may not solve all such cases, this example illustrates how individual, self-care, preventive steps can make a difference to the incidence of disease. Susan's doctor, by the way, was practicing medicine as it is taught. His focus was entirely on the biological causes of her illness, and he offered effective treatment. But he was unable to give any real help in preventing a recurrence of the infection, because medicine, with all its chemicals, technologies, and therapies, often doesn't address the underlying causes of illness. He didn't endorse the self-care steps Susan wanted to try, because they've never been scientifically validated. The fact is, most preventive strategies, just like most medical therapies, have never been properly evaluated. Why is this?

Vaccination   There are two major areas where preventive medicine has had a definite impact on improving health, and they deserve praise. The first and most important of these is immunization to control certain infectious diseases. The second involves screening for disease to detect it at an early and treatable stage. Some vaccines have been around for a very long time — the one for smallpox, for example, was developed almost 200 years ago.* Smallpox was a devastating disease that killed almost everyone who contracted it, and left the few survivors scarred and sometimes blind. No vaccine in history has been as successful as the smallpox vaccine; in fact, no case of the disease has been recorded since 1977, and in May 1980 the World Health organisation declared the eradication complete. This is the *only*

---

*Edward Jenner developed this crude but effective vaccine in 1796 from cowpox, a related cattle infection which caused few ill effects among humans. About 80 years earlier, Lady Mary Wortley Montagu had introduced "ingrafting" to England — a practice she had observed in Turkey, in which patients were infected on purpose with a mild case of smallpox to ensure future immunity.

disease ever to be wiped out completely, and we owe it all to prevention.

A number of factors contributed to this success story. First, the smallpox vaccine was very effective. It even helped people who had already contracted the disease, provided they were vaccinated early in the incubation period. Also, smallpox was very easy to diagnose, and its victims became infectious only a short time before the distinctive rash appeared. This meant you could track down contacts quickly and vaccinate them. It also made it possible to isolate infected individuals to contain the spread of the disease. Prevention had still another thing going for it — the nature of smallpox itself changed over time. Toward the end of the 19th century, a much milder strain appeared, one with much lower mortality rates. There were, of course, some risks associated with the vaccine itself. The most common complications were encephalitis (brain inflammation), and serious skin conditions, which sometimes occurred among individuals with a history of eczema. But these complications were very rare — in 1963 they accounted for only 6 deaths out of 14 million vaccinations in the United States.[6] These characteristics of the vaccine and the disease, as well as a massive worldwide cooperative effort, made it possible to wipe a terrifying disease off the map.

Other vaccines, while not as successful as the one for smallpox, have at least been "minor miracles." For example, the Salk polio vaccine was the answer to many parents' prayers when it was released in 1955. Within six years, North American rates of paralytic polio had decreased by over 90%.[7] The rubella (German measles) vaccine may eventually eliminate congenital rubella syndrome,* a cluster of birth defects associated with infection in the mother while she's pregnant. The vaccine against hepatitis B (so-called serum hepatitis) works against the infection, and also prevents a type of liver cancer that is a long-term complication of the disease in some people.

Still, other vaccines haven't managed to accomplish similar victories. Less favourable characteristics of both the individual disease and the vaccine available to combat it have hindered their

---

*A syndrome is a group of symptoms and signs, which, when considered together, characterize a disease or lesion.

success. One example is measles. Virtually everyone who isn't vaccinated for it is susceptible, although people who *have* contracted it are afterwards immune for the rest of their lives. Like smallpox, measles is primarily a childhood disease — and probably the most infectious one we know. It can also be very dangerous — the possible complications include pneumonia, mental retardation, deafness, and even death. Because the disease is so extremely infectious, about 95% of the population would have to be immunized in order to prevent its transmission. But at the same time, the measles vaccine isn't nearly as effective as the one for smallpox. Even under ideal conditions, it produces immunity in only 90 to 95% of vaccinees.[8] All of this means that we stand very little chance of eradicating measles the way we did smallpox.

Screening and Early Detection: Doing Good and Harm
Screening to detect illnesses at their earliest and theoretically most treatable stage is the other major focus of preventive medicine. Here you have to judge success as a function of outcome in order to get the complete picture. It's true that with some diseases, early detection can offer a better chance for cure; for example, finding cancer of the cervix early with a Pap smear definitely does improve a woman's likelihood of survival. But sometimes early detection merely exposes the patient to risky treatment without improving the chances for survival at all; for example, finding most types of lung cancer early doesn't improve the patient's odds for survival.

The esteemed British epidemiologist Dr. Archie Cochrane says it's more important to prove the benefits of a screening test than to prove the benefits of a treatment.[9] He explains that there's an ethical difference. When patients arrive at a doctors' office with symptoms, they're asking for help. But it's quite a different matter when a doctor, or a cancer society, or a shopping mall offers a screening test, because in doing so they're all implying that the benefit of testing outweighs the harm. The problem is we can't jump to such a conclusion without first subjecting each screening test to evaluation. Careful study is necessary to avoid some of the statistical traps that can make a test look better than it really is.

For example, suppose we start a screening program for lung cancer, and take sputum samples and chest X-rays from all heavy smokers every six months. Undoubtedly this kind of program is going to turn up a number of lung cancer cases earlier than they would otherwise have been discovered, by diagnosing some patients who haven't yet begun to experience symptoms. Now consider that survival for these patients is generally measured from the time of diagnosis. By moving back the date of diagnosis, the statistics from our program might well make it appear that we've actually improved their length of survival. But this conclusion is wrong, and here's an example to show why: Suppose Uncle Gene was fated to be diagnosed with lung cancer in June and to die in December. But instead he enters our screening program and is diagnosed as having cancer in March, three months earlier. Uncle Gene still dies in December, but it *appears* as if we've increased his length of survival after diagnosis by 50%.[10] In reality, his life span remains exactly the same. Our screening program has added to his time of *dying*, not to his time of *living*. This is why all new screening programs need to be carefully evaluated. The following list of questions can help to determine whether a screening program does more good than harm:

1. Has the program's effectiveness been demonstrated in a randomized controlled trial?
2. Are there efficacious treatments available?
3. Does the burden of suffering warrant screening?
4. Is there a good screening test?
5. Does the program reach those who could benefit from it?
6. Can the health care system cope with the screening program?
7. Will those who screen "positive" comply with subsequent advice and interventions?[11]

Bearing these criteria in mind, let's look at screening for cancer of the colon. Colon cancer can sometimes be identified at an earlier stage by testing stools for microscopic amounts of blood. But we don't know whether early detection of colon cancer increases length of survival, or whether the benefits of screening justify the costs of testing; an RCT is underway now to evaluate these issues (question 1). Beyond this objection lie concerns about the accuracy of the test (question 4 above), the effectiveness of treatment for "positives" (questions 2 and 7), and the resource implications of mass screening (question 6). These constitute the principal arguments against instituting such a program.

In fact, some experts suggest that a mass program to screen for bowel cancer might do more harm than good.[12] This is because the test is not a particularly effective way of finding cancer. Many people whose stools test positive for blood have hemorrhoids or some other benign condition. Merely enjoying a rare steak the night before the test can invalidate the results. In fact, we know that over 95% of the people who screen positive on the test for blood in the stool will *not* have cancer at all. Still, on the basis of a positive test, they will be subjected to needless investigations, some of which carry small but significant risks. Even if they suffer no physical damage from subsequent testing, these "false positives" and their families may have to endure weeks or months of anxiety before being told they have no cancer.

Despite these drawbacks, some cancer surgeons are advocating mass screening for everyone over the age of 40 or 50. Their position got a big boost when former President Ronald Reagan underwent successful surgery for colon cancer in 1985. Now in the United States, public service announcements and advertisements are promoting this test for everyone over 40.

The stakes in this debate are very high. To understand why, we need to look at a common investigation used to follow up a positive test for blood in the stool — the colonoscopy. This rather uncomfortable procedure involves passing a flexible tube through the six feet of the large intestine to look for abnormalities. Dr. John Frank, who teaches at the University of Toronto's Department of Preventive Medicine and Biostatistics, estimates that if North America opted for mass screening of blood in the stool, this would create an annual demand for an extra million colonoscopies, 95% of which would be totally unnecessary! Dr. Frank published his views on this subject in the *American Journal of Preventive Medicine*; an editorial in the well-regarded British journal, *The Lancet*, supported his position. But he came under fire from some surgeons and gastroenterologists.[13]

If all Canadians over the age of 40 were screened annually, we could end up doing an extra 100,000 colonoscopies every year.

As of March 1988, the Ontario Health Insurance Plan fee for a complete colonoscopy in a doctor's office was nearly $180. If we applied this figure to all provinces, the increased cost to Canadians for these colonoscopies alone would be $18 million — all for a test with no proven benefit.

In contrast, screening for hypertension (high blood pressure) has been more successful in identifying and treating at-risk patients. Most of this screening has been done in doctors' offices. Cross-sectional surveys show that more and more people with moderate and severe high blood pressure have already been identified by physicians, told about their condition, and been given treatment, with which most have complied. Most experts now agree that screening the general population would *not* turn up many more people who could benefit in a major way from medication. That is to say, they don't believe general screening will reveal many people with moderate to severe hypertension (question 5). What *is* likely is that mass screening would turn up lots of people with *mild* high blood pressure. But among this group the returns for the screening effort are vanishingly small, since there's less evidence that people with mild hypertension benefit from long-term drug treatment (questions 2 and 7).[14]

Medicine, by its very nature, can make only limited contributions to the prevention of sickness. The fact that medicine is practiced on a one-to-one basis restricts these contributions to only a few areas: immunization, screening, and patient counselling. None of the factors which cause most illness — personal behaviours, social relationships, the environment, and income — is really within medicine's scope. An American physician, Dr. Irving Zola, tells a story that has become almost as famous among prevention workers as the one about John Snow. It perfectly summarizes the dilemmas of practicing medicine:

> You know, sometimes it feels like this: There I am, standing by the shore of a swift-flowing river, and I hear the cry of a drowning man. So I jump into the river, put my arms around him, pull him to shore, and apply artificial respiration. Just when he begins to breathe, there's another cry for help. So I jump into the river, reach him, pull him to shore, apply artificial respiration, and then

just as he begins to breathe, another cry for help. So back in the river again, reaching, pulling, applying, breathing, and then another yell. Again and again, without end, goes the sequence. You know, I'm so busy jumping in, pulling them to shore, applying artificial respiration, that I have no time to see who the hell is upstream pushing them all in.[15]

This is how most doctors feel at the end of the day — completely exhausted by the side effects of our society and culture. It's time we started looking at what's pushing us in the water. Since most of the factors influencing our health status are beyond the scope of medical practice, it seems only wise to focus our efforts elsewhere — on other types of preventive measures, that hold greater promise for success.

Focussing Upstream

Dr. Milton Terris, a tireless American public health doctor and editor of the *Journal of Public Health Policy*, points out that the doctors' office is not the place to look for effective prevention.[16] "Secondary prevention, that is, trying to do something effective *after* a person falls ill, is very expensive when you consider its modest benefits." Early detection, he says, works for only a few things. He stresses that once disease occurs, if there's no effective treatment, it's too late. "Modern medicine cloaks its ignorance with terms like idiopathic [of unknown origin], degenerative, and psychosomatic — fancy ways of describing whole groups of illnesses it can't treat successfully." At the same time, he notes that six of the major causes of death are all preventable, at least to a certain extent. In fact, heart disease, other types of cardiovascular disease, many cancers (including lung), accidents, chronic lung diseases like emphysema, and chronic liver disease are much more amenable to prevention than to treatment. The key to preventing them, however, does not rest with the health care system at all.

Dr. William Haddon, an American epidemiologist and noted expert in the field of injury control, has helped to change how many people look at prevention. He showed how the strategies for preventing car accidents, for example, are conceptually very similar to those for preventing oil spills, or the spread of infectious diseases. What follows is Dr. Haddon's hierarchy of prevention strategies:[17]

1. Prevent the creation of the hazard in the first place. *Examples:* prevent production of plutonium, thalidomide, LSD.
2. Reduce the amount of hazard created. *Examples:* reduce speeds of vehicles, lead content of paint, mining of asbestos.
3. Prevent the release of a hazard that already exists. *Examples:* pasteurizing milk, bolting or timbering mine roofs, impounding nuclear wastes.
4. Modify the release of the hazard from its source. *Examples:* brakes, shutoff valves, reactor control rods.
5. Separate the hazard from that which is to be protected. *Examples:* isolation of persons with communicable diseases, walkways over or around hazards, evacuation.
6. Separate the hazard from that which is to be protected with a material barrier. *Examples:* surgeon's gloves, containment structures, childproof poison-container closures.
7. Modify relevant basic qualities of the hazard. *Examples:* altering pharmacological agents to reduce side effects, putting up breakaway roadside poles, making crib-slat spacings too narrow to strangle a child.
8. Make that which is to be protected more resistant to damage from the hazard. *Examples:* immunization, making structures more resistant to fire and earthquake, giving salt to workers under thermal stress.
9. Counter the damage already done by the hazard. *Examples:* rescuing the shipwrecked, reattaching severed limbs, extricating trapped miners.
10. Stabilize, repair, and rehabilitate the object of the damage. *Examples:* post-traumatic cosmetic surgery, physical rehabilitation, rebuilding after fires and earthquakes.

A listing like this is revealing in a number of ways. First, notice how most medical interventions don't really come into play until well down in the latter third of strategies. Notice as well that by using this orientation and focus, undesirable outcomes can be avoided *without exhaustive knowledge of their exact causes.* This is an important point, because medical research spends a disproportionate amount of time and money on painstaking investigations with precisely that goal — exhaustive knowledge — in mind. Dr. Haddon suggests, quite rightly, that prevention doesn't always require such specific and intimate knowledge. (John Snow didn't need to know about the cholera bacillus in order to stop the epidemic.) Medicine, when you view it this way, seems to limit the possibilities for prevention rather than expand them.*

Community Wisdom

John McKnight, a professor in the Center for Urban Affairs at Northwestern University, goes even further in outlining the limitations of our health care system.[18] He says it actually tends to hide important information about health from the very people who could use it most effectively. Like many others in the prevention field, he's a great believer in the wisdom of communities, and in the health payoffs possible when communities are strengthened. He tells about working with a small group of residents from a low-income housing project in Chicago. This group was tackling social and economic problems in their community — like unemployment, crime, and overcrowded and decaying housing — but they were also interested in health. Like many city neighbourhoods, theirs had undergone various transformations, and the composition of the population had changed. Many people had moved out to other neighbourhoods, and poorer people had moved in. The "health" problem, as they first saw it, was that their local hospital was continuing to serve former residents with whom strong ties had been made, but wasn't serving the newcomers to the community. So they formed a small deputation to lobby the hospital administrators, and in a short time the problem was resolved.

Five years later, the group was reviewing their progress when one of the members stood up and said, "I know we're getting served by the local hospital now, but it seems to me that people around here are just as sick as they ever were. How come?" They speculated that perhaps their hospital was substandard. So they hired McKnight, and his team of graduate students, to monitor

---

*We might take slight issue with Dr. Haddon's rank of 8 for all host-strengthening activities. For example, a healthy diet is necessary to life itself, as well to prevent infections, cardiovascular disease, osteoporosis, and many other illnesses.

the admissions to their local hospital, to try to get a handle on the quality of care it was providing, and also to see what kinds of illnesses were turning up at the emergency department. At that time, McKnight admits, "I was an expert in police brutality, and I didn't have a clue whether this would turn up anything useful."

Over the course of a month, McKnight's team carefully documented the services provided at the hospital; they concluded there was no reason to believe the hospital was worse than any other. But they also dutifully counted up all the various cases that came into the hospital's emergency department. At a subsequent meeting of the neighbourhood group, they presented the following list of health problems, in order of prevalence:

1. Traffic accidents
2. Other kinds of accidents
3. Interpersonal violence
4. Respiratory problems
5. Drug problems
6. Alcohol problems
7. Animal bites

When the group saw this list for the first time (McKnight delights in telling), they were amazed, because they realized that most of the reasons for an emergency department visit weren't *health* problems at all — they were *community* problems. And because they were community problems, the group felt they could do something about them.

The first item they decided to tackle was animal bites. They weren't sure about the rest, but they *knew* what was behind all those animal attacks. People in the neighbourhood were always buying big dogs for protection. When they found they couldn't handle the animals, they turned them loose to roam the streets. It meant that packs of stray dogs, hungry and untrained, were wandering around terrorizing young and old alike. "Can you imagine anybody at a hospital finding out the cause so quickly?" asks McKnight impishly. He goes on to describe what the community decided to do about it. "I thought they'd just give the city pound a call, but they came up with their own idea." They established a five-dollar bounty and offered it to any citizen who reported sighting a stray dog to the community centre. They had a budget and a vehicle and decided to round up these dogs on their own, and then turn them over to the pound. The result was astonishing. For the first time kids in the community, attracted by an opportunity to earn some cash, got drawn into the group in an active way. Riding around the neighbourhood on their bikes "like the original urban cowboys," in one week they managed to bring in 200 dogs. Subsequent reports on hospital admissions showed the incidence of dog bites had plummeted.

Thus encouraged, the group decided to tackle the most prevalent cause of hospital emergencies — traffic accidents. In this case, they used data from the city's traffic control agency to plot a map of the neighbourhood, using blue Xs to indicate where injuries had occurred, and red Xs for fatalities. Once again, the group's intimate knowledge of the inner workings of the neighbourhood helped them zero in on the underlying causes of some of these accidents. For example, they knew that at one intersection where there had been a number of accidents, a hydrant was responsible. Kids from the area used to open it on hot summer days to cool off in its spray. As water flooded the streets, cars turning the corner were unable to brake in time to avoid hitting them. "Can you imagine traffic controllers or city planners coming up with *that* explanation for traffic accidents?" asks McKnight.

At another location, an unsafe parking lot entrance for a local department store had caused a number of injuries and fatalities. So the group organized a deputation, which went straight to the store manager and told him, in no uncertain terms, that his parking lot entrance was killing their neighbours. Here, McKnight emphasizes the efficiency of local action. "They saw the 'accident' map on Monday, went to the manager on Tuesday. By Wednesday the unsafe entrance was closed, by Friday a new and safer entrance was in place. The manager responded quickly because these people were his customers — it was a good business decision. But can you imagine how long it would take to effect even a small change like a new parking lot entrance, if you had to go through City Hall?"

The point is not simply that this group was successful in finding innovative ways to prevent injuries. The real benefit they derived from their actions was a new sense of power and control. And they attained it by working together to identify problems and find solutions. Community development workers like McKnight argue that when you empower people who, for reasons of low income or education, rarely experience any sense of control over their lives, they reap health benefits that actually exceed those that result from their activities. "When you're doing this kind of work, the goal is not for health, the goal is for a stronger community. Better health just happens to be one of the beneficial side effects of a stronger community. But it needn't be tied to a health activity — it may come from a housing activity or some other area altogether. But if you're building a stronger community, you're building a healthier community." The corollary to this holds an important lesson, too. "It is impossible," says McKnight, "to produce health among the powerless." But it *isn't* impossible to transfer the tools, budgets, and authority to those who suffer the "malady of powerlessness," and thereby create a context for health.

This strategy — transferring tools to the powerless, and not just services — is consistent with the rapidly expanding research findings concerning the effect of social networks on health. As we've already discussed, having some control over your environment, and feeling connected to others, can actually improve your health. This effect may be indirect, or may be directly related to observable changes in brain chemistry. Either way, it isn't hard to understand. An elderly grandmother who gets lots of attention from family and friends, and manages to retain her independence, is likely to be happier even if she does live alone. Her positive attitude will be reflected in her health in a number of ways. For example, she may be more inclined to eat better and to have minor health problems attended to before they become more severe. Her autonomy is supported by her social contacts, rather than compromised. In short, her happiness is helping her stay healthy.

A Garden of Eden in Regent Park

Canada has its own examples of projects that illustrate this idea of "empowering the community." Five years ago a group of sole-support mothers living in Regent Park, a low-income housing project, approached Toronto's public health department; they were worried because they couldn't afford to buy many of the foods — particularly fresh fruits and vegetables — recommended for a healthy diet. "Mother's Allowance wasn't large enough to feed our children properly," said one of the mothers in the group.

Together, they made plans for a community garden. Also helping them were the local parks department, who tilled the land, and local greenhouses, who donated seedlings and fertilizers. Today the garden continues to thrive, and is generally unmolested in an area noted for vandalism. "The garden has proved to be much more than just a source of fresh food," says Ron Labonte of Toronto's health department. "It's become a focus for the whole community. We have a large and diverse ethnic population living here, and the residents organized potluck dinners where they prepared recipes from their native lands. A series of international banquets gave people an opportunity to try new foods prepared in new ways. It was a tremendous sharing experience." Organized trips to "pick-your-own" farms was another spinoff activity that resulted from this focus on food and nutrition. The local housing corporation arranged for a bus so that people could head off to the country for the day and see how food is grown commercially. Now the community is looking at the feasibility of growing enough produce to generate income. Similar experiments of this type have been tried in the Bronx in New York City, using rooftop greenhouses — market gardening on downtown farms.

The point here — just as it was in the Chicago example — is to give people who are disadvantaged the power to improve their own situation. The ultimate aim is to create economic incentives and opportunities as well. The link between low incomes and ill health is well established. It's not unreasonable to assume that strategies to improve incomes are likely to have major health payoffs.

One thing is clear. It's better to stay healthy than to depend on the limited abilities of modern medicine to treat illness. The old adage that an ounce of prevention is worth a pound of cure makes more than just good economic sense — it's common sense as well. Unfortunately, for every dollar we spend treating illness, less than a nickel goes toward health promotion and disease prevention. The enormous opportunity to promote health through non-medical approaches is scarcely recognized. The skewing of our system toward treatment and cure, and away from prevention, only succeeds in leading us further and further away from the real solutions to illness.

Chapter 9

Housecleaning
Health Care

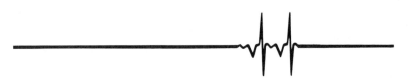

BY NOW IT SHOULD be very clear that we can't expect a significant improvement in Canada's overall health status without major social and economic reforms. Higher-quality sickness treatment, on its own, will not contribute very much to Canada's better health. But that doesn't mean quality health care's not worth pursuing — when we fall ill, we need competent, caring and compassionate treatment. We pay top dollar for our system; we have every right to expect high quality and efficiency from it.

The first half of this book may have left you with the impression that there's no way to prevent unnecessary tests, surgeries, and prescriptions. That waiting lists are inevitable. That the misuse of institutional beds is unavoidable. In short, you may doubt whether we can do anything at all to improve the quality and efficiency of Medicare.

Cheer up. Now we're going to look at some alternatives that should leave you feeling more optimistic about the prospects for reform. These examples* are relevant for two reasons: first, they illustrate how others have managed to overcome some of the problems that continue to trouble our system; and second, they demonstrate what *can* be done when services are planned, organized,

---

*We by no means suggest that these are the only models worth studying. They are simply a few illustrations of what we found works well in other settings.

and financed differently. They're not theoretical models. Their very existence, and the research backing their claims, proves that they're do-able in the real world.

Now for a caveat. No single alternative presented below offers solutions to all the problems we outlined in earlier chapters. None deserves to be adopted as the *ultimate* model. We don't see this as a major drawback, however. For too many years our system has been dominated by one approach to funding, organizing, and delivering health care. You've seen the result: long-range planning has been virtually non-existent, and the primacy of the patient has given way to the primacy of the provider. To turn this around, Canada needs to test a number of alternatives.

Lessons from America: Consumer Power

The United States doesn't have a universal system of national health insurance. Those who are elderly or poor enough do qualify for government assistance with their medical expenses.* But the majority of Americans must make their own arrangements for coverage, in the private sector.

One result is that the U.S. marketplace boasts a bewildering variety of alternative health plans. Individual consumers, and those corporations that pay for their employees' benefits, are beginning to demand hard evidence from competing health plans — evidence about the quality and cost-effectiveness of their operations. They want to be able to compare the performances of hospitals, health plans, and even individual providers; they want data that identifies suspiciously high rates of surgery and mortality, and overly long hospitalizations.

Sophisticated computer systems are making it much easier to separate the wheat from the chaff. Professor Harold Luft, an economist from the University of California at San Francisco, says that today, "you can get hospital data on diagnoses and procedures, by age, sex, charge, and whether or not patients died,

---

*The program insuring the elderly is called Medicare; the one that insures the poor, Medicaid. However, almost 40 million Americans have no health insurance at all. Typically, these uninsured are working but have no health benefits from their employers. While they're too "wealthy" (or too young) to qualify for government assistance, they're nevertheless too poor to afford the cost of coverage.

for the entire 3.5 million hospital discharges every year [in California], and the tapes cost only 800 dollars.''

For big businesses like General Motors, which spends more on health benefits than it does on steel, and Goodyear, which once calculated that the cost of health care for its employees was adding two dollars to the cost of a 57-dollar tire, this kind of information is a real bargain.[1]

And for the individual consumer, making an informed choice is getting easier all the time:

- Washington DC's *Consumer Checkbook*, a popular magazine rating all kinds of products, recently compared all the hospitals in its area. It then ranked them according to different criteria, which included mortality rates, Caesarean section rates, quality of staff (as rated by nurses and doctors in each hospital), and normal lengths of stay for particular procedures.

- In Portland, Oregon, a newspaper supplement in October 1987 summarized similar information about hospitals and health plans in its area. Typically, U.S. consumers voluntarily lock themselves into health plans for one-year periods. At year-end, such information is in high demand as a basis for deciding whether to stick or switch.

- In 1986, *The Los Angeles Times* reported on the performance of local hospitals in treating eight frequently fatal medical conditions. (Heart failure, shock, and heart attack were three). The article then listed the ten best and ten worst hospitals in the area.

In the United States there are professional review organizations (PROs). These are private, entrepreneurial companies that are contracted by government, private insurance companies, and sometimes individual hospitals to monitor and improve efficiency. They have unrestricted access to medical records and hospital information systems. They also sometimes publish their findings, and as such have become an important source of useful data.*

---

*Readers will remember that comparisons between groups of patients who have not been randomly allocated are potentially biased. Nevertheless, these data can be useful and techniques are being refined to make comparisons more valid.

Consumers have come to recognize that competition on the basis of quality is *healthy* competition.

Canadian consumers have no access to this kind of information. Neither do most health ministries. Neither do most hospitals. Isn't it time they did?

Lessons from America: The HMO

Health maintenance organizations are the fastest-growing health care alternative in the United States; they had enrolled over 31 million subscribers as of June 1988.[2]

HMOs have become popular because they offer consumers comprehensive health services at the lowest price. They're able to do this because they're very efficient; on average, the cost of care is 25% less than traditional insurance coverage.[3] Research has shown that HMOs realize their greatest savings by using hospital services — the most expensive form of care — more judiciously. On average, HMO subscribers use 40% fewer hospital days than those covered by third-party insurance.[4]

Unfortunately, HMOs are badly misunderstood in Canada. Asked about their potential application to the Canadian scene, one provincial assistant deputy minister bristled with annoyance, exclaiming, "We don't have anything to learn from the United States."

We beg to differ. Any system that delivers quality health-care services so efficiently merits careful study.

So what is an HMO? It's an organization that provides health care for a fixed, predetermined, periodic payment.[5] Enrolment is voluntary; the enrollee is covered only for those services provided by or approved by the plan. A typical HMO plan covers drugs, hospitalizations, and office visits to doctors. Some plans also offer mental health services, physiotherapy, and treatment for drug or alcohol dependency. The services available to HMO enrollees are as comprehensive as the ones Canadians get under Medicare.*

What distinguishes HMO coverage from traditional, third-party insurance is that *HMOs are at risk for the costs of services they*

---

*HMOs do not typically cover the costs of long-term care, however.

*provide.** If the physicians in an HMO determine that a patient needs to be hospitalized, the HMO pays. If they recommend surgery, the HMO pays. If they prescribe medication, the HMO pays. Because all of these medical decisions have a direct financial impact on the organization, health personnel in an HMO are more likely to behave conservatively. The "more is better" attitude is brought under control.

Professor Alain Enthoven, from Stanford University's School of Business, is quick to point out that efficient care is very compatible with high-quality care. "The most economical thing to do when a patient is sick," he says, "is to make the right diagnosis promptly, and put the patient into the hands of an appropriate practitioner, who will do an appropriate procedure proficiently and without error." Mistakes can be very costly. "If a patient gets complications," he goes on, "or needs to be operated on again because the first surgery was bungled, those added costs should come out of providers' pockets, not some third-party payer or the consumer." And that's exactly what happens in an HMO. The organization is responsible for the cost implications of its decisions.

This kind of financial accountability means that an HMO has an incentive to keep its members healthy. Typically, HMOs place more emphasis on preventive care, to reduce the need for more expensive services, particularly those requiring hospital stays. It also means that every HMO has a strong incentive to measure and improve its own clinical and financial performance. In other words, HMOs have a vested interest in being right.

Some critics of HMOs have claimed that their greater efficiency is achieved at the expense of their members. They accuse HMOs of underservicing. In particular, they suggest that HMOs keep people who ought to be in hospital, out, and discharge hospitalized patients too early.

But research on HMOs doesn't bear this out. If underservicing were common, you'd expect to find poorer health among HMO enrollees, as well as a lot of dissatisfied customers. In his review of all the research on HMOs, published in 1981, Profes-

---

*Some, however, require a co-payment or deductible from users for certain types of services, and so are only partially at risk for costs.

sor Harold Luft found "no evidence that HMOs do anything that produces less favorable health outcomes than the fee-for-service community."[6] Studies done since then have confirmed these findings. And Enthoven notes that "anyone who isn't happy with the care they receive in an HMO can always choose to join another plan. Consumer choice is a powerful restraint against underservicing."

HMOs have also been accused of "skimming the cream," that is, of maximizing their efficiency by limiting membership to the healthiest people. Healthy members are likely to use fewer medical and hospital services, and critics say that's how HMOs are able to keep their costs down. This criticism may be more justified. Enthoven told us about a for-profit HMO in Florida that tried to attract "healthy" senior citizens by holding a "get acquainted" promotional dance on the third floor of a building with no elevator service. "They figured that anyone who made it up the stairs and was still able to dance was a good risk!"

But not all HMOs operate the same way. Some skim, some don't. Some are strictly non-profit; others are for-profit, even to the extent of offering publicly traded shares. They differ in how they're organized as well. For example, in some HMOs the physicians work in groups either as salaried employees or as partners; in others, doctors in solo practice contract with the HMO for referrals and then are paid on a fee-for-service basis by the organization. Some HMOs own and operate their own hospitals, others merely purchase hospital services from existing facilities. With this kind of diversity, it's very important to be clear about *what kind* of HMO is being discussed.

Today, two out of three HMO members belong to a type known as the prepaid group practice (PPG). In this model, physicians work together in a group and are paid either by salary or by capitation (a set amount per enrollee per month).[7]

Skimming is much less likely in this type of model. In fact, non-profit PPGs actually seem to have a higher enrolment of families with chronic illnesses than commercial insurance companies do.[8] And there's a good reason for this: People with chronic illnesses might be expected to look for the most comprehensive health care package they can find. PPGs tend to offer the widest coverage for the lowest cost.

From now on, our discussion of HMOs will deal only with non-profit PPGs, and two of those in particular: the Group Health Cooperative of Puget Sound (GHCPS) and Kaiser Permanente, Inc.

Lessons from America: Group Health Cooperative of Puget Sound

The GHCPS serves about 320,000 people in 20 clinics, all of which are located in and around Seattle, Washington. It's run by a community board elected by its consumer-members, and as such is perhaps one of the outstanding examples of participatory democracy in the country. Once a year, some five to six thousand of the plan's members assemble to vote in the next board. The whole process resembles a political convention, as candidates give speeches, lobby for support among various interest groups, and shake a lot of hands.

The single largest study in the history of health-service research was the Rand Health Insurance Experiment. It compared the performance of GHCPS with that of traditional, fee-for-service practice. This study, which was commissioned by the U.S. government, took nearly ten years to complete and cost almost $100 million [U.S.].[9]

In the main part of the experiment, nearly 1,600 individuals were randomly assigned to either local fee-for-service doctors or GHCPs for their health care. This is what the investigators found:

- Costs for the HMO group were 25% lower than for the fee-for-service group. These savings were largely the result of the HMO patients using 40% fewer hospital days.

- Overall, there were no differences in health between these two groups of patients.

Readers may recall from Chapter 6 the study that compared Manitoba's use of hospital services with that of GHCPS.[10] Even when the analysts gave Manitoba the advantage, by eliminating that province's elderly patients and obstetrical cases from the sample, it still turned out that Manitobans used 60% more hospital days per capita.

Results like these indicate that it's perfectly possible to provide high-quality health care at much lower costs. But there must be an incentive to do so.

Growing competition from other local health plans is encouraging GHCPS to become even more efficient. Dr. Turner Bledsoe, a senior researcher and former medical director at GHCPS, says, "We've always been good at reducing hospitalizations, but others have learned how to do that as well." Now Dr. Bledsoe's team is looking at ways to make outpatient services more efficient. "We're particularly interested in finding better ways to manage chronic illness," he says. "And we're asking the medical chiefs in our clinics to assume more responsibility for managing their doctors." To support this effort, his research group is compiling data about the performance of doctors at GHCPS. With access to information about their staff's prescribing habits, and rates for performing various procedures, physician-managers can take steps to improve their performance.

The organization as a whole is also moving toward greater decentralization. Traditionally, GHCPS has funded its activities using a capitation rate based on the total use of services by all of its members. Now it's looking at treating its 20 clinics separately by funding each one on a capitation rate specific to its own costs. Managers at GHCPS hope that this approach will encourage better decision-making at the local level.

Lessons from America: Kaiser Permanente

Kaiser Permanente is one of America's oldest HMOs. Today it serves over 5 million people. "We have a real sense of mission here," says Dr. Paul Lairson, the liaison officer for Kaiser's 12 regional physician groups. "We feel that ours is a better way to provide health care — it's a better way for physicians to practise and a better shake for the consumer."

Kaiser's track record is impressive, particularly when it comes to using hospital services: its overall annual utilization rate is consistently less than 400 bed-days per 1,000 members. (Canada's is 1,200!) Kaiser members over the age of 65 use 1,600 bed-days per 1,000, which is well under the U.S. national average (2,400), and astonishingly lower than in Canada (about 5,000).[11] For over 40 years, Kaiser Permanente has kept costs down by emphasizing preventive health services, and by creating economic and professional incentives that encourage its doctors to avoid unnecessary interventions.

Consumers have responded positively; Kaiser's Northern California Region, for example, serves 2.2 million people, many of whom are second- and even third-generation members. It's easy to see why — at a monthly cost of about $65 [U.S.] per member, Kaiser offers the broadest package of services for the lowest cost.*

What's more, even though Kaiser uses one-third to one-half as many hospital beds as we do in Canada, and has a much lower doctor-to-population ratio (about 1 for every 800 members), *there are no waiting lists for elective surgery. When Kaiser's surgeons book non-emergency operations, they're typically done within one to two weeks!*

According to Kaiser's management, the key to the organization's success lies in group practice. Dr. Richmond Prescott, assistant medical director of Kaiser's largest region — Northern California — says that group practice is the greatest guarantee of good-quality care because "the doctors see each other, see what they do and what they fail to do. There's no hiding incompetence — it's life in a goldfish bowl."

Dr. Prescott, who's both a lawyer and a physician, began his medical career in fee-for-service practice, at Massachusetts General Hospital. "The attending staff there were brilliant," he says, "but when I had to cover for them when they went on vacation, I got a real eye-opener. Some kept terrible records, and that was bad enough, but some of the things they wrote down were just plain dumb — bad practice. The entire experience has made me extremely mistrustful of the fee-for-service world in terms of quality."

Dr. Prescott is quick to point out, however, that the kind of monitoring that goes on in a group practice is friendly and supportive. "Anybody can make a mistake, that's only human. But in a group practice you stand a better chance of finding out about your mistakes in a non-threatening way. There's a lot of pressure to do well." He adds that a doctor in solo fee-for-service

---

*Most of Kaiser's members join the plan through their place of employment, and members can continue coverage after retirement. However, it is also possible to join on an individual basis.

practice "is all alone in his office and he's the only one who sees his records. Only he knows what he's doing with his patients — except the patients, of course, and they don't understand."

Kaiser's doctors, like those at GHCPS, are paid on salary. This changes the incentives, says Dr. Lairson. "Here we do the bulk of our diagnostic work on an outpatient basis, rather than in hospital. And when we do hospitalize patients, it's because they're sick, not because there's a financial incentive to put them in hospital."

He elaborates: "If, as a practising internist, I have eight patients in hospital, I have to get up at five a.m., get to the hospital by six a.m. to see all my patients before I go to the clinic at nine a.m. And I may have to return to the hospital at noon and again at five p.m. Now as a salaried doctor, I get no more money for doing that."

At Kaiser, just as at GHCPS, doctors receive benefits in addition to their salaries. They include regular time off to participate in continuing medical education. Those physicians who go into management are still required to spend one day a week in clinical practice. "It's not just to keep up clinical skills," says Dr. Prescott. "It's really so that our doctor-managers can maintain credibility with their peers. I also think it's essential [for] a healthy perspective."

At Kaiser, new doctors are placed on three-year probation, during which time their performance is regularly evaluated. Those who are successful become "shareholders" in the organization, and eligible for bonuses.* Today, the financial significance of these bonuses is much less than their symbolic value. But Dr. Prescott notes that withholding a bonus is a sure way to get a doctor's attention.

For example, in one of Kaiser's hospitals — the chief of psychiatry was about to distribute bonuses. But a review of his department's quarterly productivity figures revealed that one of his doctors had only added two new patients in the entire three-month period. "That's just not acceptable in a program like ours," Dr. Prescott stresses. "Doctors must make room in their schedules to see new patients." In this case, the doctor was refused

---

*Regions that manage to come in under budget get to keep the surplus, which is distributed in the form of bonuses to the doctors of that region.

a bonus and told in no uncertain terms to improve his performance.

Kaiser's organization is highly decentralized. As well, its physicians are encouraged to feel a sense of ownership and control over its direction. Dr. Lairson notes that many doctors today feel they're losing out to administrators who neither understand nor seemingly care about clinical concerns. "Our physicians don't have to contend with that," he says. "Clinical decisions are theirs to make, albeit they *are* scrutinized by others in the group who are familiar with the particulars of the case." And when it comes to allocating resources, doctors are full participants in the decisions. At both the hospital level and the regional level, the decision-making authority is shared 50-50 by the administrator and the chief physician or medical director. "If one says yes and the other says no, there's no decision. They must resolve these conflicts themselves."

Kaiser's decentralized structure — every region and every hospital has a great deal of autonomy — is an effective spur to innovation. Dr. Lairson told us about a physician from the Colorado Region who conducted a controlled experiment at his hospital to see if hernia surgery could be done on an outpatient basis. "It seemed to work fine. Then he started encouraging other surgeons in his region to try it, and now it's a regional standard there." By offering its staff this freedom to initiate and test new ideas, the organization as a whole has benefited.

To serve its members better, Kaiser Northern California is moving toward even greater decentralization. Its marketing manager, Anita Gryska, explains that Kaiser wants to change its monolithic image, that "we want a more personal touch." So the region is planning to reorganize its outpatient clinics into small, tightly knit units composed of three or four doctors, a couple of nurses, and a receptionist. "That way," says Gryska, "when a patient's personal physician is away on vacation, she'll be able to see a doctor that's known to her."

Kaiser's information systems are helping to identify new ways to improve quality and efficiency. In particular, these systems help to monitor drug prescribing and laboratory tests. In Kaiser's Portland Region, for example, a detailed drug formulary, one that lists products according to their cost and effectiveness, is helping to improve the quality of prescribing and reduce medication costs.*

From our perspective, one of the few weak spots in Kaiser's operation is its overreliance on specialists, and relative neglect of non-physician personnel.** Primary care at Kaiser is delivered by internists or pediatricians rather than by family physicians or general practitioners. While this may inspire patient confidence, the evidence suggests that it's an inefficient way to use personnel. And within Kaiser, doctors wield much more authority than nurses. The savings that could be achieved if nurses were used to their full potential have largely been ignored.

Scott Flemming, a senior vice-president at Kaiser and a former lawyer, has been with the program since the early 1950s. A committed free-enterpriser, he believes that competition is critical to stimulating quality and efficiency. Anita Gryska says that in selling the program, Kaiser emphasizes its commitment to both. "We come right out and say that our doctors have no incentives other than to help people get better," she says. "This is medicine practised out of conviction, not economic coercion."

Lessons from America: On Lok Seniors' Services

Mrs. C. is 83 years old and lives in San Francisco's North Beach area. A widow for the past 20 years, she tries to make ends meet on a pension that brings in less than $600 a month. Like many others in her neighbourhood, she rents a room in a small, broken-down hotel. Mrs. C. has heart disease complicated by diabetes. She suffers from arthritis as well, and for the past year has used a wheelchair to get around. It's impossible for her to manage on her own. She needs help with her personal care, and must eat a balanced diet to keep her diabetes under control. Throughout North America, there are hundreds of thousands like her who

---

*Many large HMOs operate their own pharmacies, stocked with products from the manufacturer that the HMO purchases directly. This gives the HMO considerable leverage in negotiating bulk purchases at a good price.

**To a somewhat lesser degree, this same criticism applies to GHCPS. They do employ nurse practitioners, but not in large numbers.

live in nursing homes. But Mrs. C. doesn't. She gets whatever help she needs to stay at home through a remarkable program called On Lok.

Three or four days a week, a wheelchair-accessible van brings Mrs. C. from her home to On Lok's day health centre on Powell Avenue. On any given day, she might see a nurse, social worker, physiotherapist, chiropodist, audiologist, doctor, or some other type of health care worker. Or she might decide to play cards with her friends, enjoy a Chinese lunch, or participate in a crafts session. On the days she stays home, On Lok's skilled assistance comes to her: her meals are delivered, she gets help with bathing and housekeeping. In addition, staff from the centre keep in touch by phone to make sure she's all right.

Shortly after joining the program last year, Mrs. C. slipped and broke her hip. She spent two weeks in an acute care hospital, where On Lok staff monitored her progress. After that, instead of going to a nursing home to convalesce, she spent a month in one of On Lok's on-site respite care units. She was able to continue her rehabilitation in the day health centre and see all her friends.

None of these services costs Mrs. C. a cent.* On Lok is responsible for all the costs of her care, including hospital and nursing-home services should those be required. Today Mrs. C. is back home, but she continues to come to the centre regularly. She's back in the community, seeing her friends and maintaining her independence.

Independence is the goal of On Lok Senior Health Services. This non-profit organization for the "frail" elderly has been in operation since 1973, when its first day health centre opened in a renovated Broadway nightclub. Today, On Lok serves 300 high-risk seniors out of three such centres, one of which also features a housing unit with 54 apartments.

On Lok's participants are very elderly — their average age is 81. They're also very frail — on average, they have between five and six serious medical conditions each. Three-quarters are incon-

---

*Mrs. C., being both poor and elderly, qualifies for both Medicare and Medicaid assistance.

tinent; the same number have some degree of motor disability. Poverty and isolation add to their risk — 41% are poor enough to qualify for supplemental pension benefits, and two-thirds live alone.

To become a participant at On Lok, applicants must satisfy very strict criteria: they must be over 55, and be medically assessed as needing nursing-home care by an independent state representative. Instead of going to an institution, however, On Lok enrollees receive whatever services they might require to remain in their own familiar surroundings for as long as possible.

The result? On Lok's overall institutionalization rate is *only six percent*. At any given time, five percent are in nursing homes, and one percent in acute care hospitals. When you consider how infirm On Lok's members are, this low rate is positively astounding! (For the sake of comparison, nearly ten percent of all Canada's seniors, many of whom are much younger and healthier than those at On Lok, are housed in institutions.[12])

How does On Lok do it?

Rick Zawadski, research director for the program, explains On Lok's unique approach to managed care. "When someone has to be hospitalized with a broken leg because she fell off a chair trying to change a light bulb, or when someone gets admitted when his diabetes flares up because he hasn't been eating properly, our program is responsible for those costs. A single day in an acute care hospital costs us 700 dollars. So we have a strong incentive to prevent those kinds of mishaps from occurring. When you have a global budget and a good team, you can offer any number of specialized services. And we've found that when you do, the rate of institutional use drops."

To help participants remain in the community, On Lok will do whatever's necessary, provided the participant wishes it and stands to benefit. Zawadski explains, "We'll send a driver who may have to literally carry them out of their homes to transport them to the day health centre — seven days a week, if they want to. And we'll provide a 24-hour attendant to stay with them at home on days they don't come in." Sometimes, however, institutional care is necessary. Participants who are so confused they have no idea where they are, or those with extremely heavy care needs, are placed in nursing homes. But Zawadski stresses that "the issue for us isn't cost, it's quality of life. As long as our participants can enjoy the activities at our centre and are willing to make the effort to come, we're happy to oblige."*

On Lok's organization is truly distinctive. It uses a multidisciplinary team composed of 15 various health care professionals and para-professionals: nurses, doctors, and social workers; physical, occupational, and recreational therapists; and dieticians and drivers. Every week, the team meets to assess the changing needs of its participants, and to plan and monitor the delivery of care. Everyone on the team is an integral player with valuable information to contribute. Doctors don't dominate these meetings, Zawadski notes. When the problem is medical, their input is critical, but medical care is only one component of On Lok's integrated service package. "Our staff need input from *all* the members of the team to make appropriate decisions," he says, and offers an example: "One of our drivers who was delivering meals noticed a pile of unopened meal cartons in one participant's home. By alerting the team, we were able to keep this problem from becoming acute. A social worker and dietician made a home visit to find out why the man wasn't eating. They recommended a psychiatric work-up, suspecting depression. Ultimately the problem was traced to an adverse drug reaction. The doctor changed his medication and the problem was resolved."

Zawadski is very proud of the effectiveness of this approach. According to his research, On Lok has almost eliminated hospitalizations due to flare-ups of chronic illness. To him, this is strong evidence that careful monitoring and appropriate servicing can dramatically reduce the need for institutional care, even among the very infirm. But he admits with a smile that On Lok hasn't had much impact on reducing trauma. "If anything, injuries due to accidents like hip fractures are a bit higher than for others in this age group. But that's because our people are up and about, walking around, tripping over things. If they were in a nursing-home bed, they couldn't break a hip, could they?"

---

*On Lok offers a dazzling array of services, including technical and emotional support to family members who are involved as informal care-givers. Every year, the program will provide up to two weeks of respite care so family caregivers can take a well-deserved break.

On Lok's financing is also creative. Convinced their approach would work, they sought capitation funding from the state and Federal government, asking for 95% of what government would have spent through Medicaid and Medicare for traditional nursing-home services. Since all On Lok members qualify for nursing-home care, this was a very good deal for the government. In 1987, this formula provided On Lok with about $1,900 [U.S.] per month per participant. This is comparable to the monthly cost of care in an Ontario nursing home.

The financial risk On Lok accepts is much greater than the one faced by HMOs.* Its participants, once accepted, cannot be refused coverage. For example, if they become seriously incapacitated due to a stroke or Alzheimer's disease, On Lok must pay for their hospital and nursing-home care for the rest of their lives. Despite this heavy burden of risk, On Lok has always operated in the black.

Today, both political parties in the United States advocate the On Lok system of care in their national platforms. The U.S. Congress is so impressed with the group's track record that it has approved funding for up to ten more On Lok-style programs in other parts of the country. And it has put On Lok in charge of selecting the sites.

Only one thing bothers Zawadski about replication: quality assurance. "We're a non-profit organization," he says, "and we have a committed and caring staff here." But he worries about the vulnerability of the people being served. "Many elderly people are confused; they don't know where they are or what they're doing. In a for-profit system, there'd be plenty of room for abuse."

Zawadski ends his summary of the On Lok program on a philosophical note. "In some ways this is really like a long-term hospice program, only we care for people during the last 1,000 days of their lives, instead of the last couple of hundred. Our purpose is to create options for people and to recognize that at this point in their journey, for many the issue is quality of life, not quantity."

---

*HMOs typically do not offer coverage for long-term care.

Lessons from America: Wisconsin's Mental Health Program

In the 1970s in Wisconsin, community groups, legislators, and mental health professionals working for the state devised a totally new approach to caring for their most seriously disturbed citizens. Dr. Leonard Stein, professor of psychiatry at the University of Wisconsin, says that "the hallmark of this model is that the dollars follow the patient."

Here's how it works. The state gives a fixed yearly payment to each county based on a capitation formula. This becomes the county's mental health budget, out of which all the county's mental health services must be paid. They're at full risk.

The state leaves it up to each county to develop an appropriate network of community mental health services. If a county fails to do this, and any of its residents require hospitalization, the financial penalty is explicit: the county has to pay the cost of this expensive institutional care. This financial responsibility gives each county a strong incentive to make appropriate and efficient treatment decisions.

Under this unique funding arrangement, Dane County,* Wisconsin, has put in place a comprehensive network of community mental health services that are second to none in North America. These services, which include a day treatment program, vocational services, and supportive housing arrangements, have helped chronic mental patients return successfully to community life. As a result of these services, many of them are now functioning as productive citizens.

But the cornerstone of Dane County's program, and what really makes it unique, is its crisis intervention service (CIS). At any hour of any day or night, CIS staff are ready and able to go anywhere in the county to help people in crisis. What's more, Dane County has given CIS a lot of clout; mental patients can't be admitted to a hospital ward without their authorization. Routinely, CIS's mobile community treatment team arrives at the emergency department, does an assessment, and finds a way to avert hospitalization. The result? Over 75% of those about to

---

*Madison, the state capital, is in Dane County.

be admitted, never are. Instead, the team intervenes and puts the client in touch with more appropriate services.

To appreciate this phenomenal success, you need to understand that in the United States and Canada about 70% of mental health dollars go to hospital services. This leaves very little money for community care. *But Dane County spends only 17% of its mental health budget on inpatient care.* The remaining 83% goes directly toward community programs.[13]

We can only conclude that Dane County's reallocation of resources, encouraged by appropriate incentives, has resulted in a far better quality of life for those in its population who are mentally ill. And this model didn't require a lot of new money. As Dr. Stein says, "Nationally, there's sufficient money already in the system to provide good care, if only that money were more rationally distributed. Having the dollar literally follow the patient is crucial in making it all possible."

Back to Canada

If at this point you're wondering whether Canada does *anything* right, it's time to give a resounding yes! There are some outstanding alternatives right here.

Let's begin with some quickies:

- Foothills Hospital in Calgary has a value improvement program (VIP) to improve efficiency. By means of this program, it has decreased the average length of stay for patients with uncomplicated heart attacks from 10.8 days to 6.7 days. And for complicated cases, average stays are down from 14.2 days to 10.2.[14]

- Manitoba's home care program is world-famous. It uses a multidisciplinary team approach that makes it much easier for seniors to get appropriate care as their needs change. The program is also noteworthy for the way it supports and complements existing volunteer initiatives in each community.

- While Canada doesn't yet have any HMOs, the Toronto Hospital Corporation is doing a feasibility study about how they might adapt this model to the Canadian scene. And

governments in both Manitoba and Québec have expressed
a similar interest.

- Alternatives to fee-for-service medicine are quite rare in
  Canada, but there are some encouraging exceptions. The
  Women's Health Clinic in Winnipeg, for example, has
  responded sensitively to the demand for a less medicalized
  approach toward women's life-cycle changes.*

When it comes to large-scale innovation in Canada, however,
the first place to look is Québec. Why single out *la belle province*?
Because Québec has done more to develop a rational plan for
its health care system than any other province in Canada.

Lessons from Québec: Expert Advice

The effects of the so-called "quiet revolution" in Québec have
been dramatic.** During the 1960s, powerful egalitarian ideas —
like democratization, participation, and self-determination —
began to transform social policy. These concepts inspired
Québec's health care system to take off in startlingly new
directions.

The Castonguay-Nepveu Commission, conducted in the late
1960s, spurred major changes.[15] The province asked the commission to undertake a broad review of the health care and social
service system and make recommendations. The commission
returned with a call for two major reforms: first, it urged the
province to decentralize planning; second, it called on Québec
to develop a network of primary care facilities that would offer
both medical care and social services.

Now here's something truly remarkable: Québec actually followed this advice! It's worth emphasizing just how rare this is.
There's barely a province in the country that didn't conduct a
major review of its health care system at some point during the

---

*Other Canadian alternatives to fee-for-service care are discussed later in this
chapter.

**As just one example, Québec went from having the highest birthrate in the
country to the lowest in a single decade. Now the government is trying to reduce
that trend by offering parents a lump payment of $3,000 for having a third child.

1970s or 1980s. But little has changed as a result. The reports, praised or condemned, have tended to end up on the shelf, gathering dust.

That's not what happened in Québec, however. Its government decentralized the planning process by setting up eleven regional authorities, known as CRSSS; (Conseils régionaux de services sanitaires et sociaux). And it embarked on an ambitious strategy to develop a network of community health and social service centres, known as CLSCs (centres locaux de services communautaires), throughout the province. Today there are more than 160 CLSCs. Each is run by a community board, and each has salaried (not fee-for-service) staff.

In February 1988, the province released its second major review of health services, conducted by the Rochon Commission. After a three-year inquiry, which cost the province $6 million, this commission largely endorsed the present system, pronouncing decentralization and CLSCs a qualified success.[16] Nevertheless, the commission did offer some specific advice. It said the system needed to be more explicit about its goals and priorities. As well, it noted that patients tended to get lost in the bureaucracy, and urged the system to refocus on the needs of individual consumers. It also identified the need for an independent assessment centre that would evaluate the cost-effectiveness of new and emerging technologies. None of these recommendations was particularly controversial, and the minister of health and social services, Madame Thérèse Lavoie-Roux, publicly agreed with them.

She was less impressed, however, by some of the other recommendations in the Rochon Commission's report. She didn't agree, for example, that there was a need to redefine medical services with new legislation. The commission felt this was necessary in order to make the most efficient use of non-physician personnel.

And the minister rejected a set of recommendations addressing the issue of decentralization. The commission noted that decentralized planning had only been partly implemented, that the province still retained most of the executive power. The commission recommended that the regions become fully responsible for deciding how to allocate spending for all health and social services in their areas. To balance this increase in regional power, the commission suggested two ways to ensure public accountability: first, elected representation on regional boards and second, limited powers of taxation at the regional level. The latter would give those regions who went over budget the means to make up any shortfall. The former would allow local taxpayers to express at the polls any displeasure at how the system was being managed.

Although the minister agreed in principle that more regional autonomy was desirable, she concluded that these recommendations amounted to establishing a new level of government — something she wasn't willing to endorse.

Apart from these questions about decentralization, Québec's minister of health and social services has largely endorsed the Rochon Commission's assessment, and has announced her intention to implement many of its recommendations. This willingness to act in accordance with expert advice is nothing short of remarkable. It only seems to happen in Québec.

The government displayed similar wisdom in its reaction to the Brunet Committee's report on CLSCs.[17] As the Castonguay-Nepveu Commission originally conceived them, CLSCs were meant to become the main source of primary care in the province. But a number of problems hampered their development. According to the Brunet report, one of these was the fact that since 1981, their funding had been drastically reduced. Newer CLSCs were struggling to get by with only half the per capita amounts that had been available to those developed between 1972 and 1977. While the older ones delivered health care and social services, and were involved in various prevention activities like occupational health and safety, some of the newer ones couldn't even afford to hire medical staff.

And this aggravated a second problem identified by the Brunet Committee: many people in Québec had only a hazy idea of what CLSCs were supposed to do, and who they were supposed to serve. Were they just for poor people? For radicals? What was the difference between a polyclinic* and a CLSC? In 1986, 20% of Québec's population had received at least one type of

---

*Many physicians in Québec were opposed to the idea of salaried practice. They responded to the development of CLSCs by establishing polyclinics, in which fee-for-service doctors shared facilities. Most of these were not true group practices, however, since the physicians working there were independent and not subject to any peer scrutiny.

service from a CLSC, but only five percent had received a health care service. This was a far cry from the original vision.

In only one area was the public's perception of CLSCs firmly established. Everyone knew that they were the place to go to arrange for home care. As the Brunet report stated, "This is perhaps where CLSCs as a whole have been able to demonstrate their particular expertise in integrating social, health and community approaches."[18] The Brunet report noted that on average, CLSCs devote one-quarter of all their working hours to home care. Multidisciplinary teams coordinate nursing care, physician house calls, and homemaking and housekeeping services. Home care is available to anyone who needs it, but seniors use it most frequently. In 1985, more than 12% of those over 65 living in areas served by a CLSC, took advantage of the home-care services offered.[19] Would some of these seniors have otherwise ended up in nursing homes?

Saul Panofsky, director general of the CLSC at St-Louis-du-Park in Montreal, says that waiting lists for nursing-home beds in his area have shrunk tremendously. Other studies have confirmed that the demand for nursing-home beds is lower in those areas served by CLSCs.[20] This appears to be having an impact on long-term care facilities. Staff report that as more and more of the clientele they used to serve are having their needs met at home, those entering institutions are sicker and need more care. Panofsky says that, far from being undesirable, "this is exactly the sort of effect you'd hope for. There's no point having hospitals full of people who could be at home. If we're reversing that trend, I'm glad."

Jean-Pierre Bélanger is one of Québec's most respected sociologists. He's also assistant executive director of the Federation of CLSCs and president of the Quebec Public Health Association. "Our goal is to have 15 percent of the population using CLSCs on a regular basis," he says, "and to have 15 percent of our general practitioners working at CLSCs." To accomplish that, however, CLSCs will have to become firmly established in the public's mind as a source of high-quality primary health care.

That's why the Brunet Committee's report, which the province endorsed, recommended that all CLSCs be required to offer the same core programs in primary health care and social services.

In addition, it singled out three target groups as needing special services: children and families at risk; troubled youth; and a third group to be determined by individual CLSCs according to local priorities.*

Terry Kaufman, executive director of a newly chartered CLSC in Montreal's Notre-Dame-de-Grâce, is very encouraged by this response. "Establishing core programs for every CLSC will give a tremendous boost to us. People will know what to expect. As long as we get the money to offer these services, our future is secure."

Lessons from Québec: The Rural CLSC

Many people we interviewed pointed out that the public's understanding of CLSCs is greater in rural areas. So we decided to visit one. CLSC Arthur-Caux operates in a farming community about 30 kilometres from Québec City. Paul Coulombe, its director general, agrees that the rural location adds a special dimension. "We know one another; it makes it easier to cooperate and collaborate." He describes how they've managed to integrate with the community and encourage local initiatives:

"For 14 years we've been providing home care, but we also work closely with a committee representing local community groups. This has helped us to involve many people who like to volunteer. With their efforts, we can offer a much broader set of services to our seniors." For example, the centre hired a physical-education instructor. But his job wasn't to give exercise classes to the community, says Coulombe. Instead, he began to train seniors so they could become instructors themselves. Today, about 50 of these seniors, trained and monitored by this CLSC staff member, run their own exercise programs in a variety of locations. It's been tremendously popular; those who participate get out of the house, forget their troubles, and improve their fitness all at the same time. "Of the 3,000 elderly living in our catchment area," Coulombe says, "600 to 700 take these classes at least once a week."

CLSC Arthur-Caux also delivers primary health care with its

---

*The ministry also expects to add a further target group in the near future: adults with mental-health problems.

salaried staff of doctors and nurses. What's it like to be a doctor there? "I prefer it," says Dr. Sylvie Leclerc, the director of medical services. "I like to see patients from a more global perspective, and I enjoy having the chance to do more health promotion." She says that fee-for-service "doesn't pay you to take the time to teach a mother how to take her baby's temperature, or to explain to someone who's unemployed that headaches can be caused by stress." Being on salary encourages her to spend more time with her patients. And as a mother, she appreciates having paid vacation and maternity leave.

Dr. Leclerc also prefers working in a group. "I think it's draining to work alone, without the chance to consult with colleagues."

CLSC Arthur-Caux belongs to a farming community. The centre spearheaded an innovative approach to farm safety that was so successful it's been adopted as a provincial model. "We found that the best way was to involve the community directly," says Coulombe. They began by convincing the best farmers in the area to help out. Together, they worked on putting together a package of appropriate audio-visual aids and written materials. Those who had participated in developing the program then went on to conduct it themselves, often holding meetings for their neighbours in their own barns. After participating, one farmer told Coulombe, "Whenever I'm on the road now and see a tractor, I automatically look to see if the yellow identification plaque is there. I check if any children are playing around. If the cabin is properly secured. If it looks in good condition generally."

Coulombe attributes part of this success to the high quality of the instructional materials. But he gives most of the credit to those farmers who conducted the program. "It worked because these guys had a tremendous level of credibility among their peers. When they started talking health promotion, everyone paid attention.

"These people have become *preoccupied* with health and safety. This is much better than when a health professional intervenes, because these guys are the specialists now."

Lessons from Québec: Acute Care at Home

Paul G., a third-year engineering student, has a deep-seated infection in his arm that requires two weeks of treatment with intravenous antibiotics. Ordinarily, he'd have to enter a hospital to receive this kind of treatment. He'd miss a lot of school. Luckily for him, there's an alternative. Thanks to Verdun's Hospital in the Home program, instead of going to the hospital, the hospital comes to him.*

This innovative program started in the fall of 1986, and has helped some 400 patients to avoid or shorten their hospital stays. With a $2 million annual budget to cover salaries and overhead, the program can serve 45 patients at a time.** Teams of nurses and doctors working out of three hospitals are available day and night to respond to scheduled and emergency calls.

Louise Roy, the program's head nurse, describes how they were able to accommodate Paul's class schedule. "He had classes every other day, which meant that if he'd been hospitalized, he wouldn't have been able to continue his studies. But we were able to work around his timetable and still give the necessary treatment. Even when he was on the IV, he was still able to study at his desk and have access to all the books and materials he needed for his work."

About 60% of the patients served by this program require intravenous treatment. "We could be serving people with many other types of problems," says Dr. Carole Santerre, one of the program's physicians, "but it's taking a while to gain the confidence of our hospital's specialists." She says that respirologists, nephrologists (kidney specialists), and internists are more likely than surgeons to refer patients. Louise Roy adds that at one of their hospitals, the team couldn't convince pediatricians that babies and mothers could safely be discharged 24 hours after an uncomplicated delivery. "We've still got to do some public-relations work to establish a good image," says Dr. Santerre.

An evaluation of the program is being conducted now. According to David Levine, Verdun Hospital's executive director, early results indicate that it's saving the hospital money. "We're show-

---

*New Brunswick also offers a program called the "Extramural" Hospital, which provides acute care services to patients in their homes.

**These 45 patients are served from three locations: 15 from the Verdun Hospital, 15 from the Lasalle Hospital, and a further 15 from the Ville-Maisoneuve Hospital.

ing that it's possible for some people with pelvic fractures to go home after 24 hours, or at the most after 72 hours, by taking advantage of our service," says Roy. For some types of patients, access to this program means they can go home right from the emergency department without ever being admitted. "People are happy to go home," she adds, "once they realize that we can send a nurse out as often as five times a day if necessary. And our patients see a doctor every day to start out with and, as they improve, once or twice a week or whenever the nurse thinks it's necessary. We coordinate our services with those provided by the CLSC and wind up with a package that suits everyone."

Speaking personally, Roy is delighted with her job. "It's much more fun than regular hospital work. I've been in nursing for 15 years, working in acute care hospitals as well as in a long-term care facility. I was on the point of giving it up altogether when this program got started." Asked to describe the difference, Roy answers without hesitation: "The nurses here are more autonomous — there's a more collegial relationship with the doctors rather than the traditional hierarchy you find on the wards. And there's a big shift in the power relationship between patient and provider when you start delivering services in the patient's home. When you're in someone's house, that's *their* turf, you have to show more respect. That translates into a better quality of service."

Lessons from Québec: Palliative Care

In 1987, the Palliative Care Unit at Montreal's Royal Victoria Hospital moved to a new wing. Specially designed to be non-institutional, it features a family-sized kitchen, a glass-walled sun-room complete with piano, and 14 rooms for patients, most of which are private. Each bedside table holds a radio-tape deck. But the homelike decor isn't the only thing that distinguishes this unit from a typical hospital ward. Depending on when you arrive, you might enjoy a live concert, a glass of wine at the weekly happy hour, or a friendly chat with one of the program's volunteers.

The people working here are preoccupied with offering a high *quality* of life to those for whom *quantity* is in short supply. "Our patients come to this program for help with their suffering," says Dr. Balfour Mount, who helped to found the unit. "We take this very seriously as a goal.'' Sometimes it's as simple as changing the medication, or teaching the patient other techniques to improve pain control, while ''other times it means working with the whole family as they try to deal with the emotional pain that death often brings.'' Head nurse Irene Corbett says that's why ''for us, the family is the unit of care.''

The ward has room for 16 patients, but the vast majority of the people it serves are at home. Indeed, some never enter the hospital at all. ''Many people want to die at home,'' says Corbett. ''Our service means that this is a viable option.'' In February 1988, the program, with its team of nurses and doctors, was looking after about 100 home-care patients. The palliative care staff work very closely with the home-care staff at the CLSC to arrange services to suit the circumstances of individuals. ''I can't tell you how much this support means to our patients,'' Corbett adds. ''Much of the time their desire to remain at home conflicts with their fears about not having access to care when they need it. We can help them feel much more secure.'' Patients and their families can call in for help anytime. There's always a nurse on hand to pick up the phone, and a doctor available for backup.

One of the most fascinating aspects of this program is the way in which music therapy is used to help the dying. Music therapist Deborah Salmon is enthusiastic about its potential. ''Music is very flexible,'' she told us. ''It can be used in so many different ways. It can help patients gain some control over pain and anxiety. It can promote relaxation. Even when patients are barely conscious, music therapy can help. When someone's having trouble breathing, I try to match their respiratory rate with guitar chords, and then gradually slow the rhythm down. Sometimes this helps to ease their breathing rate.''

Music is very potent therapy, Salmon says. ''It can get through to the heart with astonishing impact.'' The ward boasts an extensive collection of taped music, and patients are encouraged to select and listen to their favourites. Sometimes Salmon also makes special tapes that have personal meaning. One woman recalled that her happiest memories were of early-morning fishing expeditions with her husband. With Salmon's encouragement, she remembered in great detail the rocking of the boat, the birds breaking into song, and the sensation of cool air on her skin.

"In this case, just listening to a tape of birds singing was enough to evoke in this woman a strong feeling of well-being."

The Royal Victoria Hospital's Palliative Care Unit is by no means the only one available in Canada.* But there are still too few to meet the demand. While most people today die in a hospital, it's usually on a regular ward, where staff have little time to offer the kind of emotional support terminal patients and their families desperately need.

We're all going to die someday. If palliative care were widely available, we could exercise more choice about how and where we do it.

Lessons from Ontario: The Sault Ste. Marie Group Health Centre

In the 1950s and early 1960s, steelworkers and their families in Sault Ste. Marie, Ontario, were having a tough time finding economical primary care. These were the days before full Medicare. Ontario residents were covered for hospital services, but not for any visits they made to the doctors' office, and private insurance was expensive. And in this northern Ontario community, doctors — particularly specialists — were in short supply.

Then in 1963, despite fierce opposition from local fee-for-service doctors, the Sault Ste. Marie Group Health Centre (SSMGHC) opened for business. This labour-sponsored facility, featuring a multispecialty group practice, gave people in the Soo a less costly alternative to third-party insurance. Funded on capitation and paying its staff on salary, SSMGHC is similar to an HMO except that it only delivers and pays the costs of outpatient care.

Today the centre, known as a health service organization (HSO), serves 40,000 people, about half the Soo's population. Its track record for quality and efficiency is well established. Patients there consistently use fewer hospital days than those cared for by fee-for-service doctors. Between January and June 1987, for example, the centre's hospital utilization rate was 1,106 bed-

---

*The first unit in the country was developed in 1974 at St. Boniface Hospital in Winnipeg.

days per 1,000. The rate for Algoma District as a whole during the same period was 1,494 bed-days.[21]

Ontario's government offers a bonus to HSOs if they use hospitals at a rate less than the regional average. So far, SSMGHC has always qualified.

Before 1971, residents of the Soo had an economic incentive to join the centre: it cost less than private insurance. But after that year, with the introduction of full Medicare, this incentive disappeared. Fred Griffith, executive director at the centre, says that all the same, its patients have remained very loyal. "We do our best to make sure that people can get in to see a doctor promptly, and that our service is friendly. These are important factors in keeping patients happy."

Griffith believes strongly in involving doctors in the decisions that affect their work. "If we don't have provider satisfaction," he told us, "there's no hope of making the patients happy." That's why planning and budgeting at the centre are joint activities: the medical director and the executive director work on proposals together, then bring them to the board's Joint Management Committee. This bilateral arrangement closely resembles that of Kaiser Permanente.

When it comes to clinical decisions, Griffith is convinced that group practice is the way to go. "Doctors frequently disagree about how a particular patient should be treated," he says. But working in a group tends to even out variations in individual styles. An American-trained physician, he told us, tends to be "gung-ho to order every test, doesn't trust his intuition much, and isn't inclined to listen." The British-trained doctor, on the other hand, tends to "look at high-tech equipment as a hoax, and prefers intuition. He bases his judgments on careful physical examination and listening to the patient's history, and uses the lab merely to confirm what he already knows." But it doesn't take long for the group as a whole to moderate these extremes in behaviour.

The centre also encourages its doctors to keep up with medical advances. Every year, its physicians receive one week's paid leave to participate in continuing education. They're expected to take it, too. The centre even subsidizes their subscriptions to the best journals.

If Canada's health care system as a whole may be characterized by inefficiency, this HSO's 25-year track record of fiscal
responsibility can be seen as an exception. John Barker, the grade-
school drop-out who started the centre, was fond of saying,
"Don't let your bleeding heart run off with your bloody head."
This may be close to "mill" language, admits Griffith, but it
should be "engraved in stone over many of our social institutions. Eventually things have to be paid for."

Lessons from Ontario: Nurse Practitioners

Dozens of studies have shown that nurses do as well as or even
better than physicians when given the opportunity to work to their
full potential. During the 1960s and 1970s, government tried to
expand the role for nurses by launching training programs for
a new profession: nurse practitioner. It was expected that this
additional training would make it easy for nurses to become the
first line of contact for patients seeking primary care. But it didn't
happen that way; the oversupply of doctors got in the way and
today there's little support for nurse practitioners.*

South Riverdale Community Health Centre is an exception to
this rule. This centre, which opened in 1976, today serves nearly
6,000 people in a working-class community in east Toronto. Since
the early 1980s, patients at the centre have been receiving health
care from doctors and nurses. Both the centre's board and its
staff believe that each profession has a valuable contribution to
make. They think that patients get better-quality health care when
they have access to both.

Staff at the centre are organized into three teams, each with
a family doctor and a nurse. Figuring out who does what depends
on who is the most *appropriate* provider for each particular
patient visit.

Nurses, because they receive more training in patient counselling and health education than doctors, are responsible for most

---

*Of course, nurses do function like doctors where and when doctors don't want
to work. Nurses in northern Canada, for example, take on many responsibilities usually assumed only by doctors. (See: Marilyn Dunlop, "Nurses: a Matter of Life and Death in the North," *Toronto Star*, February 29, 1988)

of the "well person" care. They do the prenatal care, well-baby visits, PAP smears, and physical examinations on healthy patients. Nurses at the centre are also more likely to do the follow-up care for patients with stable chronic illnesses. They monitor the blood pressure of hypertensives and check the blood sugar and diet of diabetics. And when these patients are unable to come in to the centre easily, it's the nurse who makes the house call. Doctors, on the other hand, perform those duties most appropriate to their training. Diagnosing and treating illness is their responsibility, because that's their area of expertise.

Although most patients and nurses are enthusiastic about this division of labour, physicians typically need more convincing. Their initial apprehension is perfectly understandable: it takes time to develop a trusting relationship. But once the doctor has had a chance to appreciate what nurses can really do, many of these tensions resolve themselves.

Dr. Nancy Harris, a general practitioner in private practice, happens to be a patient at South Riverdale. She gets most of her care from Marianne Cheetham, a nurse at the centre, and is delighted with the arrangement. "I only wish everyone in Canada could have a nurse and a doctor for their primary care," she says. "It's so much better for the patient."

Lessons from Saskatchewan: The Saskatoon Community Clinic

Canada's first steps toward Medicare began in Saskatchewan. When that province implemented the Saskatchewan Medical Care Insurance Act on July 1, 1962, more than 90% of its doctors went on strike. Saskatchewan residents fought back by organizing community clinics and flying in British doctors to staff them. That's how the Saskatoon Community Clinic got its start.

Today, the clinic is the largest of its kind in the province. (There are six others.) It serves over 15,000 regular patients with 14 doctors and a complement of other personnel: nurses, therapists, counsellors, pharmacists, nutritionists, optometrists, lab technicians, and support staff. The clinic also has its own pharmacy, X-ray department, and optical dispensing service.

Here, too, patients are encouraged to get involved in the process of developing new policies and programs by running for the clinic's community board. And there's a member-relations officer on staff, a kind of ombudsman who deals directly with any patient complaints and gives feedback to the providers.

Smokey Robson, a Nova Scotia native, came to Saskatchewan in 1940 to train pilots for the Royal Canadian Air Force. He's been the clinic's Mr. Everything since its earliest days; he served a long stint as its administrator, bracketed by two periods as chairman of the board, a position he continues to hold today. Like his counterparts in other group-practice health care organizations, he's convinced that "this model is the wave of the future."

Dr. Robert Ackroyd, the clinic's Oxford-trained medical director, agrees. "I have more time for patients than if I were in private practice and my patients have the convenience of easy access to physical therapists, social workers, and other health care personnel."

Judith Martin, the clinic's administrator, says that having so much on-site expertise means better-quality care for patients. "If a depressed woman sees one of our doctors, it's so much easier to refer her directly to an appropriate counsellor, right down the hall."

The clinic is efficient, too. A careful evaluation done in the early 1980s showed that overall costs were 17% lower for patients attending the Saskatoon Clinic than for those treated in the fee-for-service system. The clinic's patients had 24% fewer hospital admissions, and those who were hospitalized stayed, on average, nine percent fewer days. Drug costs at the clinic were 21% lower. This study, the most scientifically rigorous investigation ever conducted on community health centres, was initiated by the NDP while they were still in power. We obtained its results unofficially because Grant Devine's Conservative government has refused to make them public. What are they afraid of?

Lessons from B.C.: James Bay Community Health Centre

It's an unseasonably warm October evening in the James Bay neighbourhood of Victoria, British Columbia. Ten people around Dr. Rick Hudson's kitchen table are in the midst of an animated debate about Canada's health care system. Suddenly the phone rings and Dr. Hudson, a family physician at James Bay Community Health Centre, jumps up to answer it. A minute later, he apologizes to his guests, grabs his medical bag, and flies out the door. When he returns, before launching into another diatribe about the way our health care system treats seniors and doctors, he pauses to explain that his patient is going to be fine. In the drawling accent of his native Australia, he admits he probably didn't need to go out, but "with 94-year-olds, you don't take chances!"

Victoria is Canada's favourite retirement community. Almost 20% of its citizens are over 65. Dr. Hudson estimates that about 40% of his patients are seniors, and that a significant proportion are over 80. Finding a doctor who's willing to do house calls is "very important to their sense of security about remaining in the community," he says. At James Bay Community Health Centre, the house call is an understood part of the service.

But Hudson's years of experience with elderly patients convinced him that many needed a lot more than just medical care. They needed help to overcome the isolation, loneliness, and depression that so frequently accompany aging. He knew only too well that a visit from the doctor could do little to alleviate such problems. So, together with mental health professionals, social workers, and residents of the community, he helped to launch a new kind of program: a peer counselling service run for and by seniors themselves. Those who volunteer for this work attend a short course in basic counselling techniques, and then are encouraged to build their own caseloads. Today, many who might have gone to the doctor with their day-to-day troubles, are choosing instead to share them with a sympathetic and supportive peer counsellor. Inevitably as the program developed, Hudson reports, a friendly rivalry sprang up between the counsellors and the doctors at the centre. But he doesn't mind. "They're doing a great job keeping their clients out of my clutches."

House calls and peer counselling for seniors are only two of the "extras" available at James Bay Community Health Centre. Staff there also run a counselling program for young teens, a legal clinic, and a community information service. The centre, one of five health and social-service centres started by Dave Barrett's NDP government, opened in 1974. When the Social Credit Party regained power in 1975, the new government tried to close it down. No fear. The centre's administrator, Rob Dill, and its community board knew how to use political clout. They were popular in the neighbourhood and respected by the media. The government backed down.

Quality of Care — Opening the Black Box

The reality of our Canadian health care system is that alternatives to fee-for-service medicine are not well developed. Despite evidence that HSOs and community health centres provide high-quality care at a lower cost, provincial governments have neglected them in favour of the status quo. Most doctors work in solo practice and are reimbursed by fee-for-service. Isn't there anything that can be done to improve the quality of medical care under these circumstances?

The answer is yes. As an example, we want to talk about the work of Dr. David Sackett, chief of medicine at Chedoke-McMaster Hospital in Hamilton, Ontario. Dr. Sackett, a teacher, author, and physician, is irrepressibly enthusiastic about how much better we've become at evaluation. "In 1965," he says, "there were arguably only two people in Canada capable of conducting proper randomized controlled trials. Now there are lots of us."

He admits there's still a "huge amount of stuff that I do every day as a clinician that hasn't been properly evaluated," but adds it's getting better. More research is being done all the time and, increasingly, the results of that research are being put into practice. As an example, Dr. Sackett points out that the worldwide number of EC-IC bypasses performed has dropped by 80% since the negative results of the trial on that procedure were published.* "I'm much more optimistic now than I was ten or fifteen years ago."

Dr. Sackett's budding career as a research physiologist in Chicago was interrupted when he was drafted into the army right after the Cuban Missile Crisis. He was sent off to Buffalo, to

---

*Readers will recall from Chapter 3 that the extracranial-intracranial bypass (EC-IC) is a type of brain surgery that was used for years as a preventive against strokes. Results of an RCT published in 1985 proved it was totally worthless.

work with a group of public-health epidemiologists who were doing population-health surveys. His job was to conduct studies on hypertension and coronary artery disease.

Back then, Dr. Sackett recalls, "I hated epidemiology and biostatistics." But he adds that it didn't take long before "I began to recognize that the research I'd been doing in renal tubular physiology was trivial compared to the things I could do in an area like hypertension, with these new tools of epidemiology and biostatistics." Besides, he goes on, it was really quite a bit of fun. "That's where I first got the idea of applying epidemiological and biostatistical strategies to clinical problems, instead of just to public health and population problems."

At the age of 32, Dr. Sackett came to Canada to found the department of clinical epidemiology and biostatistics at McMaster University's newly created medical school. In 1981/82, while on sabbatical, he returned to the topic that had first captured his imagination in Buffalo — the possibility of making clinical medicine more scientific. The result was a critically acclaimed and highly readable textbook called *Clinical Epidemiology*, which he wrote with two colleagues at McMaster. Its premise is that you can become a better doctor by learning and applying some of the principles of epidemiology and biostatistics to clinical problems.[22]

"And when I finished," he told us, "I decided it was time to put my money where my mouth was." So at the age of 50, David Sackett went back to medical school, as a resident (a post-graduate student) in internal medicine — "to retread my skills in acute care," as he puts it. But becoming a student again did much more than that. By arranging to see the most patients and take the most call, he gave himself a wonderful opportunity to test ways of applying academic medical knowledge to clinical practice.

When it comes to teaching, Dr. Sackett employs two strategies. "The first is to show [students] how to evaluate clinical evidence which comes from a patient's history, physical examination, laboratory investigations, or medical journals, according to some simple applications of biostatistics and epidemiology. The second, is that I try to avoid an old problem. Medical students want to be doctors, not epidemiologists or biostatisticians. So I keep that in mind and focus on how these tools can help them be better doctors.''

Part of this involves teaching doctors how to appraise articles in the medical literature. Thousands of academic papers are published every year. Busy practitioners need some way to select those articles that are both relevant to clinical practice and methodologically sound. In other words, they must be able to distinguish the best research from all the rest.

There's nothing magical about this, Dr. Sackett says. ''It doesn't mean you have to penetrate the mysteries of advanced algebra. We showed in a trial here, that we could take a practising clinician *and in four hours* not only show him how to evaluate articles about diagnosis and therapy in the medical literature, but in fact, if he was a tutor in our undergraduate medical program, he could teach it to the medical students. And they in turn showed substantial improvements in their ability to evaluate clinical journals.''

And some of the journals themselves are making it easier to separate the wheat from the chaff. For example, Dr. Brian Haynes, another internist and clinical epidemiologist at McMaster, convinced one of the most authoritative journals, *Annals of Internal Medicine*, to institute a structured abstract to improve the efficiency of reading. Details about the methodology, typically the least interesting part of a paper and consequently rarely read, are now included in the abstract as a matter of policy. This is a major time-saver, says Dr. Sackett. ''It's set up so that just by reading the abstract, you can apply the critical appraisal guidelines, without having to read the whole paper first in order to see if it's up to scratch.''

This policy is also having an impact on how papers submitted to *Annals* are reviewed. Now authors must draft the first version of the structured abstract, which is then reviewed and revised by experts in clinical epidemiology. The *New England Journal of Medicine*, the world's most prestigious journal, is another example of how the medical literature is becoming more rigorously scientific. On its editorial board are a distinguished statistician and two respected epidemiologists. ''Of course, the real question is, to what extent do clinicians read *any* journals?'' asks Dr.

Sackett. "And if they do read any, are they these kinds or the throw-away journals?"*

Dr. Sackett is encouraged by the potential of computer information systems to make the clinician's job easier. Computers are making it possible to access the most recent and best medical evidence about what works and what doesn't."

As an example, Dr. Sackett explains how Dr. Haynes once used this resource to make a better decision concerning a patient who had come into the emergency department with a rare neurological disorder called Guillain-Barré syndrome. A neurologist was consulted, who said, "If she's really bad, we should do plasmapheresis."** But the doctors wanted to make sure the patient really stood to benefit, since plasmapheresis is a very expensive procedure that means calling in the Red Cross for both the equipment and the special technicians needed to run it. "It puts the patient through quite a bit too, since the process involves some rapid fluid shifts," Dr. Sackett explains. Using the computer, the team keyed in "Guillain-Barré," "plasmapheresis," and "RCT." The National Library of Medicine immediately responded with the citations for two trials. Then, using another program called "Colleague," they printed the articles and read them on the spot. In this case, the trials showed that plasmapheresis therapy can markedly shorten the length of time a patient has to be on a respirator. "The differences in overall mortality were too close to call, but in terms of quality of life, the results indicated that patients are very much better off having the therapy."

It's hard not to be impressed. These doctors were able to get the specific information they needed to make the best decision possible. This kind of technology is in place now. As physicians come to realize how valuable these resources are to their clinical practice, standards of care will change. Quality will improve as it becomes easier to offer patients the most appropriate care.

---

*Canadian physicians routinely receive 10 to 15 periodicals free of charge. The production and mailing costs for these publications are covered by drug-company advertising.

**The Red Cross uses plasmapheresis to separate the specific components in donated blood. For example, this is how the missing blood factors needed by hemophiliacs are obtained.

Putting "Caring" Back into Health Care*

More than a million people in Canada work in health-care-related occupations. They want to do a good job, but too often our straight-jacketed system gets in their way.

Gail Donner, executive director of the Registered Nurses' Association of Ontario (RNAO), describes how frustrated she felt when, as a young nursing graduate in the early 1960s, a hospital's rigid, hierarchical policies compromised the care she felt one patient needed and deserved.

To save money, the hospital where she was working permitted only one change of bed linen per day. Fresh sheets and pillowcases were kept in a locked storage cupboard, and only the ward's head nurse had the key. Donner explains that one of her patients was "a young, very large woman with terminal cancer. Her perspiration-soaked sheets needed to be changed more frequently than once a day for her to be comfortable. The head nurse, however, refused to break the rules. The next day, when both Donner and this head nurse were standing in front of the open storage cupboard, the latter was called away to the phone. Donner, feeling "like a thief," grabbed what she needed and stashed the extra linens in the patient's locker.

Putting patients first is essential to quality care. How a health care system is planned, financed, and organized can help or hinder this goal.

The alternative approaches to health care offered in this chapter are strong examples of how we could be doing a much better job meeting the needs of patients. Here are some key elements found in these alternatives:

- *A strong corporate culture*, in which providers see the organization's goals and objectives as a *mission*.
- *Financial and professional incentives* that encourage the appropriate use of personnel and resources.
- *A decentralized organization*, in which the authority to make decisions is tempered by accountability at every level.
- *Strong mechanisms to ensure high quality*, so that patients only receive services that stand to benefit them.

---

*This title of this subheading is a paraphrase of an excellent submission to the Health Services Review in 1980 made by the Canadian Nurses Association. Their title was "Putting 'Health' Into Health Care." (CNA, February 1980.)

To achieve high quality and efficiency, we'll have to reorient our sickness treatment system with these elements in mind. The details about how to do it will follow, in the last chapter. But first, we want to look at how other reformers have succeeded in bringing about other kinds of healthy changes.

Chapter 10

Healthy Public Policy

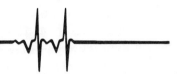

DR. TREVOR HANCOCK IS a British-trained physician who came to Canada in 1975. "But not to escape England's National Health Service," he quickly points out. After two years in a fee-for-service practice in rural New Brunswick, he moved to Toronto. There he worked for two years on salary at a community health centre before joining Toronto's Public Health Department, where he eventually became the city's Associate Medical Officer of Health. A founding member of the Medical Reform Group, and a former president of the Ontario Public Health Association, he now works as a private consultant to a number of groups, including the World Health Organization (WHO). It was Dr. Hancock, a "practising health futurist," who first coined the phrase "healthy public policy."

Healthy public policy can be defined as any policy that creates and encourages a context for health. By now it should be very clear that people can't be healthy unless they have the basics: food, shelter, income, and social equality. But our health stands to suffer as well if we destroy our ecosystem and use up all our resources. So ecological stability and resource sustainability are prerequisites for health, too.* What this means, of course, is

---

*These prerequisites are based on a statement from the European region of WHO, which has been endorsed by 35 nations.

that policies governing labour and business, the environment, income, transportation, agriculture and food, and so forth have important health implications. We need such an all-inclusive list because our health is really a reflection of the social, economic, and physical environment in which we live. How well we manage these environments, and how much we, as a society, are willing to pay for their management, indicate our values.

Federal health minister Marc Lalonde's 1974 report, *A New Perspective on the Health of Canadians*, officially recognized that these "other" factors are more important in safeguarding our health than doctors and hospitals. Twelve years later, in 1986, health minister Jake Epp's report, *Achieving Health for All: A Framework for Health Promotion*, reaffirmed this conclusion: "Our system of health care as it presently exists does not deal adequately with the major health concerns of our time." Epp's report set out a three-pronged strategy for moving beyond the laboratory, the doctors' office, and the hospital to tackle the real present-day health challenges. To promote health it recommended that we:

1. Foster public participation
2. Strengthen community health services
3. Coordinate healthy public policy

Also in 1986, an international conference in Ottawa sponsored by WHO, Health and Welfare Canada, and the Canadian Public Health Association produced the *Ottawa Charter for Health Promotion*, which contains a strikingly similar list of strategies:

1. Build healthy public policy
2. Create supportive environments
3. Strengthen community action
4. Develop personal skills
5. Reorient health services

These strategies, of course, form an implicit hierarchy. We need *healthy policies* to create the kind of *supportive environments* that are conducive to *strong communities*, which in turn will demand that we *reorient health services*. But they are also circular, in that the strongest communities will also push for healthy public policies. So it's not exclusively a top-down process, with all the leadership coming from government. There's plenty of room for action at the local level.*

Until now we've implied that these ideas are fairly new, and perhaps even revolutionary. But in fact, they're not new at all; many were well understood even in ancient times. They've been there all along, only waiting to be rediscovered.

The ancient Greek physician Hippocrates is probably best remembered today for his famous oath, which is still solemnly recited by graduating doctors. But Hippocrates had much more impact in his day through his advocacy of healthy public policy. One of his contributions was a textbook called *Airs, Waters, and Places*, in which he set out advice for town planning. His suggestions included that soil be tested for fertility, and that housing be located on high ground, well away from marshes and the malaria they bred. As Greek civilization spread east and west, colonists followed these and other principles from Hippocrates' book when locating and building their new settlements.

This fundamental connection between the environment and health was well understood in ancient times, and not just by "health" professionals.

A few centuries later, the Roman architect, Vitruvius Pollio, recommended that livestock be sacrificed at potential development sites, and their livers examined carefully to determine "the health of the land."[1]

Of course, doctors and other health workers have also had a long-standing and profound influence on the development of healthy public policy. For example, almost 200 years ago a German public health advocate, Dr. Johann Peter Frank, fought for state-supported maternity leave to improve the health of mothers and children. Sounds rather modern for the late 18th century, doesn't it?

Public Health in the 19th Century

Public health — which, while important, is still only one aspect of "healthy public policy" — had a renaissance in Britain in the

---

*Another noteworthy aspect of these strategies is that only one of the eight — "Develop personal skills" — is directed toward the individual.

early 19th century.The Industrial Revolution — which started earlier in England than anywhere else — had already been underway for a generation, and was transforming the nation. Growing urban industries were hungry for labour and looking for ways to fill their factories, but most of the population still lived in the countryside, as tenant farmers. Mounting pressure from industry led Parliament to pass various "Enclosure Acts," which succeeded in driving peasants off the land but failed to bring them into the cities. The "Poor Laws," which dated from Elizabethan times, were the obstacle. These laws made it possible for the able-bodied poor to subsist on alms from poorhouses and workhouses, which meant that many could and did remain in their own communities. To Adam Smith and many other economists of the day, this form of state subsidy was anathema. They argued vehemently that the Poor Laws were interfering with the "free" labour market they believed in. On the recommendation of a Parliamentary Royal Commission in 1834, these laws were soon amended. Once state support for the able-bodied poor had been substantially decreased, large numbers of peasants were forced to seek employment in industrial towns. This migration had an enormous impact on English life: in 1801 only 17% of Britons lived in towns; 60 years later the figure was nearly 40%.

But the industrial cities of England were ill-prepared for such rapid expansion. Factories and housing were erected wherever the developer owned land, without planning and at the cheapest possible cost. There were no municipal by-laws against overcrowding, so thousands of working families slept more than four to a bed. There were no indoor toilets, which meant that communities were quite literally choking on their own filth. In 1841, 70% of Liverpool's 223,000 citizens were industrial workers; almost two in three of these workers lived in conditions described as "crowded, dirty and unsanitary."[2] One area of Manchester had only two privies for 250 people. Another district had just 33 tubs (known then as "necessaries") for 7,000.

Obviously, such neighbourhoods were perfect breeding grounds for disease. Virulent epidemics of infectious disease killed thousands. As the Industrial Revolution spread to the continent, the United States, and Canada, the pattern repeated itself: vile living conditions, epidemics, and death.

Yet it took a long time for British politicians, or the British public, to tackle these threats to health. The effort began in Manchester, England's first "industrial city," where the world's first "modern" board of health was established in 1796. Its first recommendation, which was passed into law by Parliament in 1802, sought to improve the unspeakable conditions for children working in factories.[3]

About 40 years later, an inquiry was conducted into the living conditions of the "labouring population." It made full use of the epidemiological tools being developed at the time in England and the continent.[4] The subsequent report showed clearly that areas with working-class populations and unsanitary living and working conditions had the highest death rates. A full generation ahead of Pasteur and his "germ theory," Edwin Chadwick, the principal author of this landmark report, was firmly convinced that environmental conditions and the lack of clean water were responsible for these high mortality rates.[*] His recommendations, which were very radical for the times, clearly mesh with our definition of healthy public policy:

> The great preventives, drainage, street and house cleansings by means of supplies of water and improved sewerage, and especially the introduction of cheaper and more efficient modes of moving all noxious refuse from the towns, are operations for which aid must be sought from the science of the Civil Engineer, not from the physician, who has done his work when he has pointed out the disease that results from the neglect of proper administrative measures, and has alleviated the sufferings of the victims.[5]

So much for the "sickness treatment system."

During the 1840s, various pressure groups brought about a swift succession of legislative reforms. One of the most vocal of these early lobby groups was the Health of Towns Association, founded by a friend of Chadwick's, the physician Southwood Smith.

---

[*] Edwin Chadwick was *the* civil servant of his day. Between 1830 and 1854, he was the main author of most reports on social and health conditions in Britain. But over the years, he made a number of enemies, and although he lived to an old age (1800-1890) he was "deposed" from public life in 1854.

Smith's group used the same political strategies developed 50 years earlier by John Howard, the great prison reformer: first, they educated the public; then, using public pressure to get attention, they convinced legislators to pass remedial laws (which the reformers had often drafted themselves!). Of course, Dr. Smith's political success was likely helped by his close association with many of England's nobility. But his upper-class connections didn't stop him from pointing an accusing finger at those in power:

> For every one of the lives of these 15,000 persons who have thus perished during the last quarter, and who might have been saved . . . those are responsible whose proper office is to interfere to stay the calamity — who have the power to save but will not use it. But their apathy is an additional reason why you should arouse yourselves . . . . Let a voice come from your street, lanes, alleys . . . that will startle the ear of the public and command the attention of the legislature.[6]

The reform movement reached a crescendo in 1848. These were revolutionary times: Marx and Engels had just published *The Communist Manifesto*; there were rebellions in Europe, particularly in the German states. The most enlightened members of the English ruling class knew that harsh conditions for the poor was just as likely to breed revolution as disease.

News that an impending cholera epidemic was sweeping through Europe helped ensure the passage of the Public Health Act in Britain that year. Cholera is a bacterial disease[*] spread by contaminated food or drinking water, or by unsanitary contact with infected individuals. It can kill young, healthy people within hours of their becoming ill. During one cholera outbreak in London, there were over 10,000 deaths in a single three-month period.[7]

Chadwick and Dr. Smith had been hoping for stronger legislation. But all the same, this law did establish a General Board of Health with powers to initiate surveys and investigations, and to appoint local health boards. These local boards, in turn, had

---

[*]Caused by *Vibrio cholerae*.

some authority over water supply, sewage control, and certain aspects of occupational health and safety.

In its first six years, the General Board of Health was quite effective in getting municipalities to set up local boards to improve water quality and sanitation. Their authority, however, was resented, and the reformers made many enemies, particularly among vested interest groups. Private businesses, in the name of individual freedom and property rights, typically opposed measures to ensure a safer water supply and better sewers. (Later in this chapter you'll read how similar arguments are still being used today against health care reform.)

In 1854 came yet another cholera epidemic. This time the public health movement suffered a setback. Parliament failed to renew the Public Health Act, and the first National Board of Health, at least for a time, ceased to exist. The Earl of Shaftesbury, an ardent reformer of the day, blamed vested interests for its temporary demise; he singled out the private water and sewer companies, the local councils (which were often dominated by property developers and their friends), and even the College of Physicians, whose members chafed at being less effective against cholera than local medical officers of health. Ultimately, Parliament did restore the national health board, perhaps because it agreed with London's first medical officer of health, Dr. John Simon, who said that "the physical strength of a nation is among the chief factors of national prosperity."[8]

The reform movement gained credibility thanks to the pioneering work of Dr. William Farr, the statistician. The reports he wrote in the middle and late 19th century were full of strong ammunition for the fight against disease. They must have been readable as well, because politicians regularly quoted from his data, referring to the death rates in their own ridings to underscore how healthy — or unhealthy — their constituents were.

Public Health in Canada

The development of public health agencies in Canada followed the British example; here, too, the threat of cholera provided the impetus for legislative reform. The first cholera outbreak on this continent occurred among Irish immigrants in Québec in 1832.

From there, its devastation spread throughout North America. Upper Canada — which is now the province of Ontario — responded by passing a Public Health Act in 1833. Although this legislation authorized a health board, its powers were limited — it only dealt with infectious diseases, when and if outbreaks occurred.

It would be 50 years before Canada's first *permanent* board of health was established in Toronto. Dr. William Cannif was Toronto's first medical officer of health. With a team of six policemen, he set up a household sanitary inspection program. He also hired health inspectors to examine food, especially milk, for contamination. Dr. Charles Hastings, Toronto's fourth medical officer of health, was particularly skillful at influencing public policy. He followed the same strategies as Dr. Southwood Smith and the other 19th-century British reformers. Toronto newspapers regularly featured his health promotion messages — messages designed to educate the general public and to create support for reform. As public pressure mounted, Dr. Hastings presented politicians with appropriate legislation that he and his colleagues had carefully drafted themselves. In 1910, for example, his initiatives resulted in laws requiring the pasteurization of milk and chlorination of water. During and after Dr. Hastings's tenure, Toronto was widely regarded as one of the healthiest cities in the world. No one doubted that public health activities had contributed heavily to this achievement.*

But during and after the Second World War, public health initiatives were eclipsed in prominence by new developments in curative medicine. New "miracle" drugs, like penicillin, were taking the credit for reducing the death rates from infectious disease, when the accolades should have been going to healthy public policies. As subsequent advances in medical technology attracted more and more admiration, people shifted their expectations and trust. They began to believe that doctors and hospitals were the safeguards of health, and the stature of public health declined further.

Part of this fall from grace was deserved; many public health

---

*In 1934, for example, Toronto was the first large city without a single death from diphtheria.

departments had lagged behind the times. They hadn't adapted to address modern "outbreaks," like heart disease and cancer. Dan Leckie first came to Toronto's Board of Health as a freshman school trustee in 1973. He says the way the city's health department was organized at the time didn't seem to reflect modern health concerns at all. For example, there was little tuberculosis in Toronto, yet the health department maintained an active TB division. There were serious public and medical concerns about the dangers of lead pollution, yet no one in the health department had expertise in environmental health.*

Even today, public health still lags behind, partly because it has forgotten how to capture the public's imagination. Modern health campaigns focus almost exclusively on raising money to support new technologies for *diagnosing* and *treating* diseases — not *preventing* them. Communities lobby for C-T scanners, not more social housing. They hold fund-raisers for new cardiac wings, not better workplace safety. Why should governments take action if there's no public pressure? It's better to win a few votes by opening a new hospital wing, than to offend economic interests by taking on industrial polluters or the powerful tobacco companies. It's much easier by far to issue episodic warnings about health risks than to deal directly with the manufacturers of illness.

In 1854, the business community accused John Snow of interfering with free enterprise when he insisted on closing the Broad Street water pump to stem a London cholera epidemic. To them, this was economic revolution. In 1964, the tobacco industry voiced a similar complaint when the U.S. Surgeon General released his report identifying cigarette-smoking as a major health problem. Indeed, the mammoth struggle over tobacco regulation is a good illustration of how little has changed in the intervening years.

The Smoke Ring

British journalist Peter Taylor became so incensed about the tobacco industry that he wrote a book about it. He called it *Smoke*

---

*Readers will be relieved to learn that Toronto's Public Health Department today is very involved in a variety of health advocacy and health promotion activities, including plans for a community heart-health program. Resources have accordingly been reallocated to programs that address our most pressing modern health problems, like family planning, and AIDS.

Ring because he was struck by all the connections between the tobacco industry on the one hand and government, unions, organized sports, the arts, and other powerful sectors of our economy on the other.[9] Everyone knows that tobacco is very dangerous *when used as directed*, yet the industry has made sure that each sector gets its payoff — enough to keep them from taking the offensive.

Canada's smoke ring encloses an impressive number of prominent people. For example, until recently it included Paul Martin, Jr., whom many expect will be the next leader of the national Liberal Party. He served on the Board of Imasco Ltd. until 1988. Imasco owns Imperial Tobacco, Canada's largest tobacco company. Former British Columbia premier Bill Bennett is another Imasco director. So is Murray Koffler, the pharmacist and philanthropist. The Ontario Medical Association awarded him its Centennial Medal in June 1988. Koffler founded Shoppers Drug Mart. He also established one of the larger anti-drug-abuse organizations in Canada, the Council on Drug Abuse (CODA). Is it a coincidence that CODA never mentions tobacco products or alcohol in its work, or that a representative from the alcohol industry sat on *its* board? Until 1987, Mila Mulroney served on the board of the du Maurier Council for the Arts; Ontario's former lieutenant-governor, Pauline McGibbon, chairs this council today. What do these connections mean? Are they important? Read on and judge for yourselves.

Tobacco's connections to power and influence go way back to the 17th century, shortly after Sir Walter Raleigh introduced the plant to England from America. Britain's James I despised smoking as "a custom loatheful to the eye, hateful to the nose, harmful to the brain, dangerous to the lungs."[10] He tried to eliminate the habit by instituting a 40-fold hike in tobacco taxes. And it worked — smoking rates plummeted! But alas, even for an anti-smoking activist like James I, it worked a bit too well. As sales fell, so did tax revenues. He finally lowered the rate to 12 times the original tax, and revenues poured in to fill his coffers.

Of course, James I did have alternatives. He could have levied an income tax to produce equal or even greater revenues. After all, as king he didn't have to worry about facing the polls every four or five years! But even he recognized the value of an addictive product. What could be more reliably profitable?

Winners and Losers   It would be hard to name an enterprise more profitable or more concentrated than the tobacco industry. Today's world tobacco market is controlled by just six companies. This is an extraordinary degree of concentration. And the profit levels are about what you'd expect from an addictive yet legal product. In 1987, the *Globe and Mail* estimated that the industry profit on each pack of cigarettes sold was 35%[11]. This high profit margin has furnished the companies with ample resources to diversify their operations. For example:

- Imasco controls Canada Trust, Shoppers Drug Mart, United Cigar Stores, and several thousand Hardee's restaurants in the United States.

- Rothman's controls Star Oil.

- RJR MacDonald, the smallest of Canada's big three tobacco companies, is owned by the American company R.J.R. Nabisco, recently taken over by a New York consortium. R.J.R./Nabisco controls Del Monte, Canada Dry, Sunkist, Kentucky Fried Chicken, General Foods, and Nabisco.

All this expansion has been made possible by a product that U.S. Surgeon General Everett Koop says is more addictive than heroin. Every time you eat a bowl of Shreddies or head off to your local Shoppers Drug Mart, you're helping to enrich some of the largest marketers of death on the planet.

Canada's governments are also big winners in the tobacco sweepstakes, and haven't forgotten the lessons learned by James I. They've come to count on tobacco tax revenues, which in 1987 dropped $4.1 billion into federal and provincial coffers. Governments know that even after they've paid the health costs from tobacco-related disease, they still come out well ahead. Health and Welfare Canada estimates that in 1982 the cost of tobacco-related disease to Canadian society was over $7 billion.[12] But the estimated cost to government of providing hospital care and physician services for smoking-related illness that year was just a little over $1.5 billion.[13]

These health expenditures are what economists call "direct costs." But most of the costs of tobacco-related illness are indirect — that is, they affect society as a whole by reducing productivity, and the individual by lowering income potential. And then there are the intangible costs, like the pain and suffering to tobacco's victims and their families.

Even if governments did act to reduce tobacco-related illness, they'd stand very little chance of recapturing any health-care dollars. And they know it. From earlier chapters, you no doubt already understand that the cost of our health care system bears little relationship to the actual amount of illness in our society. If we had fewer lung cancer cases, doctors would simply devote more time to their other patients, and fill in their schedules by performing other types of services. Besides, when people die prematurely because of smoking-related illness, governments don't have to pay as much in pension benefits. The way things stand, government comes out ahead by just sitting back, like James I, and letting all the money roll in. Provincial and federal treasurers are unlikely to kill "the goose that lays the golden eggs."

Meanwhile, between 30,000 and 50,000 Canadians every year are the big losers when it comes to tobacco — they lose their lives.* Here's a summary of what we know about smoking:

- Cigarettes are the major cause of mortality in Canada, causing between one-seventh and one-third of all deaths.

- Nicotine, one of the hundreds of chemicals found in cigarette smoke, is extremely addictive.

- Most smokers would like to stop.

Here's how the industry behaves:

- The tobacco industry targets its promotion to the young. They know their addictive product will hook many young people into becoming lifelong customers.[14]

---

*See Chapter 7.

- Tobacco manufacturers install many prominent, well-connected people on their boards. They're also major supporters of artistic, cultural, and sports activities, sponsoring, for example, the Royal Canadian Golf Association, Tennis Canada, and the Royal Winnipeg Ballet.

And how governments behave:

- Canada's governments rarely, if ever, enforce laws that forbid the sale of tobacco products to minors.

- Provincial and federal governments take in more money through tobacco-tax revenues than they spend on the health costs of smoking-related diseases.

The principal barrier standing in the way of saner tobacco policies is, of course, the power of the industry itself. Michael Daube, from Western Australia's health department, notes that most of today's board members and senior management joined the tobacco industry when the dangers of smoking were already well-known. He describes these people as more ruthless, cynical, and tough-minded than their predecessors;[15] he adds that they know how to use their power over government. For example, in the past decade the industry has got one British health minister fired, and similarly disposed of an outspoken health secretary in the United States.[16]

The tobacco industry is really engaged in a mass strategy to hook the population on a drug that's as addictive as heroin and much more dangerous. If this makes it sound like some South American drug cartel, remember that the tobacco industry dwarfs the illegal drug business both in size and political influence. On health grounds alone, there's far more reason to ban tobacco than heroin.

What's a politician to do? What would *you* do if you were prime minister, or a minister of finance or health? Here are a few suggestions:[17]

1. Enforce the laws prohibiting tobacco sales to minors.
2. Ban advertising and promotion of cigarettes.
3. Increase tobacco taxes.
4. Restrict smoking in public areas and in the workplace.
5. Assist smokers who want to quit.

6. Develop incentives for tobacco farmers to switch to healthier crops.
7. Develop a labour strategy to redeploy tobacco workers.

Hurray for Canada After a slow start, Canada has actually implemented a few of these strategies. The political spur to this change of heart at the federal level was Lynn McDonald, until recently the NDP member of parliament for the Toronto riding of Broadview-Greenwood.

McDonald said she had no particular opinion at all about the tobacco issue when she was first elected in 1982. No opinion, that is, until she "nearly died" from all the tobacco smoke at her first caucus meeting. Even though NDP leader Ed Broadbent is a devoted cigar smoker, it didn't take long for the caucus to enact a no-smoking policy at Ms. McDonald's urging. Her success was widely publicized in the media and she soon began to hear from many Canadians about their own problems with "second-hand" smoke. Gradually, her interest in the tobacco issue grew and she became a forceful advocate for saner policies.

After the 1984 election, McDonald introduced a private member's bill to control tobacco products in Canada. It found little support in the Conservative-dominated house. Health minister Jake Epp maintained at the time that we didn't need legislation. He believed that the tobacco companies would voluntarily tone down their promotion and implement better product warnings. Judging by their silence, the Canadian Cancer Society, the Lung Association, and other "health" groups must have thought so, too.

But as time passed, it became abundantly clear that the industry wasn't prepared to do very much on a voluntary basis. So McDonald drafted a second bill. This time she proposed an amendment to the Hazardous Products Act, Bill C-204, noting that tobacco is currently the most hazardous product on the market not yet regulated under this legislation. By now the health groups had given up on Epp and the tobacco industry, and fully supported the new bill.

Finally, in 1987, amid mounting public pressure, Epp took a courageous step and introduced Bill C-51 to eliminate all advertising and promotion of tobacco.

Of course, the tobacco companies simply hated this idea. They claimed that a ban against promoting and advertising their deadly product violated their right to free speech.[18] They fought hard to derail the legislation, relying on their vast connections in the business and political communities. They hired Bill Neville, a former close adviser to Prime Minister Brian Mulroney, to lead their lobby. And they called on all the diverse sporting and cultural groups they sponsor to protest its passage. Canadians witnessed the bizarre spectacle of athletic organizations and dance companies — which, presumably, are concerned about health and fitness — defending the tobacco industry's right to peddle death.

Who was on the other side? You might have expected strong leadership to come from the organizations of health professionals, who see the effects of smoking every working day — groups like the Canadian Medical Association, the Canadian Nurses Association, and the Canadian Public Health Association. And since smoking causes over one-third of cancer and heart disease deaths, and two-thirds of respiratory deaths, you might also have expected the Cancer Society, the Heart and Stroke Foundation, and the Lung Association to be prominent in supporting this legislation. The annual budgets for these three voluntary organizations total more than $100 million. Yet until very late in the day, the battle against tobacco was waged largely by a group whose annual budget is only $400,000.

This "David" in the struggle against the giant tobacco industry is the Non-Smokers' Rights Association (NSRA). Garfield Mahood, its executive director, and David Sweanor, its legal counsel, are widely regarded as the most effective one-two lobbying tandem in the country. Dr. Alan Blum, former editor of the *New York State Medical Journal*, says that the NSRA has had more impact than any other anti-smoking organization anywhere. And the *United States Tobacco Reporter*, an industry trade paper, called them one of the fiercest lobby groups in the world!

And no wonder. The NSRA's impressive track record — which includes everything from getting smoking banned on short-distance flights, to the passage of Toronto's workplace and restaurant anti-smoking by-laws — testifies to their formidable political clout. The secret of their success is that they don't give ground, they don't give up, and they use the media more skillfully than other groups a hundred times their size.

From his small, cluttered office in downtown Toronto, Sweanor describes his organization as the shock troops in the fight against tobacco. It isn't easy, he says, to get governments to take the tobacco issue seriously. He's particularly upset with Ontario, which proposes launching a province-wide public-education program on the dangers of tobacco with a budget of only $375,000. "That level of funding," says Sweanor, "is tantamount to sending out one man with an axe and a bucket to fight a forest fire."

But Ontario's Ministry of Health isn't the only backslider. Its Ministry of Correctional Services routinely hands out rolling tobacco and cigarette papers to juveniles in detention. When the NSRA found out about it, they made an official complaint, to which the government has yet to respond, despite provincial laws that expressly forbid distributing tobacco products to minors. Indeed, according to Sweanor, defenders of tobacco are found in many government departments. Senior bureaucrats and politicians in ministries of finance, labour, education, and even health have been reluctant to view tobacco's adverse effects as a matter for public policy. Sweanor, like the reformers from the Victorian era, believes that government must take action to control a private industry that "profits from addiction and death."

More traditional health groups tend to blush at this forceful language, but the NSRA and their companion group, Physicians for a Smoke-Free Canada, have been instrumental in bringing many of these organizations into the fray. While Sweanor speaks charitably about their participation, it's pretty clear that their "medical model"* orientation and a shyness about entering the political arena delayed their involvement. For example, persuading the Canadian Cancer Society (CCS) and the Canadian Heart and Stroke Foundation to regard smoking as an issue hasn't been easy. Both organizations want to reduce the incidence of disease. But their philosophies have been shaped by the physicians who advise them and sit on their boards. As already noted, doctors tend to be more concerned with sickness treatment, with caring for their present patients. This bias has led many health groups

---

*The term "medical model" refers to an orientation in which the biological causes of illness receive more attention than social and environmental factors.

away from preventive strategies, particularly those whose benefits only occur 20 or 30 years down the road.

That's why the CCS deserves a great deal of praise for changing its philosophy and taking a more long-sighted view. Doug Barr, the CCS's executive director, says it was the NSRA that spurred the society into action. In 1986, the society set up an office of public issues. It's active on about 40 fronts, but tobacco is its number-one issue.

This office, with a tiny budget of only $150,000 — compared to CSS's overall budget of $60 million — and committed full-time staffer Ken Kyle, gained considerable stature during the Bill C-51 debate. Recently, John Ronson, a lawyer with the firm of Blake Cassels & Graydon, has become the new chairman of the Public Issues Committee in Ontario's division of the CCS. Ronson is no stranger to controversy. He served as executive assistant to Murray Elston, when he was Ontario's health minister, during the turbulent years 1985 to 1987. (Readers will no doubt remember the bitter work stoppage Ontario doctors staged in the summer of 1986.) Ronson represents a new breed of anti-tobacco lobbyists. He's politically sophisticated and very well connected — he wears all the establishment trappings. He admits that he hesitated at first before accepting the chair of this committee because he doubted it would be active enough on the prevention front. But now he's thoroughly convinced that the CCS has changed, and that it will increasingly use political action strategies to achieve its goal of preventing cancer. Doug Barr agrees; although he isn't prepared to use his door-to-door canvassers for political advocacy, he does predict more political action against smoking.

The NSRA and CCS, along with the other groups brought into the tobacco debate, have together created a potent force for change. In the fall of 1987 and winter of 1988, the gloves came off between the pro- and anti-smoking forces. The Tobacco Manufacturers' Council hired Bill Neville to lead their lobby. The NSRA and supporting groups took out full-page newspaper ads attacking his appointment and criticizing him for accepting money from the industry. The CCS sent black-edged postcards to members of parliament reminding them of the thousands of Cana-

dians who die every year from tobacco-related illnesses. When
Simcoe South MP Ronald Stewart spoke out against Bill C-51,
a coalition of health groups sent letters to each of Stewart's constituents, reminding them that Stewart was in the wholesale
tobacco distribution business.

In spite of all this effort, health minister Jake Epp was forced
to tone down Bill C-51. The ban on advertising would still be
implemented, but with a delay. And the ban on promotion and
sponsorship would only apply to new activities — existing con-
tracts would continue. Epp admits that even in its weakened form,
he had a tough fight on his hands eliciting support from his cabinet colleagues. But he believes that the industry made a tactical
error when it chose Bill Neville to champion its cause. Neville's
former close association with the prime minister turned out to
be a liability rather than a bonus, in that any government retreat
would have compromised the prime minister's integrity.

This tale has a happy ending. Bills C-51 and C-204 were passed
in the summer of 1988. Today, Canada has some of the tough-
est anti-tobacco legislation in the world.

The credit for this success belongs to many, but chiefly to a
tenacious opposition MP, to a courageous federal health minister
who stuck to his principles, and to the Non-Smokers' Rights
Association, the fierce little lobby that wouldn't let go.

Lessons from the Tobacco Fight   What can we learn from the
tobacco fight about the prospects for healthy public policy? First,
that the stakes are often very high. Healthy public policies often
threaten powerful economic and political interests. Winning
against these forces requires a very careful strategy. And that's
the second lesson: to develop public support, you have to involve
a wide array of interest groups — in other words, you have to
build a coalition for reform. This brings us to the third lesson:
you don't have to be big to make waves. The larger, more traditional health organizations in Canada devote little time or money
to promoting healthier laws. It's the small groups from the grass
roots, like the NSRA, that have proven themselves very effective as health advocates. The fourth and final lesson is this:
governments won't move in a vacuum. Their chief business is
to get elected and, once in power, to stay there. When it comes

to the health of Canadians, politicians are the original pragmatists. It's very easy to win votes by opening a new cancer or cardiac wing; much harder to act against the products that ensure a steady supply of patients. All the same, government did act, which proves it's possible to pass laws to protect our health in spite of fierce opposition from business. Are Canadian politicians finally discovering the vote potential of healthy public policy?

Getting the Lead Out

No story better illustrates how much impact neighbourhoods can have on public policy, than the saga of South Riverdale's fight against lead pollution. But first here's a bit of background on lead.

Lead is a highly toxic substance. Even very low blood levels of lead can affect the hearing, learning, growth, and mental development of children.[19] In fact, some scientists today say *there is no known safe level for lead.* This is quite a change. In the 1960s, levels of 60 micrograms per decilitre were considered tolerable. During the 1970s and early 1980s, the "safe" level was revised downward several times, to 40, then to 30, then to 25. By 1986 major American and Canadian reports were simply advising that children's blood lead levels should be as low as possible.[20]

It's been known since antiquity that lead is poisonous, but people have continued to use it through the ages because it's so useful. Historians today blame *sappa*, a sweetener made by heating grape juice and honey in lead vessels, for hastening the decline of Imperial Rome.[21] Because it doesn't corrode, lead seemed a natural for water pipes. But lead plumbing in older buildings can be a significant source of poisoning. This conflict between the health hazards of lead and its usefulness remains the crux of the problem today.

Lead is a very dense substance. Even very tiny particles of it, when released into the air, eventually fall to the ground and contaminate the soil. Lead in the soil gets tracked into homes and becomes incorporated into house dust. Children are particularly at risk for lead poisoning because they're always putting their hands in their mouths and because they absorb lead more readily than adults.

Spreading the Lead Most modern lead pollution comes from two 20th-century sources: paint, and automobile emissions. Until fairly recently, lead was used as the pigment in most white and grey paint. And leaded gasoline* was hailed as a great discovery when it was introduced in the 1920s, because it prevented "engine knock." Over the next 50 years more lead was spewed into the environment than had been released by human activity in all the previous centuries.

From the start, public health and occupational health and safety workers lobbied hard against leaded gasoline, against adding millions of tons of lead to the environment from car exhaust. They tried to highlight the health risks. But their voices couldn't prevail against the twenties ethos that "the business of America is business."[22] Of the two studies conducted at the time about the safety of leaded gasoline, one was heavily influenced by the industry producing it, and the other, in retrospect, had major design flaws.[23]

By the early 1980s, people living in large cities had as much as a 1,000 times more lead in their bodies than would have occurred naturally.

Public health advocates tried again in the 1950s and 1960s to warn those in authority that children living in inner-city communities, particularly those in homes near lead smelters, were in danger. But strangely, changes in public policy to reduce lead pollution came from a different quarter. Air pollution was the issue of the day during the 1960s and 1970s. Most Western governments responded by restricting automobile emissions — but sulfur dioxide and nitrous oxide were the targets, not lead. To comply, the car industry began installing catalytic converters in their new vehicles. Because lead deactivated the catalyst, these new cars had to use unleaded gasoline.

The results were astonishing. Within a decade, air lead levels fell by more than 80%.[24] Between 1976 and 1980, children's blood lead levels in the United States fell by 40%.[25]

Governments have gradually responded to pressure from health

---

*The lead in gasoline is tetraethyl lead (TEL).

advocates by restricting the lead content of food and paint as well. All of these measures mean that by the early 1990s, Canada's urban children will likely have blood lead levels one-third to one-quarter those their parents had as city kids.

The Battle in Riverdale   South Riverdale is a densely populated working-class neighbourhood in Toronto's east end. It's also home to Canada's largest secondary smelter, the Canada Metal Company.* During the 1960s, residents of the community became alarmed about the lead issue when children living near another Toronto smelter in the Niagara neighbourhood were admitted to the Hospital for Sick Children with lead poisoning.

Their fears were confirmed when scientific studies in the 1970s showed that South Riverdale's air and soil had much higher lead levels than other parts of Toronto. Soil immediately adjacent to the Canada Metal plant has several thousand parts per million of lead. This level falls to 500 to 1,000 ppm a few hundred metres from the plant. For comparison, most other parts of Toronto have lead levels around 100 ppm, and in rural areas soil lead levels are rarely above 20 ppm. There was also some evidence that blood lead levels among the neighbourhood's children were dangerously high as well, particularly among those living closest to the Canada Metal Smelter.** Cathy Walther was a young mother with toddlers at the time. Her house was only 300 metres from the plant. "I was horrified when I learned about the health effects of lead," she says. "I was afraid to let my kids play in the yard."

A number of community groups formed to pressure the company and the government to reduce lead emissions and remove poisoned soil from their front and back yards. It was slow going. All along, provincial action fell short of community demands. In 1974, for example, Ontario's Ministry of the Environment adopted emission standards that allowed much higher levels than

---

*A secondary smelter retrieves lead from manufactured materials, like automobile batteries.

**The average blood lead level among South Riverdale's children in the early 1970s was 28 micrograms per decilitre.

the community felt was safe. And in 1977, the ministry set a stand-ard for removing contaminated soil two-and-a-half times *higher* than its own junior officials had recommended.

Meanwhile, the lead industry was working hard to fight controls. The International Lead and Zinc Research Organization (ILZRO), the industry's lobby, pressed their case in the courts. In 1974, it won an injunction that prevented the CBC from airing a documentary about lead on *As It Happens*. It also brought lawsuits against 70 journalists and three members of Toronto's health board, including its chair, Anne Johnston, to discourage them from pursuing the issue. Johnston, for example, wound up with a legal bill for $28,000. But, once the city, with provincial approval, agreed to cover health board members' legal costs, these suits were dropped.

Because lead poisoning was a health issue, the neighbourhood groups tried to get the community's doctors involved. None would cooperate. There were very few family doctors in South Riverdale, and a number of community groups, including one involved in the lead issue, were also working to get a neighbourhood health centre.

South Riverdale Community Health Centre opened for business in 1976, in an old police station only a kilometre from the Canada Metal plant. Though it was established to provide primary care for residents in the area, it also took action on the lead issue. Its community board established an environmental health committee in 1979 to lobby for tougher regulations and to educate health centre staff and residents about the lead problem.* With help from Toronto's public health department, this committee published and distributed pamphlets explaining how to control dust, and which vegetables could safely be grown in contaminated soil.

Two unrelated events in June of 1979 boosted the committee's efforts. An article in the *New England Journal of Medicine* estab-

---

*Father Jim Webb, a Jesuit priest with a strong faith in social justice and community development, chaired this committee for many years. In 1985, he left Toronto to minister to a poor community in Kingston, Jamaica, but he never lost hope that the community would win in the end.

lished there was a link between behavioural problems and IQ deficits, and blood lead levels previously considered "safe."[26] And in the same month, an equipment failure at the Canada Metal Company led to a massive one-day release of lead. This prompted Ontario's environment ministry to secure a court order forcing the company to clean up its act.

Better emission controls and an effective public education program helped reduce the blood lead levels of South Riverdale's children during the 1980s. But they still remained higher than levels found in other Toronto children. Both the health centre's committee and the city's public health department lobbied harder for the neighbourhood soil to be removed. Success came in 1987, when James Bradley, the environment minister, announced an $8 million soil removal and replacement program, jointly sponsored by the province and the city. As many as a thousand properties in the area were eligible, and the project got underway shortly after the announcement.

Maureen McDonnell, a nurse and a mother of three, had been chairing the health centre's environmental committee since 1985. "When Curtis and I first discussed having children," she says, "we were seriously thinking about moving out of the neighbourhood." But they didn't. "It's our home and our community. I'm glad we decided to stay and fight."

Lessons from Lead The story of South Riverdale teaches many of the same lessons we learned from the tobacco fight. Healthy public policy threatens economic and political interests. Leadership from traditional health organizations is unlikely: the Canadian Medical Association, the hospital association, and similar groups were completely uninvolved in South Riverdale's fight against lead. But you don't have to be big to win; small grassroots organizations, like community health centres, can be very effective health advocates, and can find strong allies in municipal public health departments. Finally, improvements to health don't always come from health-sector organizations. The decision that required manufacturers to install catalytic converters — which were responsible for most of the general decline in lead emissions, as well as other pollutants — came from the Department of Transport, not Health and Welfare.

Community Heart Health

From Chapter 7, you already know a lot about the various factors that contribute to Canada's major cause of death: coronary heart disease. These include smoking, diets high in saturated fats and cholesterol, high blood pressure, obesity, diabetes, social isolation, and stress.

What's the best way to reduce these risks? Is it better to focus on individual treatment, using doctors, nurses, and other health professionals? Or are community-wide strategies for prevention more effective? Some studies comparing the two approaches to preventing heart disease find the latter more promising.

Here's one reason why. It's clear to all health researchers that the *average* cholesterol reading for Canadians is far too high. By merely singling out those individuals with the highest levels and spending lots of money trying to get them to change their habits, we'd be missing a lot of people who are also at risk. It would be far more effective to lower the *average* cholesterol levels by starting programs to reduce overall community risk. By lowering the average, everyone would benefit, because we'd also find fewer people with extremely high levels.[27]

Perhaps an analogy would help to clarify this. Suppose on one street it's been proven that speeds above 60 kilometres an hour are unsafe, but that on average, motorists on that street drive at 80 km/hr, which is the legal speed limit. Among all drivers, about 20% drive at speeds between 100 and 120 km/hr. Police are kept very busy ticketing this top 20%, but accidents are still occurring even at lower speeds. Wouldn't it make more sense to use a community approach, and lower the legal speed limit to 60 km/hr? Wouldn't you expect to find fewer people driving at 100 to 120 km/hr in a 60-km/hr zone?

Two of the better-known examples of community-wide programs aimed at preventing heart disease come from California and Finland.* The California study was done by Stanford University in the early 1970s. Researchers there selected two areas

---

*Other large community-based projects outside of Canada have been launched in Minnesota and Rhode Island, as well as in several European cities.

of the state that were served by different mass-media networks (that is, different television and radio stations, newspapers, and so on). In the study area, investigators used public service announcements and mailings to educate residents about risks for heart disease. The other area received no particular intervention and served as the control group. The results of the study found that both groups reduced their risks for heart disease, in keeping with a downward trend throughout North America, but that the average risk reduction in the targetted area was 23% *greater* than in the control group.[28]

In the 1950s and 1960s, the eastern part of Finland had the world's highest death rates from coronary heart disease. North Karelia, a county in east Finland, asked its federal government for help with this "epidemic" in the early 1970s. Thus was launched the "North Karelia Project."[29]

Researchers began to collect baseline data about risk factors for heart disease in two counties: North Karelia, the study group, and a neighbouring county, Kuopio, the control group. Using the mails and the media, they promoted risk reduction to residents of North Karelia. Their interventions also involved a number of "healthy public policy" initiatives. Existing smoking restrictions were enforced. Grocery stores were encouraged to promote low-fat dairy and meat products. Farmers were encouraged to produce more vegetables. The study carefully avoided targetting high-risk individuals for attention; the researchers reasoned that if the lifestyle of the entire community was the problem, then the target had to be the whole community. The results reported reductions in blood pressure, serum cholesterol (men only), and smoking (men only) among North Karelia's population. Ten years after the project was first started, it was found that death rates from heart disease in Finland as a whole had declined, by 12% for men and 26% for women. But the corresponding decreases in North Karelia were far greater: heart disease deaths fell by 24% for men and 51% for women.*

---

*Methodological problems in evaluating community-wide interventions create almost insurmountable difficulties in assessing their effectiveness. However, even the most skeptical evaluator would find the results of the Stanford and North Karelia studies worthy of replication and further investigation.

Heart Health Comes to Canada   Canada has its own example of how community-based prevention can reduce heart disease. In 1986, the Ottawa-Carleton Public Health Department launched Heartbeat, a program designed to raise the profile of prevention by involving businesses, governments, and the media. Even though the annual budget for Heartbeat *is less than the cost of one heart transplant operation*, its achievements have been very encouraging.

Dr. Geoff Dunkley, associate medical officer of health for Ottawa-Carleton, compares most traditional public health programs to "selling refrigerators in the Arctic" — no one wants them. But with Heartbeat, he says, it's just the opposite: everybody's jumping on the bandwagon. For example, CJOH, the city's largest television station, supported Heartbeat's "Quit and Win" contest.* Residents in the region who quit smoking for a designated length of time were eligible to win a trip to the Bahamas, donated by a local travel agency. CJOH undertook to distribute brochures explaining the contest to over 100,000 homes in the area. Talk about participation! And Heartbeat is helping to reinforce existing programs, too, including anti-smoking activities in Dr. Dunkley's public health department. Partly thanks to this program, he expects that several municipalities will soon institute workplace smoking by-laws.

But it hasn't all been smooth sailing. When Heartbeat asked the retail food industry and local restaurants to begin marketing food on the basis of its effect on heart disease, they got a warm reception. But they ran into a snag because Canada's Food and Drug Act prohibits food promotions from making health claims. Kellogg's ran into similar problems, and had to scrap a planned collaboration with the Canadian Cancer Society. They had wanted to advertise high-fibre foods as a way to prevent colon cancer; the law said they couldn't.

This raises an interesting point: should we encourage food

---

*The "Quit and Win" idea came from the Minnesota Heart Health Project.

producers to compete on the basis of how healthy their products are? Nutritional labelling is one thing, but allowing a manufacturer to promote bologna as a "good source of protein," without mentioning its high fat and salt content, is very misleading. Obviously, certain controls are necessary to protect consumers.

All the same, free enterprise can be a boon to healthy public policy, and vice versa. Dr. Dunkley says he's quite willing to work with media outlets that want to cooperate with Heartbeat, even if their ultimate motive is to increase their market share. Why not? If healthy public policy is good for business, so much the better.

Canada now has a national Heart Health Network. Its momentum is picking up as more and more health workers, civil servants, and politicians recognize the potential of community-wide strategies. On March 2, 1988, Jake Epp announced that the Health Services and Promotion Branch of Health and Welfare Canada would assist any province that wanted to start community heart programs. He made this announcement from Nova Scotia, where he and representatives of that province had just agreed on a $2 million project.

We're starting to get the message that you can't deal with the epidemic of cardiovascular disease by treating sick individuals. Targetting high-risk groups for prevention isn't enough, either. The prospects for healthy public policy have never been better. Dr. Harold Colburn from Health and Welfare Canada says community heart health is "an idea whose time has come."

Victory over Violence

As recently as 1982, some politicians found wife abuse funny. Many members of parliament laughed out loud when they were told that one in ten women were beaten by their husbands. But those MPs, and Canadian society as a whole, have learned a lot since then about the extent of family violence. Today we fund more services for its victims, and there are more hostel beds offering safe though temporary refuge. But it's still not nearly enough.

The Canadian Advisory Council on the Status of Women estimates that one million women are beaten — at least to some extent — every year.[30] If even one-tenth of them began demanding services and protection, it would cost billions more than we spend today to treat the afflicted women and their tormentors.

The real answer to this society-wide problem rests with a community approach. According to Linda MacLeod, author of *Battered But Not Beaten*, we have to focus on the long-term goal of societal prevention. We need economic policies that promote equality between the sexes. We need a society that values mothers and children. We need a society that will not tolerate violence in intimate relationships. In short, we need healthy public policies.

Lessons from London   For a long time London, Ontario, has been demonstrating how individual treatment and community prevention strategies can be combined to achieve these objectives. Its package of programs against family violence is world-famous.

London's police department has been a key player in this movement, and is unique in a number of ways. It had a policy of laying charges against wife-batterers long before federal and provincial governments required all police forces to do so. London police have long held that the threat of legal action is vital to the offender's rehabilitation. No excuses about paperwork here!*

Way back in 1972, London's police force set up a Family Consultant Service (FCS) to help officers intervening in violent domestic situations. The FCS is staffed with social workers, clergy, and other professionals, and is available around the clock to offer advice to police by phone, or to do on-the-spot, immediate crisis counselling. They even follow up potentially dangerous cases.

When this pilot program was evaluated, researchers found that the number of "core families" — that is, those with a record of calling the police frequently for help in violent situations — had been reduced by 20%.[31]

---

*In Chapter 7 we discussed how some police fail to lay charges because of the time it takes to fill out forms.

Meanwhile, London has a Coordinating Committee on Family Violence* (CCFV) active on other fronts:

- In 1978, a new shelter for abuse victims was opened, the Women's Community House.

- The Crown attorney's office took over a victim-witness protection program, previously run by the Salvation Army.

- The London Battered Women's Advocacy Clinic was set up as a source of legal advice.

Marion Boyd, the director of this clinic, thinks it's time society changed its attitudes about wife abuse. "This is a serious issue," she says, "with serious repercussions."

Research has shown that children who witness family violence are at greater risk for a variety of psychiatric and social problems.[32] We have to teach children, and in particular boys, that violence has no place in intimate relationships.[33] The CCFV has made sure that children from violent families get treatment. But services aren't enough. Sheila Cameron, who chairs the CCFV, says it's essential to change the way children are taught to follow rigid sex roles. In that light, perhaps the most important of all the CCFV's achievements is that it got the issue of family violence onto the public-school curriculum. The fact that Dr. Peter Jaffee, director of the Family Court Clinic and an expert on family violence, was on the school board no doubt helped to get this healthy public policy adopted.

London's programs and policies tackling wife abuse are both changing and reflecting the changes in society's attitudes toward violence. Rosemary Broemling, service coordinator for the FCS, says they're the result of "the right mix of people, in the right place, at the right time."

---

*The Solicitor General of Canada commissioned Dr. Peter Jaffee (now director of the London Family Court Clinic) to conduct a research study on wife abuse in 1979. After this study was finished, the advisory committee to this research project decided to stay together as the London Coordinating Committee on Family Violence. CCFV does not operate services but has coordinated their development.

More Success Stories

Healthy public policies have a proven track record:

- In areas where it has been introduced and enforced, compulsory seat belt legislation has saved many lives.[34] In fact, buckling up has probably saved more accident victims' lives than all the trauma units in the country combined.*

- Laws requiring motorcyclists to wear helmets have been passed, over the objections of those who feel they infringe on personal freedom. With these laws, head injuries as a result of motorbike accidents have dropped by 60%![35]

- In the United States, researchers have found that the newer sections of the interstate expressway system have 20% fewer fatalities.[36] Improved pavement surfaces, and the building of median barriers and wildlife and pedestrian crossings, are believed to be factors in the improvement.**

- Canada's gun-control legislation is another lifesaver. It's certainly one reason why there's a four-fold difference in per capita homicide rates between this country and the United States.[37]

Your Money or Your Health?

Several of our examples of healthy public policy in this chapter may have left you with the impression that economic health and human health are inherently incompatible. The business philosophy that pitted the private water and sewage companies against the reformers in the 19th century, and the tobacco and lead industries against community lobbyists in our own time,

---

*Much of the credit belongs to all the individual doctors and medical associations who campaigned to get these laws passed.

**Using headlights during the day as yet another way to reduce road carnage is now a matter of public debate in Canada. Another is whether we should insist on equipping cars with "air bags," which inflate on impact, protecting drivers involved in head-on collisions, from being run through by the steering column.

seems to suggest that private enterprise has little to gain from healthy public policy.

This is dead wrong. After all, what could be better for a healthy economy than a healthier and therefore more productive population?

All the same, if government and communities really want to protect *everybody's* health, then unhealthy industries must not be phased out at the expense of people working in those industries. We need to create a win:win scenario, one that doesn't penalize one group to save another. For example, if we take steps to restrict the tobacco industry, we also have to do something to protect the livelihood of tobacco farmers and the workers who manufacture tobacco products. A creative labour strategy with appropriate incentives and opportunities for redeployment must accompany these reforms.

Phasing out the tobacco industry needn't bring the dire economic consequences its apologists would have us believe. Just because people quit smoking and therefore stop spending $1,000 a year or more on tobacco, doesn't mean that this money will be pulled out of the economy. It will be spent on other things, that's all — most likely on products far less dangerous to health. And if poor people stop smoking, it's a safe bet that the money they used to spend on cigarettes will go toward much healthier purchases, like food and housing.

There are plenty of powerful incentives for businesses — and governments — to actively support healthy public policies. The insurance industry, for example, has an obvious economic interest in a smoke-free society. Airlines are going to save millions in maintenance costs thanks to the smoking ban on short-haul flights. Health is good for business in many ways. For more examples, let's look at what's happening in two modern industrial nations whose political orientation could not be more diverse: Japan and Sweden.

Lessons from Economic Competitors   Probably no nation in recent times has been singled out more often for its economic performance than Japan. Its spectacular successes in the automotive industry and in the world of high technology hardly need mentioning here. What we want to tell you about instead is how Japan solved a serious social problem that was threatening to undermine its industrial expansion.

Dr. Fraser Mustard, head of the Canadian Institute for Advanced Research, explains what happened. "In the early 1970s, many of Japan's brightest 40-year-olds, the people being groomed to take over senior management positions in the key industries along the Tokyo-Osaka corridor, were leaving their jobs and going back to their regional communities. Why were they leaving? To look after their aging parents. In the Japanese culture, people must look after their parents or the 'loss of face' is profound."

To resolve this problem, the Japanese set in motion a massive reorganization of their major industries. To retain their most valued employees, many companies decentralized their facilities. "The Japanese," says Dr. Mustard, "have no misunderstanding about the importance of science and technology for their survival in the future." They built high-technology centres in 18 key cities. Satellite linkage means these centres can talk to one another easily. Each city is either already served by an airport capable of handling jumbo jets, or is being retrofitted to accommodate them. It's an example of how business can benefit by being responsive to the social and cultural needs of its employees.

Sweden, too, has an economic and social performance that's the envy of much of the modern world.* Sweden's economic strategy is based on full employment. During the early 1980s, while Canadian unemployment rates rose to double-digit levels, Sweden's remained at less than five percent. This small country, with a population less than Ontario's, exports many world-class products; Ikea, Saab, and Volvo are household names in our country. How many Canadian manufacturers do you suppose a Swede could name?

Health is at least part of the rationale behind Sweden's full-employment policy. We know that when people stop being active in the labour force, they deteriorate intellectually, psychologically, and physically. That's why when Swedish workers are laid

---

*It's true that Sweden spends a higher percentage of its GNP on health than we do; wasteful spending on useless and inappropriate medical services is no less common there than here.

off, they're immediately enrolled in retraining programs. Some companies have a policy under which a former employee can continue to come to the office after being laid off, to work on community projects of interest to both the worker and his or her company. That way, the former employee maintains contact with colleagues in the working world, and has an opportunity to develop newer and more marketable skills in the process.

Full employment also means that the Swedes manage their labour market. At any given time, they know that a portion of their work force will be on parental leave — maternity *or* paternity. They even have a policy that encourages workers to take time off, with no loss of seniority or salary, to look after a "friend" in need. This means that if your neighbour, your best friend, your aging parents, or other family members need help at home because of illness or disability, society as a whole will support you as a care-giver. A policy like this explicitly recognizes that formal systems of care can never be more efficient than informal ones.

Sweden's society differs from Canada's in many ways. For example, 80% of that country's work force is unionized, so tripartite approaches involving labour, business, and government are far more common there. Dr. Mustard went to Sweden in 1982 to look at its occupational health and safety policies. "Sweden opted not to create a large bureaucracy within its Ministry of Labour to deal with these issues. Instead, they put labour and management together and said, 'You create the policy.' " The document that resulted from this collaborative effort was ultimately redrafted into formal law. The result — 26 regional occupational health and safety boards with equal representation from management and labour, funded by contributions from employers (through taxation) and employees (through wage transfers). As a footnote, Dr. Mustard adds that in 1982, Sweden's labour ministry employed about a hundred people; Ontario's, that same year, employed about 1,700.

The Swedes' commitment to social equity and a happier work force is not at cross-purposes with their efforts to remain competitive in world markets. A number of economic policies in their country encourage the private sector to be entrepreneurial, and to maintain high standards. The Swedes are far less likely than Canadians, for example, to bail out failing industries. Instead, they maintain their competitive edge by supporting the development of new products and new skills. Sometimes health concerns have featured in this process. For example, Sweden has a nationwide program to promote *ergonometric* progress. (Ergonomics is the study of humans at work. It focusses on the complex interrelationships between workers and their machinery, working methods, and job demands.) Dr. Clyde Hertzman, Director of the occupational health program at the University of British Columbia, gives two examples of how this program led to the development of new products.

- The footwear used by Sweden's armed forces wasn't sensible. So they designed a whole new line for their military, which is now being considered for export.

- Occupational health and safety experts found that traditional drill presses vibrated so much that workers were suffering chronic tendon and nerve disorders in their fingers, wrists, and hands. The result — a completely redesigned drill press with appropriate cushions to reduce vibration. This product is on the export market today.

Sweden's competitive edge has also been helped by a new breed of enlightened managers, who really care about their workers. In *Reinventing the Corporation*, authors John Naisbitt and Patricia Aburdene give this example:

> As a young man, Jan Carlzon made a name for himself by turning the domestic Swedish airline, Linjeflyg, into a very profitable operation. In 1981 Carlzon became president of Scandinavian Airline Systems, SAS, which at the time was losing $17 million per year. After a single year of Carlzon's leadership, SAS was earning $54 million. He did it by turning the organization chart upside down. Truly believing that SAS should be customer-driven, he put those who dealt directly with the customer in charge of the company. The rest of the company on the upside-down organization chart worked for those who dealt with the customers.[38]

So healthy *private* policy can be profitable too!

Healthy Cities: A New Focus

In 1984, Toronto hosted a major conference on healthy public policy. This was a landmark year in many ways: Toronto was celebrating its sesquicentennial, its public health department was 100 years old, the Canadian Public Health Association was turning 25, and it had been ten years since Health and Welfare Canada had released the Lalonde Report.

Immediately after the international conference, organizers held a one-day workshop to discuss how to apply the broad themes of healthy public policy at the city level. They called it "Healthy Toronto 2000." Here was a way to take ideas about health promotion, strengthening communities, and creating healthy environments, and make them concrete. It was exactly what Ilona Kickbush* of the World Health Organization (WHO) had been looking for — a way to tie all these concepts together in one neat package. WHO now has a formal project known as "Healthy Cities," with participants from all over the world, including several from Canada.

"We began," says Dr. Trevor Hancock, "by holding strategic vision workshops for health department workers." What did a healthy city mean to them? "They'd usually start with something like more bikes, fewer cars, more public transit, less air pollution, more green space, employment, housing, less congestion, parks and gardens, safe streets." A long list would be generated. "Then," says Dr. Hancock, "someone would notice that we hadn't mentioned anything about the health care system yet — maybe we should add something about that." In the context of a healthy city, "sickness treatment came up only as an afterthought."

Seattle, Washington, has its own "healthy cities" project, called Kidsplace. "Seattle's population of children has fallen alarmingly in recent years," says Donna James, an assistant to the mayor.

---

*Ilona Kickbush is now the acting director of health promotion for the European division of WHO. In 1984, she was their Officer of Health Education.

"We were disturbed that families transferred here bought homes in the suburbs and avoided the inner city altogether, as an unsafe, dirty environment."

Kidsplace, an idea brought forward by Dr. Robert Aldrich, a pediatrician and professor at the University of Washington, was originally sponsored out of the mayor's office. It began with a survey of the city's children, cleverly disguised as a contest. (The winner, drawn from all completed entries, became "mayor for the day"!) Schools were supplied with an innovative questionnaire full of boxes with adjectives like "ugly," "noisy," "dangerous," and their opposites, "beautiful," "peaceful," "safe." Children were asked to write down the places in Seattle these words brought to mind.

The results gave city planners some good ideas about where to begin improving Seattle's image — at least from a child's perspective. For example, heavy traffic on downtown streets was almost universally denounced by kids as dangerous. The city's engineering department is working to complete a network of bicycle routes connecting all city schools with recreation facilities and parks by 1990. The children also complained that the new aquarium wasn't accessible to them. The tanks were so high they couldn't see the fish. Once again, the city responded. Ramped walkways and lower viewing windows improved the vantage points for children, as well as for other short people, and those using wheelchairs.

Because a lot of children felt insecure being downtown, the city promoted a "Safe Place" program in Seattle's business community. Many downtown windows now exhibit this slogan, which tells children they're welcome to come in and use the telephone to call for help.

Kidsplace is now a separate program, no longer attached to the mayor's office. Donna James explains that they wanted to be sure it would continue regardless of political changes. It now has an independent community board with representatives from the police, libraries, and schools, as well as social workers and parents. The board also includes children as members. "How could we justify not involving them?" asks James. "Kidsplace is for kids!" Future plans include new programs to address family violence, more pedestrian crossways, and an annual Kids Day, with lower prices at restaurants, cinemas, and other city attractions. As the program matures they intend to survey children on a regular basis. According to James, it's the best way "to keep in touch with our constituency."

Full Circle

Hippocrates and the reformers of the 19th century and early 20th century had little reason for faith in curative medicine. Instead, they understood the role that public policy played in protecting society's health. This time-tested solution is no less potent today.

To put it into practice, however, means we have to make the nation's health a high-profile public issue — one that can hold its own in the competition for dollars with funding for the curative system. That's a tall order. To find out how to fill it, please turn to the next chapter.

Chapter 11

The $12 Billion Solution

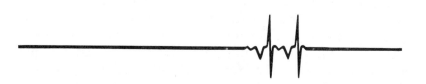

"IF YOU DON'T KNOW where you're going, how will you know when you've arrived?" asks Pran Manga, an economist and professor of health administration at the University of Ottawa. This single question lies at the heart of our health care system's woes. We need to know what we're trying to achieve with our 46 billion health dollars. We need to figure out how to allocate health spending on a more rational basis.

From previous chapters, you already know that our system is terribly inefficient and wasteful. We aren't alone in this assessment. Many doctors and health economists, and even the CMA's Task Force on Resource Allocation,[1] have come to similar conclusions. Now we want to look at how much money we could actually save by reforming our illness treatment system, and how these savings could be reallocated to produce better health. At the end of this chapter, we'll suggest how this reform agenda might be implemented.

As you'll see, a more efficient health care system would generate enormous savings, amounting to *$12 billion annually*. But it's important to understand that even if we start a reform process right now, it will take 10 to 20 years to fully realize these savings. The impossibility of achieving instant results shouldn't discourage us, however. The point is it will take time, and careful strategy, to improve the quality of care Canadians both deserve and expect. Redirecting health care is a bit like steering an oil tanker — you have to start turning the rudders well in advance.

The alternative to well-planned, long-term reform is frightening to contemplate. If we fail to act now, government will have no choice but to dismantle Medicare as we know it. And they'll do it by default. Cost-cutting, not quality, will be the objective. Canada's most popular social program — universal health insurance — will be hacked to pieces by the broadaxes governments have always employed to curb spending. Waiting lists for medical procedures will grow even longer, emergency rooms and nursing homes even more crowded. Quality will suffer and waste will prevail. It's a grim future.

But look on the bright side. We have a good idea what's wrong with our system, and some clear ideas about how to fix it. And by trimming the fat from our current system we can generate enormous savings — savings that can and must be used to make the system work better. As Canadian taxpayers, we collectively pay the piper. Surely that gives us the right to choose what music he plays.

Because the factors affecting our health are so diverse, reforming our sickness treatment system is really only one tactic among many in the fight for a healthy society. While improved living and working conditions are more important to our overall health, a more efficient health care system is also a priority for at least two reasons: first, efficiency implies higher quality, and we all want that, and second, funding for other reforms depends on eliminating or reducing current levels of waste.

In drawing our blueprint for health care reform, we were guided by six principles:

1. Patients must come first.
2. Planning, administration, and delivery of health care should be decentralized.
3. Quality assurance mechanisms must be developed and implemented.
4. The number of doctors entering our system must be immediately reduced.
5. The financial and professional incentives must be changed to encourage efficiency and quality.
6. The system needs to be community-based.

Let's begin by discussing these principles in more detail.

1. Patients Must Come First

Health care is an industry like no other. Its consumers are vulnerable because they don't have the expertise to evaluate the appropriateness of medical decisions. Patients are on the receiving end of health care's "products," the quality of which they're in no position to judge.

This is why some patients consume health care services that aren't useful to them, while others are denied those they desperately need. How is it that our system will pay, without a quibble, for ineffective treatments like chemotherapy for most lung cancers, yet offer only limited access to palliative care? Why should terminal patients be required to pay for their own nurses and homemakers, if they choose to die at home?

Ginette Rodger, executive director of the Canadian Nurses Association, believes that putting patients first is the key to a more efficient health care system. "If we focussed more attention on meeting the needs of individual patients quickly and humanely," she says, "we'd end up using our resources much more wisely."

The Ontario Health Review Panel,[2] chaired by Dr. John Evans, and Québec's Rochon Commission[3] both concluded that our current system isn't responsive to individual needs. How can we change that?

Clearly, we need better strategies for including patients in the treatment decisions affecting them. Sick people need accurate information presented in understandable terms. The question is, how can they get it? One way would be to expand the number of "agents" who interact with patients. Given their track record, we've found that physicians are often terrible at this. They lack training in patient counselling and family dynamics; they frequently resort to technical language that patients find confusing and intimidating; and they often don't schedule enough time to talk to patients.

Nurses, however, could be very effective agents if given the chance. That's why we believe that doctors and nurses should work as joint agents. The nurse/family doctor teams at South Riverdale Community Health Centre could serve as a model for this approach in a primary care setting. Within hospitals, nurses might be more appropriate as the primary agents, because they usually spend much more time with patients. And for patients with multiple problems, particularly those in long-term care settings or rehabilitation facilities, a full multidisciplinary team might be the most appropriate "agent," with one member designated as a contact person for the patient and family.

How would this new kind of agency work for a patient? For one with terminal lung cancer, for example? Well, first of all, the patient and his or her family would receive, either from the family physician or the family nurse,* careful counselling regarding the diagnosis and possible treatment options. Generally, people are in shock for several days after learning about a serious diagnosis, so a number of counselling sessions would be arranged over the next week or so. (Delaying any final decision about treatment for a few days would not jeopardize the patient's status.)

We think it's reasonable to assume that if terminal patients fully understood their condition, most wouldn't choose active treatment. Instead, they'd be more likely to opt for palliative care, including home nursing and homemaking services, perhaps family counselling, and the assurance of home visits from physicians knowledgeable about the control of pain and other symptoms.

Let's look at another example. What would happen if heart attack patients had the chance to make informed choices about their care? Imagine a patient who comes to the emergency department with chest pain. The staff quickly diagnose a heart attack and administer painkillers, an anticlotting agent, and an aspirin.[4] Our patient stabilizes. It's clear after 24 hours that his heart attack isn't serious. He and his family are counselled about his condition and offered various choices: he can stay in hospital and risk all the usual things that can go wrong there (infections, the chance of getting the wrong medication, the noise and

---

*At present, this counselling is given by a hospital-based specialist and is often cursory. Our comments, however, should not be interpreted to mean that hospital specialists should be excluded from patient counselling. Those who want to be involved in this activity would be welcome. We simply want to highlight the fact that specialists are not well-trained in this area and are *usually* not the most appropriate source.

disruption endemic to hospitals, and the like), *or* he can go home.

Of course, the patient must be reassured that it's perfectly safe for him to choose the latter option. He needs to know that if he opts to go home, for the first week or so a nurse will visit four times a day, and a doctor once or twice a day. If our patient or his family has any concerns, either can be in immediate contact with a specialist nurse at the hospital, or even a cardiologist. The patient's heart rhythm can even be checked over the telephone, if necessary. The family should be reassured that emergency resuscitation is available almost as quickly at home as in the hospital.

As the days go by, the hospital-based specialist nurse spends less time on our patient's physical problems, and more working with the family's primary care nurse and doctor to develop a rehabilitation program. The patient and his family are carefully counselled about nutrition, exercise, and sexuality. He's given the strongest support possible to quit smoking.

It's interesting that decisions about where to allocate resources within our health care system become much easier *once we allow patients to make informed choices.* We simply spend money where our patients choose. We could even allow patients, within certain margins of safety, to choose unwisely. If, after hearing all the facts, our terminal lung cancer patient still wants chemotherapy — fine, he can have it. If the heart attack victim wants to stay in hospital a few days, that's all right too. The point is that most people would make sensible decisions if they were given accurate and understandable information and were supported in their right to make a choice.

Simply offering that right could lead to huge reforms. In a system driven by patient choices, we'd have far fewer hospital and nursing-home beds, and far fewer doctors. Letting patients decide would lead to an overall reduction in the use of unnecessary services. This, in turn, would greatly reduce waiting lists, and thereby enhance access to the system for those who urgently require care. At the same time, we'd see a rapid expansion of community-based services, including palliative care, and jobs for many more nurses. Indeed, nursing as a profession would rise in status as new opportunities for professionally rewarding work in community care increased. Many ethical dilemmas currently faced by doctors would be resolved. With patients and their families fully informed, and responsible for making the final decisions, physicians wouldn't have to play God.

Of course, responding quickly and efficiently to what patients need would require a high degree of integration between all the elements of the system. Cooperation, communication, and streamlined administrative procedures would be essential.

A transformation like this wouldn't require masses of new legislation or regulation — just a commitment to the principle that patients come first. Indeed, if anything, we need *less* regulation, not more, if we're going to realize effective health care reform. This is really a call for more market freedom in our system. We can begin by allowing the market to decide how to allocate health care resources. As long as our consumers are well-informed, we can trust them to make the decisions.

2. Decentralization

The principle of decentralization — that is, the granting of decision-making authority to the local level — should be applied to both the planning and the running of our system. But there's a flip side to it: those who make the decisions must be accountable for them.

We believe that our system won't be responsive to local needs until communities are put in charge of their own health. This is because those needs are bound to differ from place to place. Some provinces already have local planning councils to advise health ministries about priorities. But at the moment, except in Québec, these councils have no spending authority. Nor are they accountable to the communities they serve for their recommendations about resource allocation.

That's why we suggest changes in the roles of the provincial health ministries and regional agencies. The provinces would still set an overall budget for health care. They'd also be responsible for establishing minimum standards, interregional coordination, and for supplying the regions with the pertinent information and technical expertise they need to make wise spending decisions. Funding would be apportioned differentially among regions within the province. The amount each region received would be based on a capitation formula[*] — that is, a set amount for every person living in the region, adjusted for age, sex, the burden of illness, and other relevant socio-economic factors.[5]

In a reformed system, the province would set minimum standards for personnel and facilities. For example, a province might set a minimum ratio of 1.2 acute care beds per 1,000 population. If a region wanted to surpass the provincial standard and fund, say, four acute care beds per 1,000, they could do it, but they'd have to give up some of their community programs in exchange. In such a system, the trade-offs between one type of service and another would be explicit, not hidden like they are now.

The regional health councils would, of course, be required to meet provincial standards. But having complied with these minimum provisions, they would be able to spend their remaining resources according to their own local priorities. A community with a high proportion of senior citizens might choose to spend relatively more on programs for its elderly, on home care and seniors day-care programs. Another community might happen to have a high teenage pregnancy rate, in which case it would probably devote more funding to family planning, and parenting programs for single teen mothers.

The point of encouraging such variety is obvious. Central planning, the kind based on province-wide "averages," is insensitive to diversity. It tends to produce cookie-cutter health care services that aren't based on real needs. It leads to the overfunding of some programs and the underfunding of others. Decentralizing decision-making, and giving more clout to the regions, is the best way to fine-tune our system.

If we're going to transfer authority to regional agencies, we're also going to have to make those agencies accountable to the public for their decisions. One way would be to have elected representation on these local planning councils. We could look to the

---

[*]Obviously, large cities with a disproportionate concentration of hospitals — particularly the hugely expensive teaching hospitals — would require special treatment. Capitation alone would not be an adequate funding mechanism for these facilities. All the same, it makes no sense to penalize the rest of the country, by designing a new system to fit the special needs of these large cities.

school boards as a model and elect trustees for this purpose, as suggested by the Rochon Commission. Or we could use back-benchers from provincial legislatures as suggested by Guy Chevrette MNA, a former Québec health minister. Either way, the public must have a say in the decisions made on its behalf.

You may be wondering whether there's any role at all for the federal government within this decentralized framework. We think there is. Specifically, Health and Welfare Canada should be involved in coordinating and conducting health surveys, assessing new and emerging technologies, coordinating a more rational approach to manpower planning, and promoting healthy public policies. Federal leadership in these activities is necessary to reaffirm that our nation's health is Canada's most vital asset.

3. Implementing Quality Control

When defining medical quality using "patients-first" as the fundamental principle, we have to look at what benefits patients reap from our health care efforts. Specifically, we have to find ways to reduce the rates of overtesting, unnecessary surgery, and poor prescribing, all of which are characteristic of present-day medical practice.

Let's begin by looking at who's responsible for the quality of our health care system. Is it the provincial health ministers? The colleges of physicians and surgeons? Hospital accreditation committees? Hospital boards? In other words, who's in charge?

We put these questions to politicians, senior civil servants, and officials from organized medicine all over Canada, and never received a satisfactory answer — the overall responsibility for quality was always someone else's job. Governments have been slow to act in this area; they don't want doctors to accuse them of interfering with professional autonomy. Hospitals are similarly reluctant to impose effective quality-control mechanisms; they don't want to upset doctors, either. The result is that we have no quality-assurance programs of any consequence anywhere in the country, except in a handful of hospitals.[6] At the same time, the medical associations, which represent physicians' interests, typically deny any role for their organizations in improving the quality of medical care; it's up to the colleges of physicians and surgeons, they claim. It's true that the colleges are the official medical licencing bodies; the legal authority to establish and enforce standards of practice is theirs and theirs alone. But few are living up to this responsibility.

Dr. Adam Linton, a director of the Ontario Medical Association, says that unless the profession takes steps to improve its own practices, the government will be forced to introduce blunt cost-cutting instruments and quality of care will be even further compromised. We agree, and urge more involvement from organized medicine. Medical students and practising physicians must be taught how to apply the principles of epidemiology and biostatistics to improve their decision-making. And because the vast majority of surgeries and other non-drug therapies have never been rigorously evaluated, more money must be spent on research to determine what works and what doesn't. This must include a collective review of existing evidence by doctors, to establish new diagnostic and therapeutic standards. These standards must then find their way quickly into clinical practice.

Better-quality health care also demands strict requirements for continuing medical education among physicians already in practice. Provincial colleges of physicians and surgeons have a responsibility to protect public safety; they must insist that the practitioners they licence make the effort to keep abreast of new developments in their respective fields. The same holds true for the Royal College of Physicians and Surgeons of Canada, which certifies specialists.

Ensuring high-quality medicine also requires non-threatening, constructive processes for peer review. A major step in the right direction would be to have more doctors practising in groups.

The thrust of these reforms is not to punish doctors, but to help them be the best at their chosen profession. "My vision for a future health care system," says Dr. John Evans, "includes incentives that support upgrading doctors' skills and knowledge and incorporating them into clinical practice, not as ordained commands for performance, but as helpful encouragement to share what works."

Improving the quality of care also means determining the appropriateness of providers according to what the evidence shows about their cost-effectiveness. By doing this, we'd be freeing ourselves to decide who does what based on the training, interests, and skills of the practitioner and how well these match the needs of the patient. Under such a system, nurses would provide much of the primary care now provided by doctors. Doctors, in turn, would have more time to do what they know best — diagnosing and treating illness. Those doctors who want to see healthy people, still could (even though nurses receive more training in wellness care), but they would have to accept lower fees. The role for specialists would change as well: they'd do what they know how to do best — diagnosing and treating complicated cases. This new orientation would open the door for a number of other health and social-service professionals. Duly licenced midwives, chiropodists, physiotherapists, and the like could all make their contribution, within a scope of practice determined by evidence of their cost-effectiveness.

A firm commitment to quality care for the patient means we have to find ways to end the territorial squabbling between government and doctors, doctors and nurses, nurses and nurses' aides, and so on. "Sectarianism," according to Dr. Evans, "is part of the problem and part of the solution. Addressing it requires patience — you have to confront people with a broader view, inspire them to respond to the challenge."

Present legislation gives nearly all the decision-making power to physicians. While we could always amend the laws and regulations, what's really needed in order to establish more equitable decision-making is a new attitude — mutual respect.

4. Reduce the Number of Doctors

Once we accept the principles that patients must come first, and that we should determine the providers, as well as the therapies to be employed, according to their cost-effectiveness, we have no choice but to view our current oversupply of physicians as a monumental crisis.

That's why we have to take immediate steps to stem the tidal wave of newly trained physicians that threatens to swamp our system. The problem is actually getting worse. Between 1975 and 1981, the number of doctors in Canada increased by 2.7% per year. But between 1981 and 1987, the number of doctors increased by 3.5% per year.[7] To maintain our present ratio of 1 doctor per 465 people, we would only need to produce 1,600 new doctors every year.* Instead, we're adding about 2,200. Just to stay even, we have to reduce that number by 30% right away.

Marc Lalonde, the one-time federal health minister, has returned to private life as a corporate lawyer. He also chairs the board of Hotel Dieu, Montreal's largest French-speaking hospital. Lalonde suggested one solution — the closing of one or more of our medical schools. but he admitted that such a decision would be extremely difficult for any politician. But suppose government did have the necessary political will, suppose we even had national consensus for closure? How could we choose which school should go? One factor to consider is Canada's uneven distribution of doctors; most have set up practice in large urban areas. Attracting doctors to remote regions is a challenge for some provinces. That's why, for starters, you'd have to protect medical schools in Newfoundland and Saskatchewan from outright closure. Without those schools, these provinces would have even more difficulty attracting and retaining specialists. Closing those facilities would also mean that students from these provinces would be forced to move away to learn medicine; how many graduates would likely return to set up practice back home after such a long absence?

On the other hand, you might well ask whether we really need the 350 new doctors Montreal's two medical schools (one French and one English) produce every year, or the 250 who enter the system from the University of Toronto. And while we're on the subject, why does Ontario need five medical schools at all? Why does Alberta need two, when British Columbia manages with only one?

Of course, there's an alternative to outright closure. We could achieve the same 30% drop in numbers by reducing enrollments in *all* medical schools. This would have a negligible effect on savings to the university; in fact, it would *increase* the per-student

---

*This calculation includes an average yearly rate of attrition of 1.87% in the physician supply (as was seen between 1975 and 1985), and an average yearly increase of 1% in the Canadian population. We haven't adjusted these figures for the aging of the population or the changing "productivity" of physicians. On the other hand, in this section we have also not included the reduction in the number of doctors possible with the appropriate use of doctors, nurses, and other health professionals.

costs of training doctors. However, politically, it's a more palatable alternative. One dean of medicine said he'd be more than willing to consider such a move, but no one from the province had ever approached him. In the end, the option selected isn't nearly as important as the decision itself — to do something right away to turn off the tap. That's why we suggest that Canada undertake a nationally coordinated strategy for human-resource planning in medicine, using the kind of needs-based methodology employed by the GMENAC study in the United States.* Of course, this strategy should be used to determine how many personnel we require in *all* health professions, not just medicine.

5. Change the Financial and Professional Incentives

Reforming health care also means changing the financial and structural incentives that now actually reward inefficiency. To do this we need to find new ways to fund hospitals, and new ways to pay health care providers.

Funding for hospitals and other institutions should be tied to the quality of care they provide, and how well they meet the acute care needs of the communities they serve. They must be able to assess their performance. This means they need a versatile cost-accounting system that integrates clinical and financial information.

To do a good job, hospitals need performance standards that relate to the decisions their doctors make about things like length of stay and surgical, drug, and laboratory utilization. But the only way to enforce these standards is to have physicians actively involved in hospital management. Sunnybrook Hospital could serve as a model. The physician-managers there are accountable for spending within their own departments. The incentive for responsible management at Sunnybrook is explicit: efficient departments — that is, those that come in under budget — get to spend part of their "savings" on new programs or equipment. (This assumes, of course, that the new service corresponds to a regionally determined "need.")

As efficiency and quality improve, hospitals and long-term care

---

*The GMENAC process was discussed in detail in Chapter 6.

facilities will face new challenges. Shorter lengths of stay in acute care, and the expansion of home-care services, will mean that the average patient in an institution will be sicker than the average one is today. That's because patients well enough to receive services at home will be discharged, or won't be admitted at all. There's no question that nursing staff, already hard pressed to meet patient needs now, will face even higher demands unless we reduce the number of hospital beds. And this is exactly what has to happen if we're going to circumvent the effects of Roemer's Law (which tells us that unless we close beds, they'll be filled). But closing beds doesn't represent any threat to health care. We've already shown how more efficient systems manage very well with far lower bed ratios; cutting back on beds has not affected the health status of their patients. And bed closure is the best way to improve the lot of hospital nurses. With fewer patients to care for, albeit needier ones, nurses will be able to get on with the job they want to do. We need to put *caring* back into health care, and nursing is an ideal place to start doing that.

When it comes to payment for health care workers, the need for reform is quite obvious. Almost everyone we interviewed agreed that fee-for-service often encourages doctors to overdo it. Vickery Stoughton, the executive director of the Toronto Hospital Corporation,* says fee-for-service doesn't create the right incentives for health care. Glenn Wilson, a professor at the University of North Carolina, and an adviser to the Sault Ste. Marie Group Health Centre since its inception, says that "a system that operates under fee-for-service is simply not manageable." Even Dr. Hugh Scully, past president of the OMA, wants government to examine alternative methods of delivering and funding health care.[8]

This doesn't necessarily mean we have to abandon fee-for-service entirely. It does mean we have to cap the overall budgets for physician services, which in most provinces are still open-ended. In addition, physicians should have the option of being paid generous salaries, with full benefits, as an alternative to fee-for-service. A survey of more than 2,000 physicians in Nova Scotia, Québec, Ontario, Alberta, and British Columbia found that

---

*The THC, as it is known, is an amalgamation of Toronto General Hospital and Toronto Western Hospital.

42% approved of a "salaried system for all physicians in hospital or group practice which included such benefits as pension and vacation and overtime payments."[9] At the very least, physician-managers, who head hospital departments, should be on salary, with the opportunity to share in bonuses as a reward for good management.

At the same time, our system needs better ways to reward other health professionals. Improved salaries, more generous benefits, and supportive working conditions are needed to attract and retain high-calibre staff. This is particularly true for nurses. Their pay-scale range must be expanded to reflect their skills, responsibilities and experience. Similarly, they deserve more status within the system. We'll have to offer them incentives like the chance to participate in management, paid leave for continuing education, and more autonomy consistent with their training and experience, if we're going to keep them in the system. Unless steps are taken to make nursing more professionally and financially rewarding, we'll continue to lose nurses to other fields. Remember Louise Roy, the nurse from Verdun's Hospital in the Home program? She was on the verge of leaving nursing altogether when she decided instead to head the nursing team for this innovative program. Today she loves her job. "It's wonderful to have the chance to make a real difference," she told us. "This is what nursing is all about."

Finally, we need to encourage patients, who are the consumers of health care, to choose the best services we can provide. In the United States, competing sources of health care are compared in the media on a regular basis. Consumers are treated to masses of statistics about the quality of various local hospitals; often included are data on surgical rates, lengths of stay, mortality rates, quality of meals, competence and pleasantness of personnel, and so forth. We need more of this kind of "free enterprise" in Canada's health care; it needn't compromise our commitment to a non-profit system. Competition in quality is healthy competition in more ways than one.

6. Make the System More Community-Based

Many people we interviewed cautioned against using hospitals to spawn new community programs. "Hospitals have a narrow focus on individuals and illness," says Ginette Rodger, "and that model simply isn't appropriate for community care.'' Most people who've been hospitalized associate the experience with a loss in personal autonomy. "A hospital has to deal with life-threatening illness," says June Callwood, who's had extensive experience launching community programs. The hospital approach encourages passivity: patients must follow orders and adhere to hospital schedules. But this authoritarian model isn't appropriate for community services. "I think they should stick to their job," says Callwood, "and let others deliver community care." Fred Griffith, executive director of the Sault Ste. Marie centre, adds that hospitals, by and large, don't have the expertise to deliver community services.

We agree. We believe reform of our health care system should begin "at the bottom," with community programs developed by and for the community. And that hospitals should be influenced by community programs, not the other way around. This reorientation will mean a relative shrinkage in hospital-based services and a dramatic expansion in community services. But we'll have to be very careful during this transformation to avoid disenfranchising hospital workers. We suggest that for health care reform to succeed, planning a labour transfer from hospitals to the community will have to follow these three principles:

1.   No net loss of jobs
2.   No loss of union affiliation
3.   No decrease in wages or benefits

And of course, retraining will be necessary to provide those now working in hospitals with the tools they'll need to deliver community care effectively. We believe the net effect of this transfer will be positive for health care workers as well as their patients. Judging by the experience of the nurses working in the Hospital in the Home program, health care workers employed in these new community jobs will find them much more professionally and personally rewarding.

How Much Could We Save?

Figure 11.1 shows that if we were to begin a reform process right away according to the six principles we've just outlined, we could

generate enormous annual savings within 10 to 20 years. It's true
that some of these savings could be achieved much more quickly
— a reduction in prescription drug costs, for instance, could be
realized almost instantly. But most savings will take one to two
decades to accrue — it will take many years, for example, to
reduce the number of doctors to a more appropriate level.

Figure 11.1 The potential for annual savings from more efficient
sickness treatment. (All numbers are in millions of 1987 dollars.)

Item	1987 Public expenditures*	Reduced by	Maximum Savings	Reduced by	Minimum Savings
Hospitals	$16,805	60%	10,083	25%	4,201
Other institutions	3,883	67%	2,602	28%	1,087
Physicians	7,225	50%	3,613	20%	1,445
Prescribed drugs	1,237	50%	618	25%	309
Totals	29,150**		16,916		7,042

*The public portion of health expenditures in these four categories is an esti-
mate based on the proportion publicly covered in 1985. (Source: Health and
Welfare Canada)

**Total health spending (private and public) for these four categories in 1987
was $33,395,000,000. (Source: Health and Welfare Canada)

Except for prescription drugs, the estimates of potential savings
in this table are based on the actual experience of many of the
innovative programs discussed in Chapter 9. In other words, *if
our system could match their level of efficiency, this is how much
we could save.* Here's how we arrived at the amounts:

Hospital Care: We based our estimate for maximum savings
on the use of hospital services by On Lok and by the Dane
County, Wisconsin, mental-health program. Readers will recall
from Chapter 9 that On Lok serves people who have already been
assessed as needing institutional care. But On Lok's innovative
program helps virtually all of its participants remain in the community. Despite the fact that they're very elderly, often have multiple medical problems, and tend to be quite poor, only one
percent of them are in an acute care hospital at any given time.

In fact, only 14% of On Lok's overall budget is spent on institutional care — a figure that includes both hospital and nursing-home services. Ontario, by contrast, spends 64% of its health care budget on acute care hospitals. If Ontario were to match On Lok's performance, it would reduce its hospital expenditures by 78%.

Similarly, both the United States and Canada as a whole spend about 70% of the money allocated to mental health on hospital care. But the innovative program in Dane County devotes only 17% of its mental-health budget to inpatient care. By matching Dane County's performance, we would reduce hospital expenditures by 76%.

In estimating the maximum potential savings in hospital care we have tried to be conservative, and so suggest that Canada could reduce its hospital spending by 60% *if appropriate community services were in place.*

For our minimum estimate, we looked at data from the Saskatoon Community Clinic, and from the Group Health Cooperative of Puget Sound in Seattle, Washington, where doctors work in groups and are paid on salary. Spending on hospital care by these two groups is 30% and 40% lower, respectively, than for patients attended by fee-for-service physicians. (The use of hospital services among patients who go to the Sault Ste. Marie Group Health Centre is similarly lower; they use 25% fewer hospital days, at a per capita cost 25 to 30% lower than that of Algoma District residents cared for by fee-for-service doctors.)

Once again, we have chosen to err on the conservative side, and have based our minimum estimate for savings on a 25% reduction in hospital costs.

Other Institutional Care (primarily nursing homes): We also used On Lok's experience to estimate maximum savings on institutional care. At any given time, only about five percent of On Lok participants are in nursing homes, even though to be admitted to the program in the first place, clients must be assessed by independent state authorities as needing nursing-home care. The institutionalization rate for Canadians in the same age group as On Lok participants — whose average age is 81 years — is about 15%.[10] This is astonishingly high, particularly when you consider that many Canadians in that age bracket live quite independently and don't require any special services at all. In other words, most 81-year-old Canadians wouldn't meet On Lok's stringent admission requirements. If we Canadians were able to match On Lok's performance, we'd achieve a 67% reduction in institutional spending — our maximum estimate for potential savings in this category.

For our minimum estimate of savings, we looked at the institutional rates[11] for seniors in Australia (5.9%) and the U.S. (5.3%), and established a target rate midway between the two (5.6%). Since Canada now institutionalizes 9.45% of all seniors, meeting this target would represent a 41% reduction. However, we felt we had to discount this figure by 30% because patients remaining in long-term care would be sicker on average than those who are there today. Accordingly, our minimum estimate calls for reducing other institutional spending by 28%.

Physician Services: We identify two major strategies for reducing the costs of physician services over time: reducing the supply of physicians, and using non-physician personnel more effectively. You've already seen how prepaid, group-practice HMOs in the United States are able to provide quality care with far fewer doctors. The Group Health Cooperative of Puget Sound and Kaiser Permanente's Northern California Region both use about 1 doctor for every 800 members. Canada's current doctor-to-population ratio is 1 for every 465. Even though the Canadian figure includes an unknown number of physicians who aren't in full-time practice, it seems reasonable to conclude that we could drastically reduce our supply of doctors with no risk to patients — especially if we acted on already existing evidence to expand the role of non-physician personnel.

For example, we already know that primary care nurses could provide much of the care that's currently being delivered by family doctors.[12] And we know that midwives attending normal deliveries perform *at least* as well as doctors.[13] And that specialist nurses could replace specialist doctors for much of the care provided in hospitals. (Chedoke-McMaster Hospital, for example, uses specially trained nurses instead of doctors in its intensive care nursery.) There's no simple way to combine these data.

But it does seem reasonable to conclude that the most rational use of personnel would likely result in a 50% reduction in expenditures on physician services. So 50% is our maximum estimate of savings. Our minimum estimate is considerably more conservative, and calls for a 20% reduction in spending.

Drug Costs: The maximum estimate for savings, which represents a 50% reduction in prescription-drug expenditures, assumes four improvements: more appropriate prescribing by doctors; the use of generic drugs instead of brand-name products, wherever possible; the substitution of cheaper but therapeutically equivalent products (for example, using aspirin as the first treatment for arthritis instead of other antiarthritic drugs, which might cost ten times as much); and bulk drug-purchasing by provincial governments. The minimum estimate simply reduces the maximum by half.

Overall, the total potential savings from these four spending categories alone range from a minimum of just over $7 billion to a maximum of almost $17 billion! For the purposes of the following discussion, we've decided to split the difference and so estimate that within 10 to 20 years we could reasonably expect to save $12 billion annually from our sickness treatment system. That's more than enough to fund an impressive reform package.

What to Do With $12 Billion Dollars: A Plan for Reallocation

Before going any further, we need to issue a word of caution. These "savings" must not be used to pay down government deficits, nor to reduce taxes, however appealing such options will be to provincial governments. They must be ploughed back into the system to make it better. The whole point of this exercise is to improve health status and quality of care, not to cut health spending. The good news is that we can fund these improvements *within existing health budgets.*

Perhaps an example would help explain why we must reallocate. When Ontario was looking for ways to reduce health spending in the 1970s, the province initiated a wide-scale closure of mental-health facilities. Thousands of psychiatric patients were de-institutionalized." What had seemed at first like a very humane policy turned sour. These emotionally fragile people were suddenly out on the streets without adequate community services to support their adjustment to independence. The government's failure to reallocate enough resources for supportive housing, job training, and crisis intervention for this vulnerable population is a well-documented disgrace.

What follows is a plan for reallocating the $12 billion worth of savings just described, in ways we believe will improve both our health and the quality of care we receive from our health care system. In preparing this agenda for reform we were guided by two firm convictions: first, that it's vital to attack the roots of ill health, instead of just treating illness itself; and second, that we must commit ourselves to a rigorous evaluation of *all* programs, as the only arbitrator of what works and what doesn't.

The first of these convictions is reflected in a number of our reform proposals — those which are specifically aimed at reducing inequality — for the simple reason that inequality *causes* ill health. All the same, we're forced to admit that we won't win the "war against poverty" — or "racism," or "sexism" — using the savings from a more efficient health care system alone. The savings simply aren't large enough to do the job. We agree with Drs. Spasoff* and Offord and many others, that Canadians also need a fairer tax system, universal and accessible day-care, and other reforms. And, like Marc Lalonde, Pauline Jewett, and others, we agree that Canada's priorities are not well-served by investing billions of dollars on a fleet of nuclear submarines. Clearly, a full discussion of these and other policies is beyond the scope of this book, but their impact on our "health" in the broadest sense should not be forgotten.

With respect to our second conviction, we'd like to alert readers that our plan reallocates over a billion dollars to research and evaluation. We've been very critical of medicine for its cavalier neglect of research that would establish the cost-effectiveness of

---

*Dr. Robert Spasoff is a professor of community medicine at the University of Ottawa. He chaired a commission on health goals for the Ontario government. Dr. Dan Offord is a professor of psychiatry at McMaster University. He was one of the authors of the Ontario Child Health Survey.

various diagnostic tests and treatments. But this criticism also applies to social and economic programs. It's time to find out what works and what doesn't. With a billion dollars, we'll have a chance to do just that.

The outline* that follows is really just a starting point for debate — we haven't crossed all the t's or dotted all the i's. At the same time, we know that some of our recommendations will have more intrinsic appeal than others. Legislators and other decision-makers may be tempted to pick out only the easiest ones, leaving the tougher reforms aside. Let's be clear that a patchwork approach will only add to the policy confusion that pervades our current system. When you change a tire, you have to tighten all the nuts, not just one or two, or the car simply won't be safe to drive. Similarly, to be effective, health reform must be implemented as a coherent, integrated package. Vague tinkering with the system's various bits and pieces won't work. We have an opportunity to have the best health care system in the world. Let's not blow it.

Charting a Course: $100 Million

It should be obvious from earlier chapters that Canada's health care system badly needs a sense of direction. Where are we now? Where do we want to go? A health-goals process is one way to address these challenging questions.**

The United States has been pursuing health goals ever since 1979, when the surgeon general's report, *Healthy People*, identified five main goals and 15 priorities.[14] Health professionals, government officials, and consumer groups consulted with each other to flesh out these goals. They came up with 226 detailed objectives, specifying targets and implementation dates.[15] The Americans have even published mid-term reviews of their

---

*A summary of this outline is presented in Figure 11.2 on page 323.

**The European Region of the World Health Organization has also been involved in a health-goals process. (See: *Targets for Health for All: Targets in support of the European regional strategy for health for all*, Copenhagen, 1985.)

progress,[16] and are now setting new goals and targets for the year 2000.*

By comparison, Canada's involvement in goal-setting has been much more timid. We've been hesitant about setting measurable targets and implementation dates. The 1984 Québec publication, *Objectif Santé*, for example, suggests goals but doesn't specify these vital elements.[17] All the same, it makes a valuable contribution in another direction by setting out an analytical framework for establishing goals. (At the federal level, Jake Epp's report, *Achieving Health for All: A Framework for Health Promotion*, is similarly helpful.) Ontario established an expert panel chaired by Dr. Robert Spasoff, a professor of community medicine at the University of Ottawa, to set in motion a health-goals process there. Its report, like the one from Québec, anticipated the need for targets and dates, but didn't establish them.

Of course, setting health goals doesn't have to be a top-down process, with all the initiative coming from senior levels of government. For example, at least two of Ontario's district health councils (DHCs are regional organizations that advise the health ministry about local priorities) have established their own goals. Mick Peters, executive director of Durham Region's DHC, is excited about the potential of this exercise to inspire reform. "Because the process is future-oriented, and does not make assumptions about the status quo remaining intact," he says, "it allows us to dream a little and think about where we would put our dollars ideally."

Durham Region's goals do set out explicit targets and implementation dates. For example, one of its goals is to have 95% of its elderly cared for at home by the year 2000. "To achieve that," says Peters, "we have to cut down on the number of long-term care beds and instead fund more community services." That's why his region is not encouraging the development of more nursing homes. They want more home care instead.

---

*In the United States, the health-goals process is viewed as a "national" rather than a "federal" undertaking. This distinction has served to protect it from partisan politics. New administrations may come and go, but the process continues.

We've earmarked $100 million for a health-goals process and for monitoring our progress in achieving those goals. Some of this money — about $25 million — would go toward a comprehensive, periodic national health survey. Such baseline data is essential for measuring our starting point and charting our successes and failures along the road to reform. With this level of funding, Canada could rise to world prominence in epidemiological research by developing new health indicators — ones that integrate social and economic factors with the more traditional measures such as mortality and illness rates. One day, Dr. Fraser Mustard predicts, we might even be able to offer the public a national "health account," figures that people "would take as seriously as they do the consumer price index or GNP today."

Putting Healthy Public Policy into Practice: $6.1 Billion

Income security, taxation, housing, energy, the environment, transportation, education, food and agriculture, labour and business . . . . We know that all of these policy areas have an impact on our health. And that all are subject to legislation and/or regulation by federal, provincial, regional, and local governments. This means, of course, that governments have important tools outside the health care system itself, that they can use to improve people's health.

That's why we suggest taking a lesson from a well-established practice in another sector: the environmental impact assessment. To safeguard our natural resources and protect fragile ecosystems from damage, our government requires environmental impact assessments for all proposed large-scale developments. This policy has led us to abandon certain projects altogether, and to modify the design and location of others.

We believe that this technique could and should be applied to address health concerns. A "health impact assessment" would review proposed policies, laws, and regulations for their likely effect on our health. If we can protect the migration routes of caribou or the spawning grounds of salmon using this strategy, surely it would be worth trying in the interests of our own health.

We believe that lawmakers will find strong public support for healthy policies. For example, a Gallup poll found that over three-quarters of Canadian adults would favour cigarette-tax increases if the additional funds were used to sponsor the arts activities previously funded by tobacco companies, to help tobacco farmers find alternative crops, to finance public-health education, or to sponsor medical research. Over 80% of those polled wanted the laws restricting the sale of tobacco to minors enforced.[18] We allocate $100 million to set up a health impact assessment process, with the amount split between the federal government and the provinces.

From earlier chapters, you already know that inequality makes people sick. Poverty, racism, and sexism are toxic agents that must be eradicated. Every major health-goals process to date has noted the wide disparity in health status between rich and poor, and has called for social and economic reforms to reduce inequality. Where do Canadians stand on this issue? Would we champion equal access to health with the same fervour we champion equal access to health care? If the answer is yes, then we must view the unequal distribution of wealth, and discrimination against women and minorities, as health issues as well as social-justice issues.

"There's no point," says June Callwood, "treating the symptoms of poverty down the road through our education, corrections, and health care systems when the real problem is too little money." Many families are unable to provide their children with an adequate level of nutrition, housing, and clothing. Not all of these families are on social assistance; many have jobs but are unable to earn enough to cover these basics. So the first strategy we suggest is to put more money in the hands of those who haven't enough to secure these essentials.

The rallying point for this initiative is the value we place on our children. Dr. Dan Offord told us that Canadians have a collective responsibility to make sure that all children have the opportunity to become productive members of society. As a nation, we simply can't afford to have one-sixth of them growing up in poverty. If there is, as Dr. Offord believes, "a massive reservoir of good will toward poor children," let's tap it. Of course, rooting out poverty among children means ensuring their parents have an adequate income.

This isn't an unattainable objective. Dr. Spasoff notes how Canada's social policies have already managed to eliminate the most extreme levels of poverty among one group in our society.

"Extreme poverty occurs among all age groups," he says, "but stops suddenly among those over 65, thanks to [the availability of supplements to] Old Age Security. I find it interesting that we've managed through this pension program to do something that works. Is it a coincidence that our elderly seem to be getting healthier, too?"

As a start, we've reallocated almost $5.5 billion to reduce economic inequality, particularly among women, who head almost all single-parent families, and native peoples, whose extreme poverty is a national disgrace. Over half this amount is for income security — but not necessarily for present social-assistance programs. Like Dr. Clyde Hertzman and others, we believe that self-esteem suffers when people don't have useful tasks to perform, and that this in itself is unhealthy. Current welfare schemes don't work. They fail to provide adequate income and at the same time discourage recipients from seeking employment. We don't have a magic solution to offer. All the same we think a better welfare system would incorporate incentives for working, a less intrusive bureaucracy, and a recognition that being a parent is the most important job in our society. That's why we'd like to see this new money used to support income in ways that empower those who are disadvantaged. That's also the rationale for funding adult literacy programs, and skills development and recreational programs for children. That's why we target funds for economic development programs for women and native peoples. It's a first step toward giving poor people the tools and the power they need to escape their poverty and become productive.

We'd like to remind our hard-nosed readers that people from middle- and upper-income brackets have already benefited substantially from programs originally intended for the poor. Dr. Marshall Jones, a professor at Pennsylvania State University, says that summer camps, schools, and hospitals for the poor were rapidly adopted by all segments of society, once their benefits became clear.[19] He adds that programs for poor children, in particular, have proven a rich source of social innovation.

Because housing is such a crucial determinant of health, our reallocation strategy also includes significant funding for both permanent and transitional housing. Low-income Canadians, as well as special groups — like disabled people, the mentally ill, and women fleeing abusive relationships — desperately need affordable housing. Thus, our provision for the construction of 20,000 new units of permanent housing every year. On top of that, we advise that the number of transition homes for abused women and children be quadrupled, and that the number of rape crisis and sexual assault centres be substantially increased.[20] Because workers in both settings are notoriously underpaid, our reallocation includes a major increase in the average level of funding for both new and existing facilities.

"Until we create true social and economic equality between the sexes," says Constance Backhouse, a law professor at the University of Western Ontario, "we won't be able to eliminate family violence." At the moment we have neither. Women continue to earn 60% of what men earn, even though they work significantly longer hours. And negative images of sexuality continue to thrive in the media. According to Backhouse, children need to be taught about the benefits of sexual equality, they need to be given the tools to cope with the negative images that pervade our culture. That's why our reallocation includes funding for prevention programs in our schools and in our media — programs to promote healthier attitudes toward sexuality. For the same reason, we set aside funds for treatment programs aimed at abusers and their victims. Attitudes are learned. They can change.

Obviously, these new programs alone aren't enough to establish sexual equality. Many others, such as universal child care, improvements in maternity and paternity leave, and the enforcement of existing anti-discrimination laws, are also basic requirements. But they do represent a step in the right direction.

To assess the success of these health-improvement strategies, we have earmarked a full three percent of all new program monies (almost $200 million) for research and evaluation.

Promoting Health: $700 Million

No, we don't have all the answers when it comes to promoting health and preventing disease. But that's no reason to abstain from action in areas where we *do* have good evidence. It's very clear from research that if we ate better, exercised more often, quit smoking and drank less, had more friends and social contacts, and had safer workplaces, we could dramatically improve our health. In fact, if we acted on this information, we could sharply reduce deaths from cardiovascular and respiratory disease, cancer, accidents, suicide, cirrhosis of the liver, and many other maladies of modern life.

Because nearly all Canadians are at risk for heart disease, we advocate heart health programs targeted at communities rather than at individuals. There's less "crash for the cash" when you screen only those individuals at highest risk. After all, most heart attack deaths occur among people considered at low or middle risk. It's our society's lifestyle that's sick, not that of only a few individuals.

To ensure that all Canadians get a good start in life, we also advocate community-based health-promotion strategies aimed at decreasing the prevalence of low-birthweight babies. Our society needs to become more aware about the connection between undersized infants and the mother's nutritional level, smoking habits, and access to social supports. Possible models include the Montreal Diet Dispensary and the Toronto Public Health Department's "Healthiest Babies Possible" program. (These programs should be considered an adjunct to improvements in primary care during pregnancy — improvements that depend on some of the reforms outlined in the next section of this chapter.)

Our reallocation also includes funding for programs that promote participation in physical exercise. Regular activity is known to prevent heart disease and osteoporosis, and also increases an individual's sense of well-being. Strategies to encourage participation could include constructing new recreation facilities, waiving existing user fees (poor kids in Toronto swim for free, in Vancouver they pay), and hiring more physical-education personnel in schools.

Our workplaces should promote and protect our health. At present, they're too often a *source* of injury and illness. Accordingly, our reallocation earmarks funds for prevention programs that would reduce occupational accidents and diseases, and for health-promotion programs that would encourage workers to get more physical exercise and quit smoking.

We also allocate funds for health promotion specifically targeted at Canada's native populations. In particular, we suggest the development of community-based programs aimed at address-ing violence, substance abuse, and prenatal care.

Even though there's already substantial scientific evidence to support most of these programs, our reallocation assumes that three percent of all new monies ($21 million) will be spent on research and evaluation. Research can be a powerful program-development tool. Funding it at this level will help to refine pro-grams so they can be even more effective.

Healing Health Care: $5.1 Billion

In deciding where to allocate over $5 billion to improve the quality of our health care system, we followed the advice of virtually every official report on health care that's come out in the last 20 years. That's why we devote most of these resources to community-based services.

We allocate $800 million to improve the network of community-based primary care. That's enough to fund 800 com-munity health centres or primary care "modules."* Within these centres:

- Both providers and consumers should have an effective voice in management and policy.

- The staff should be multidisciplinary, and include physi-cians, nurses, and rehab, social, and community workers, as well as other personnel as dictated by local conditions.

- Funding should not be based on fee-for-service (although limited fee-for-service payment may be appropriate for cer-tain staff).

- Both individual and community-based programs for prevention and health promotion should be available.

A typical centre would serve about 6,000 clients, using four primary care teams. An organization of this size is small enough

---

*Chapter 9 offered a number of alternative models for community-based pri-mary care. These centres could be autonomous or part of a larger organization.

that patients can receive care from providers they know and trust, yet large enough to handle the logistical problems associated with arranging after-hours "call."*

Each centre would offer routine primary care to anyone in its community, but would have "core" programs for the elderly, the chronically ill, and those with mental-health problems. This would require a high degree of cooperation with pre-existing community services. The object of this exercise would be to support and complement local initiatives, not to undermine them.

In addition, we've earmarked a billion dollars to establish 200 community-care programs for the elderly, modelled on San Francisco's On Lok program. A further billion would be used to set up community-care programs for the mentally ill, modelled on the Dane County program in Wisconsin.

Despite our earlier cautions about hospital involvement in community care, we've allocated a billion dollars to fund 400 programs for acute care within the home. Verdun's Hospital in the Home program is our model. These programs would be administered by hospitals and would use hospital-based staff.

Because we recognize that certain programs within hospitals *are* underfunded, we've allocated $700 million back to hospitals. Long waiting lists for procedures of proven benefit are unacceptable in a system committed to quality care. In particular, we believe this money should be used to expand programs for cataract surgery, some joint replacement operations, and transplant surgery (especially kidney transplants).

Finally, we've tagged almost $500 million to improve the management of our system. Half of this amount would establish a national technology assessment council, along with a national and ten provincial health care evaluation agencies. We've earmarked a further $200 million for training programs in health care management and evaluation. And another $70 million to improve existing quality-control and utilization-review activities.

Although we've criticized medical research for devoting itself almost exclusively to finding the biomolecular causes of illness, such work does expand our understanding. Accordingly, we've

---

*From the results of market research into patient preferences, the Northern California Region of Kaiser Permanente is now reorganizing its operation into units of the size we are proposing.

allocated an additional $150 million to basic research, with the recommendation that much of this money be used to study the social determinants of health.

Well, that's it. Figure 11.2 below summarizes our agenda for reallocation.

Figure 11.2 The reallocation of savings from the health care system.

Item	Cost
1. Charting a Course	
A process (national and provincial) to establish and monitor health goals (Including a national annual health survey)	$100,000,000
2. Healthy Public Policy	
Health impact assessments of new public policies	100,000,000
Reducing inequalities	
A war on poverty	
$1000 to each poor person who relies upon government assistance ($1000 × 1,898,500)	1,898,500,000
$800 to each "working poor" person ($800 × 1,801,500)	1,441,200,000
Additional funding for literacy programs	200,000,000
Skills development and recreation programs for poor children	100,000,000
Build 20,000 new units of social housing every year (20,000 × $60,000 each)	1,200,000,000
An attack on family violence and sexual inequality	
Fund 750 new transition houses (750 × $300,000)	225,000,000
Increase average funding of existing centres to $300,000 from $170,000 (230 × $130,000)	30,000,000
Fund 80 new rape crisis/sexual assault centres (80 × $200,000)	16,000,000
Increase average funding of existing centres to $200,000 from $50,000 (60 × $150,000)	9,000,000

Establish prevention programs in schools and through the media	100,000,000
Treatment programs for abusers and children	100,000,000
Skills development for women	100,000,000
Economic development programs for women	170,000,000

Assistance for natives

Skills development for natives	170,000,000
Economic development programs for natives	230,000,000

3. Health Promotion Programs
   Community Health Promotion

Fund 50 heart health programs (50 × $2,000,000 (average cost))	100,000,000
Prenatal health promotion (including nutrition, anti-smoking, and social support)	200,000,000
Programs to increase participation in physical exercise	100,000,000

   Workplace health promotion

New money for programs to prevent occupational injuries and illness	100,000,000
Workplace anti-smoking and physical exercise programs	100,000,000
Health promotion programs for natives	100,000,000

4. Healing Health Care
   An effective network for primary care

Fund 800 new community health centres, particularly — but not exclusively — for the elderly, the chronically ill, and those with mental illness. Each centre is designed to serve about 6,000 people. (800 × $1,000,000)	800,000,000

   Community care for the elderly
   Approximately 200 community programs
   modelled on the On Lok service

described in Chapter 9. It is assumed
that these programs would rely on community health centres for professional
services. (200 × $5,000,000)   1,000,000,000

Community care for the mentally ill
   Approximately 200 community programs
     modelled on the Dane County service
     described in Chapter 9. It is assumed
     that these programs would rely on com-
     munity health centres for professional
     services. (200 × $5,000,000)   1,000,000,000

Acute care within the home
   Approximately 400 programs modelled on
     Verdun's Hospital in the Home
     described in Chapter 9. It is assumed
     that these programs would be
     administered and staffed by hospitals.
     (400 × $2,500,000)   1,000,000,000

Funding for certain in-hospital programs,
   e.g., joint replacement surgery, cataract
     surgery, transplant surgery   700,000,000

Better management
   A national technology assessment council   100,000,000
   A national and ten provincial health and
     health care evaluation agencies   100,000,000
   Support for utilization review programs in
     hospitals   50,000,000
   Support for review programs for physician
     competence   20,000,000

Support for education and research
   To expand university training programs
     for health care evaluation and
     management   190,300,000
   Basic medical research   150,000,000

| Total | 12,000,000,000 |

Selling Health Reform

Reform may be a good idea, but how do we make it happen?

Former federal health minister Monique Bégin offers some advice about the "internal logic" of politics. "When I was just starting out as a politician," she remembers, "I felt that a good idea should be judged on its own merits. I rather naively believed that the intrinsic value of a project spoke for itself."

As a brand-new minister, Bégin says she was shocked when Allan MacEachen, a cabinet colleague, asked where the demand was for her ideas. "I didn't know what he meant. But now I understand that politics is a balance of forces and that it's strategy that makes you a winner or a loser."

The basic strategy for health reform, then, is to create a huge demand for it.

Most elected politicians clearly understand the need for reform. Here's what Dave Barrett, former BC premier (and its former treasurer), has to say about it: "The prescription for better and more affordable health is not an exponential resort to more drugs and more surgical procedures for the diseases of civilization, but a more enlightened society which realizes that by tolerating or even inducing poverty through economic and social policy, we light the fuse of an expensive-treatment time bomb. We rescue banks with millions, but do nothing [to eliminate the need] for food banks. It is socialism for the very wealthy but free enterprise for the very poor. The politician is trapped."

And Larry Grossman, former Ontario health minister, says, "Our health care system is like a car from the 1950s that's been retrofitted to operate as efficiently as possible in the modern world, but it still weighs 1,000 pounds more than 1989 cars. We've got a system that was designed for the postwar era, during a time when all the incentives were for building hospitals. So hospitals got built. The crux of the problem is that the basic health-status question must be resolved outside the traditional ministry-of-health functions."

Barrett and Grossman know health care isn't a major determinant of health. They know that every major government review has called for more money for community health initiatives, and less for institutions. Party politics didn't enter into it: the Conservatives, Liberals, New Democrats, Parti Québécois, Social

Credit — each has said they want reform. Governments are desperate to bring our system out of its present state of chaos and make it a well-administered, coherent response to the needs of our population. Why is it so difficult?

One-time Ontario health minister Frank Miller explains with an example from his own experience: "Back in 1974, I asked for a detailed plan of action to cut back on waste and duplication. Ministry staff were anxious to help and produced five big books of plans. We set targets for institutional beds, planned to close some hospitals, reallocate technology, convert some acute care beds to chronic care, and so forth. It was an ambitious, exciting plan. Three months later, [financial] constraints were put in place following the election of a minority government in 1975, and we pulled this research down off the shelf and amended it slightly and off we went. And I learned an important lesson that all politicians must heed or face the consequences: you don't close hospitals — ever!"

The point is that as long as the public associates more doctors and more hospital beds with better health, reform doesn't stand a chance. No politician is going to go against the expressed desires of those who elected him. Health reform has to seek its own constituency.

The first place to look for leadership is within the system itself. Ken Fyke was once a deputy minister of health in Saskatchewan. "Attitudes are changed by leadership," he says. "At the government level, I believe that the politician should lead public opinion and attempt to change it. By offering better services, it will change by itself."

Today, Fyke is president and chief executive officer of the Greater Victoria Hospital Society. Most of Victoria's acute and long-term care beds are under his administrative control. He describes how attitudes can be changed: "Today I was asked to speak to a patient who had cracked her pelvis slightly and was upset about being discharged. This woman felt she needed to be in the hospital. So first I reassured her that it was medically safe for her to go home, and then I asked her if she didn't believe she'd be happier in her own familiar surroundings, rather than in a hospital room. And she agreed. When it comes right down to it you've got to give the message that they can feel as secure at home as in the hospital."

Through their efforts to establish innovative programs, many hospital administrators — like Peter Ellis of Toronto's Sunnybrook Hospital, Rod Thorfinnson of Winnipeg's Health Sciences Centre, Vickery Stoughton of the Toronto Hospital Corporation, and David Levine of the Verdun General Hospital — show a strong commitment to quality and efficiency. Others could benefit from their know-how.

Nurses, too, are becoming more powerful advocates for reform. They've only just begun to exercise the considerable influence their numbers confer. No longer self-effacing and subservient, nurses are speaking out on behalf of their patients as much as for themselves.

There's even a growing constituency for reform among physicians. Until recently, reform-minded doctors were viewed as "traitors" by their own profession. But more and more mainstream physicians, like Drs. Landry, Scully, and Linton, are openly urging reforms to improve quality and efficiency.

Of course, reform won't happen without broad support from the public — the consumers of health care. Monique Bégin has some harsh words about "the schemers and the backroom boys that think the public's about five years old and pretty dumb. Well, it's not true. The public knows what it wants."

And even though Canadians as a whole have made it clear they treasure Medicare, individuals often describe their encounters with our system very negatively. It's these people, the dissatisfied users, who could create a groundswell of support for reform. Three groups in particular — women, the elderly, and those with mental illness — have a great deal to gain from health reform.

Let's begin with women. Women typically have frequent and regular contact with our system. They see doctors two to three times more often than men, but they don't always benefit from this extra attention.* Consider how many of them receive prescriptions for sedatives, or are told they need surgery for silent

---

*This isn't because women are more prone to illness, however; women have to see doctors for all sorts of concerns related to their reproductive system. Whether it's about having a baby or taking precautions not to become pregnant, *young* women see physicians five times more frequently than young men. As well, women are usually the ones who bring their children to the doctors' office, and frequently take the opportunity for a consultation at that time.

gallstones, or are rendered infertile because their doctors failed to diagnose chlamydia.

Many women complain that their natural life cycles have been medicalized, to the detriment of their well-being. Many resent the fact that normal changes in their reproductive physiology have given the medical profession an "in." Many have been alienated by their experiences with pregnancy, childbirth, and menopause. They want to know why these normal events have all become medical conditions requiring "treatments" (many of which are unproven or disproven) from physicians. They want to know why Caesarean section rates are so high, why episiotomies are still so common, why their menopausal symptoms are so badly controlled.

And our system fails women in still other ways. Women make up the vast majority of informal care-givers in our society. Looking after a frail parent usually falls to the daughter or daughter-in-law, not to the son. That's why home care, respite care, and day centres for seniors are important women's health issues.

Women also stand to benefit from a broader definition of health and illness. Reforms that explicitly identify rape, wife-battering, and childhood poverty as health issues should attract their support. For all of these reasons, we believe that organized women's groups need to put health reform high on their agendas.

Canada's growing population of elderly is a second major constituency for reform. Our system has been notoriously insensitive to their needs. Consider how our appallingly high rates of institutionalization have compromised their independence. Look at the extent of inappropriate prescribing, and its toll on their health. And why are there so few palliative care programs to make their last days comfortable? Organized senior citizens' groups could be a powerful lobby for reform. Every politician knows that seniors vote. Seniors need to tell governments what they'll vote *for*.

When it comes to the third constituency, the mentally ill, we face a problem. These people aren't well organized, as seniors and women's groups are. They have little political clout. Yet this is a group whose rights are systematically denied, and whose urgent needs are frequently ignored. Chronic mental illness is a devastating condition made worse by an uncaring society. Psychiatrists working with chronic mental patients earn half what a doctor can earn seeing patients with colds at a walk-in clinic. Other mental-health workers strain under "burnout" conditions. Urgently needed community services are regularly passed over for funding.

Chronic mental patients have trouble being strong advocates for themselves. But their families can and should be (and in some communities already *are*) educated about the waste in the rest of the system that condemns their sons and daughters to lives without dignity. As well, mental-health workers must be shown that a dollar spent on unnecessary surgery is a dollar withheld from their clients. The "mental health community" has become politicized over the past decade. Now it has to get into the broader battle to reform the health care system as a whole.

A Sunset for Short Horizons

Professor Gail Siler-Wells, a health policy analyst who teaches at the University of Toronto, has identified three major barriers to health care reform:[21]

- A universal fear of change;

- Poor understanding of the technology of social change;

- The failure of government to plan the implementation of the very policies it creates.

What Siler-Wells is really describing is a marketing failure. The same backroom politicians who are so skillful at selling a new leader or planning an election campaign, strike out when they attempt to reform health care.

During 1982/83, Ontario's health minister, Larry Grossman, tried to put together a coalition of support for reform. But when he left that ministry to become provincial treasurer, the process stopped dead. Later, during the Liberal government's tenure, the end to extra-billing and the freeze on hospital bail-outs alienated many potential supporters. The problem isn't that these policies were wrong. The problem is how they were handled. The promising coalition of support for reform disintegrated.

In 1987/88, Manitoba tried its hand at setting up a collaborative reform effort. The government involved provider groups and representatives from the institutional sector, and made great strides in achieving consensus. The reform plan agreed on included a strong fiscal management strategy to reallocate resources, as well as a special health trust fund for new initiatives, particularly in community care. But in the spring of 1988, the NDP government of Howard Pawley was defeated. And it looks unlikely that the Conservatives will pick up the ball.

A big problem is that the fruits of a major reform won't drop from the tree before election time. Even if a new government acts immediately, five years is simply not long enough. Besides, seasoned politicians try to avoid any unpopular action for about two years before an election. That's why a smart premier or health minister would have a two-pronged strategy — a slow track for long-term action, and a fast track for quick results.

Reform to improve doctors' prescribing habits is a leading candidate for the fast track. Public awareness about this problem is growing. And many doctors would champion this kind of reform. So would many pharmacists, because even though drug reform could reduce their incomes, their professional stature would increase. Only the multinational drug companies stand to lose, and they're politically unpopular anyway. Evidence from the scientific literature indicates that cost savings could be realized almost instantly. What's more, a successful campaign to improve doctors' prescribing habits would tend to promote reforms in other areas. The tactics in this campaign — public education, a focus on quality rather than costs, and a broad coalition for reform — could easily be transported to other issues.

The slow-track reforms will require extensive public education. And that means the media need a better understanding about what really makes our system tick. Public-relations departments in hospitals aren't exactly unimpeachable sources of data. Miracle technology is *not* a major boon to health. Bed shortages are *not* an indication of underfunding. This isn't to suggest that journalists are irresponsible when they repeat these timeworn myths, only that they're missing out on a much more significant story — one that could contribute greatly to what is sure to be a major national debate.

The education process shouldn't be boring. Dr. Charles Hastings, Toronto's medical officer of health from 1910 to 1929, made himself freely available to the press. And he was always good copy. Whether he was giving a medal to the child who killed the most flies, or having his picture taken in front of an unsafe tenement, he was in the newspapers every week with items that educated the public. Why not single out individual healthy children and claim their lives were saved by public-health measures? Why not lionize family doctors or community health centres that keep their patients' blood pressure under control? How about a picture of the premier giving a big gold medal to a primary care nurse for preventing a prominent person from having a heart attack? Some of the best minds in this country spend their days thinking up ways to promote products that make people sick. Let's pay them well to find ways of making illness prevention and health promotion sexy.

All major political parties in Canada have policies supporting health reform; all claim to want more efficiency and more community care. But none, except the Québec Liberals and Parti Québécois, has been able to implement these policies once in power. Health ministers talk about "surviving the portfolio." Well they might.

The fact is, health "positions" have little to do with political allegiance. For example, accusations of hospital underfunding were partly responsible for the defeat of Manitoba's NDP government in 1988. Yet in BC, the NDP is raising funds by pointing to the growing waiting lists for surgery. Political parties should call a truce on these misleading horror stories. Opposition health critics should remember that if their party becomes the government it will benefit tremendously from a reformed health system. They shouldn't make it more difficult to achieve.

In our reform agenda, we outlined a rather extensive role for the federal government, despite the fact that health care is a provincial responsibility. There are two main reasons for this. First, the overemphasis in our system on doctors and hospitals and the neglect of more appropriate and cost-effective alternatives is a federal legacy — one that evolved directly from incentives the federal government created to get the provinces to build hospitals and buy into Medicare. That's why, for starters, we believe that the federal health minister today is duty-bound to introduce a new cost-shared program to encourage community-based care. It's a moral obligation to correct past mistakes by helping provinces to achieve more rational social spending.

The second reason for more federal involvement is that the major levers for improving the health status of Canadians are under federal control: the state of our economy and our environment, the supply of affordable housing and day-care, in short, the living and working conditions of all Canadians are a national responsibility. Marc Lalonde recognized this in 1974; in 1986, Jake Epp reaffirmed it. In 1989, the challenge remains for the federal government to demonstrate its capacity for leadership and vision.

Canada's health care system owes its existence to our society's broad commitment to fairness. Because we held the conviction that access to health care was a fundamental human necessity, we were able to transform a privilege, available only to those with financial means, into a right for everyone.

Today, we face a new challenge — to test the strength of our commitment to equity. Do Canadians believe that we all deserve equal access to *health*, as well as to health *care*? If the answer is yes, can we transform yet another privilege into a new right — the right for all to a healthy life?

Appendix

IMPORTANT LIMITATIONS
TO INTERPRETING TEST RESULTS

NO TEST IS 100 percent accurate. Each test has its own characteristic sensitivity and specificity rate. The figure below shows a typical "2 by 2" table that scientists use to evaluate a test.

A-1

		Disease Present Yes	No	
Test Result	Positive	A	B	A + B
	Negative	C	D	C + D
		A + C	B + D	A + B + C + D

The sensitivity is the proportion of truly diseased people who have a positive test result. That is, $A/A+C$. The specificity is the proportion of truly well people who have a negative result. That is, $D/B+D$. Even excellent tests, like microbiological cultures, are only 98% sensitive and specific; most are less than 90%. That's how we get false positives and false negatives. The false-positive rate is the proportion of well people who have a positive test result. That is, $B/B+D$. The false-negative rate is the proportion of diseased people who have a negative test result. That is, $C/A+C$.

Most of the time we have to make a trade-off between sensitivity and specificity. For example, look at the following data for a test which measures the level of an enzyme called creatinine kinase (CK) in blood.[1] This is a common test used to diagnose patients with suspected heart attacks.

A-2

Patients Who Had a Heart Attack	CK Level	Patients Who Did Not Have a Heart Attack
35	480+	0
8	480	0
7	440	0
15	400	0
19	360	0
13	320	1
18	280	1
19	240	1
21	200	0
30	160	5
30	120	8
13	80	26
2	40	88
	0	
231		130

We can see that CK tends to be higher in people who are having a heart attack than in people who aren't. In fact, if the level is above 320 then the patient must be having a heart attack. If it is less than 40 he is almost certainly not having a heart attack. But what if it is 120? The patient might or might not be having a heart attack. If we classify anyone with a CK level above 320 as having a heart attack, we won't label anyone who is not hav-

---

[1]Adopted from: David Sackett, Brian Haynes, Peter Tugwell, *Clinical Epidemiology: A Basic Science for Clinical Medicine*, Toronto: Little, Brown and Company, 1985.

ing a heart attack as having one (high specificity, low false-positive rate) but we will mislabel many people who are having a heart attack as not having one (low sensitivity, high false-negative rate).

On the other hand, if we classify any with a CK above 40 as having a heart attack, we will label only two people as not having a heart attack when they are (high sensitivity, low false-negative rate) but we will mislabel a lot of people as having a heart attack when they are not (low specificity, high false positive-rate).

So what do we do? In the cold cruel world, we have to select the best level, which has the fewest false-positives and false-negatives. It's like tuning your radio to a distant station: you try to maximize the signal and minimize the noise.

Another complementary tactic is to use other tests to confirm. For example, with a suggested heart attack, we can perform an electrocardiogram or EKG. In fact, you can perform high-sensitivity, low-specificity tests first and then high-specificity, lower-sensitivity tests later to maximize the diagnostic accuracy. Of course there is another tactic a wise doctor should employ — skepticism. He or she should always remember that no test is perfect.

Apart from determining the sensitivity and specificity of tests, there is yet another mathematical snag for those who would like the world to be black and white. Although the sensitivity and specificity of a test will usually not vary, the overall usefulness of a test is greatly reduced if it is given to patients who have a low probability of having the disease in question. A non-mathematical analogy might help to clarify this point. Suppose you have an Uncle Fred who lives in Barrie (80 km north of Toronto). You are at the Bloor/Yonge subway station in downtown Toronto, look across the platform and see someone who looks like your Uncle Fred. Is that person your uncle? You know Fred likes to come to Toronto to shop every couple of weeks so you shout a greeting to the man. Next month you are in Montreal for business and, while using the Metro, you look across the platform and see someone who looks like your Uncle Fred. You know Fred has a sister (your aunt) in Montreal whom he visits every year or two. You tentatively wave your hand. A couple of months later you are in London, England, to see the plays and, while you and your consort are waiting for the tube, you glimpse someone across the platform who looks like your Uncle

Fred. Now, Fred has never been further east than Québec City. In fact, he is terrified of airplanes. Do you think the man across the platform is your uncle? Of course not. Even though the test (your visual inspection) was positive, you conclude that the man across the platform is unlikely to be your uncle.

Let's now look at an example of how a decreased prevalence (occurrence) of a condition decreases the usefulness of a positive result. Let's assume that we have selected a CK result of 80 international units as the "cut-off" to diagnose heart attack. Anything above we call a heart attack. Anything less we call no heart attack. Let's construct a "2 by 2" table out of the data in Figure A-1.

A-3

| | Heart Attack Present | | |
	Yes	No	
CK			
Test +	215	16	231
Result −	15	114	129
Totals	230	130	360

Predictive value of a positive test: 215/231 = 93%.
Predictive value of a negative test: 114/129 = 88%.
Prevalence (proportion with disease) = 230/360 = 64%.
Sensitivity = 215/230 = 93%.
Specificity = 114/130 = 88%.

The sensitivity of our test is 93% and the specificity is 88% — not bad actually. But the real meat is in the predictive value of the test. In this population of patients who were admitted to a coronary care unit, a person with a positive test has a 93% chance of having a heart attack and person with a negative test has an 88% chance of being free of heart attack. But what if some hot-shot cardiologist now suggests that the test is so good, it should be given to all general hospital admissions. If we apply the test to 2300 admissions when only 10 percent of them are having heart attacks, the data would look like this:

A - 4

| | Heart Attack Present | | |
	Yes	No	
CK			
Test +	215	246	463
Result −	15	1822	1837
Totals	230	2070	2300

Predictive value of a positive test: 215/463 = 46%.
Predictive value of a negative test: 1822/1837 = 99%.
Prevalence = 230/2300 = 10%.
Sensitivity = 215/230 = 93%.
Specificity = 1822/2070 = 88%.

Note that the sensitivity and specificity rates are still the same. The predictive value of a negative test is remarkable at 99 percent. However, the predictive value of a positive test has now fallen to 46 percent. A patient with a positive test is more likely *not* to have a heart attack. The predictive value of a positive test would be even worse if we started doing this test with the general public, like in shopping malls. If we have told our story properly, you should now be able to see the fallacies behind two modern medical nostrums:

1. I'm certain the patient has condition "x" but we'll run this test just to be sure.
2. I'm certain the patient hasn't got condition "x" but we'll run this test just to be sure.

A negative test when the doctor is 90 percent certain the disease is present will not rule out the condition. It simply makes it less likely, lowering the physician's certainty of diagnosis to 70 or 80 percent. Similarly, a positive result when the doctor thinks the disease is very unlikely, say a 10 percent chance, does not necessarily mean the person is sick. It merely increases the likelihood to 20 or 30 percent.

The moral of this story is that there are useful tests and useless tests but even a useful test can be useless if it is used improperly. A wise doctor with only a few tests at his disposal will do a lot more good (and less harm) than an unwise doctor with the highest of high tech.

Notes

The following acronyms are used in the end notes:

AJM   American Journal of Medicine
BMJ   British Medical Journal
CMAJ   Canadian Medical Association Journal
IRPP   Institute for Research on Public Policy
JAMA   Journal of the American Medical Association
NEJM   New England Journal of Medicine
OECD   Organization for Economic Cooperation and Development
WHO   World Health Organization

CHAPTER 1

1. R. Wildovsky, "Doing Better and Feeling Worse: The Political Pathology of Health Policy," in *Doing Better and Feeling Worse,* ed. John H. Knowles, New York: Norton and Company, 1977, p. 105.

2. Personal communication with Ursula Verstraete, Director of Nursing, Shouldice Hospital.

3. Health and Welfare Canada, *Health Sector in Canada Fact Sheets,* (mimeograph) Policy, Communications and Information Branch, November, 1987.

4. Thomas McKeown, *The Role of Medicine: Dream, Mirage or Nemesis?* Princeton: Princeton University Press, 1979.

5. David Naylor, *Private Practice, Public Payment: Canadian Medicine and the Politics of Health Insurance, 1911-1966,* Montreal: McGill-Queen's University Press, 1986, pp. 58-94.

6. Joel Lexchin, *The Real Pushers,* Vancouver: New Star Books, 1984, pp. 112-153.

7. B.K. Cypress, "Drug utilization in general and family practice by characteristics of physicians and office visits," National Council on Health Research, Report No. 86, 1983.

8. G. Carruthers, T. Goldberg, H. Segal, E. Sellers, *Drug Utilization: A Comprehensive Literature Review,* (A report to the Ontario Minister of Health.) Toronto, 1987, p. 194.

9. David L. Sackett, R. Brian Haynes, Peter Tugwell, *Clinical Epidemiology: A Basic Science for Clinical Medicine,* Toronto and Boston: Little, Brown and Company, 1985, pp. 176-177.

10. Paul Starr, *The Social Transformation of American Medicine,* New York, Basic Books: 1982.

11. Donald Trunkey, "Trauma," *Scientific American,* August 1983, 249: 28-35.

12. Statistics Canada, *Current Demographic Analysis: Report on the Demographic Situation in Canada in 1986,* Cat. No. 91-524E, (1987).

CHAPTER 2

1. Health and Welfare Canada, Policy, Communications and Information Branch, (Personal communication, 1987.)

2. See footnote 1.

3. Malcolm Taylor, *Health Insurance and Canadian Public Policy: The Seven Decisions That Created the Canadian Health Insurance System,* Montreal: McGill-Queen's University Press, 1978.

4. Health and Welfare Canada, *National Health Expenditures in Canada,* 1984.

5. Statistics Canada, *National Income and Expenditure Accounts* (1987).

6. As quoted in: Canadian Medical Association (CMA), *Health: A Need for Redirection,* Ottawa, 1985, p. 109. (A task force on the allocation of health care resources)

7. T. Hilden, R. Raaschou, K. Iversen, M. Schwartz, "Anticoagulants in acute myocardial infarction," *Lancet,* 1961. ii. 327-331. Also, United Kingdom, Medical Research Council Working Party on Anticoagulant Therapy in Coronary Thrombosis, "Assessment of short-term anticoagulant administration after cardiac infarction,"*BMJ,* 1969, 1:335-342. Also L. Goldman, E.F. Cook, "The decline in ischemic heart disease mortality rates: an analysis of the comparative effects of medical interventions and changes in lifestyle," *Annals of Internal Medicine,* 1984, 101: 825-836.

8. J.D. Hill, J.R. Hampton, J.R.A. Mitchell, "A randomized trial of home versus hospital management of myocardial infarction," *Lancet,*1978, i: 337-341.

9. OECD, *Measuring Health Care 1960-1983: Expenditure, Costs, and Performance,* Paris, 1985.

10. Ibid.

11. James O. Robinson, " Treatment of breast cancer through the ages," *American Journal of Surgery,* 1986, 151:317-333. Also, OECD, *Measuring Health Care.*

12. CMA, *Health: A Need for Redirection,* p. 25.

13. Robert G. Evans, *Strained Mercy: The Economics of Canadian Health Care,* Toronto: Butterworths, 1984, pp. 160-161. (Evans goes on to explain that after 1976, wages began to account for a bigger share of the increase in costs than service intensity.)

14. *Rapport de la commission d'enquête sur les services de santé et les services sociaux* (Rochon Commission), Publications du Québec, 1987, p. 341.

15. *The Globe and Mail,* February 6, 1987.

16. *The Toronto Star,* September 19, 1988.

17. *The Globe and Mail,* June 1, 1988.

18. *The Toronto Star,* March 20, 1988.

19. Ibid.

20. D.J. Roch, Robert G. Evans, David Pascoe, *Manitoba and Medicare,* Manitoba Health, March 1985, p. 21. (Manitoba Health is the provincial health ministry)

21. Ibid., pp. i-xiv.

22. David U. Himmelstein, Steffie Woolhandler, "Sounding board: cost without benefit; administrative waste in U.S. health care,"*NEJM,* 1986, 314:442.

23. Ibid., pp. 441-445.

24. Ibid.

25. U.S. Current Population Survey data, as quoted in Alain Enthoven, *An Introduction to Health Economics,*Oakland, California: Kaiser Foundation Health Plan Inc., February 1987.

26. CMA, *Health: A Need for Redirection,* p. 112.

27. CMA, "CMA policy summary: Health care financing," *CMAJ,* 1986, 134: 656A.

CHAPTER 3

1. Alain Enthoven, *Health Plan: The Only Practical Solution to the Soaring Cost of Health Care,* Reading, Massachusetts: Addison-Wesley, 1980, p. 2.

2. Cameron and McGoogan, "A prospective study of 1,152 Hospital autopsies: 1. Inaccuracies in death certification," *Pathology,* 1985, 133:223. Also, Kircher, et al., "The autopsy as a measure of accuracy of the death certificate," *NEJM,* 1980, 313:1263.

3. James O. Robinson, "Treatment of breast cancer through the ages," *American Journal of Surgery,* 1986, 151:317-333.

4. Eugene Braunwald, "Effects of coronary-artery bypass grafting on survival: implication of the randomized coronary-artery surgery study," *NEJM,* 1983, 309:1181-1184.

5. For a good analysis of the idiosyncracies of medical training, see Martin Shapiro; *Getting Doctored,* Kitchener: Between the Lines, 1978.

6. Schor and Karten, "Statistical evaluation of medical manuscripts," *Journal of American Medicine,* 1966, 195: 1123. Also, Sheehan, "The medical literature: Let the reader beware,"*Archives of Internal Medicine,* 1980. 140: 472. Also, S.A. Glantz, "Biostatistics: how to detect, correct and prevent errors in the medical literature," *Circulation,* 1980, 61:1.

7. David Eddy, L. Sanders, J. Eddy, "The value of screening for glaucoma with tonometry," *Survey of Ophthamology,* 1983, 28:194-205.

8. For a full discussion of bias in research, see: David L. Sackett, R. Brian Haynes, and Peter Tugwell, *Clinical Epidemiology: A Basic Science for Clinical Medicine,*Toronto and Boston: Little, Brown and Company, 1985.

9. Ibid., p. 180.

10. Thomas Preston, *The Clay Pedestal: A Re-examination of the Doctor-Patient Relationship,* Seattle: Madrona Books, 1981, p. 20.

11. Ibid., p. 21.

12. Ibid., p. 30.

13. H.K. Beecher, "The Powerful Placebo," *JAMA* 1955, 159:1602-1606.

14. D. Feeny, G. Guyatt, P. Tugwell, eds., *Health Care Technology: Effectiveness, Efficiency and Public Policy,* Montreal: IRPP, 1986.

15. Ibid., p. 64.

16. Abraham Flexner, *Medical Education in the United States and Canada,* New York: Carnegie Foundation for the Advancement of Teaching, Bulletin No. 4, 1910.

17. Lester King, "The Flexner Report," *JAMA,* 1984, 251: 1079-1086.

18. Preston, *The Clay Pedestal,* p. 95.

19. Ibid.

20. O.L. Phelps, "Retinopathy of vision loss in the United States," *Pediatrics,* 1981, 67:924-926.

21. G. Martin-Bouyer, R. Lebreton, M. Toga, "Outbreak of accidental hexachloraphene poisoning in France," *Lancet,* 1982, ii. 91-95.

22. For a full discussion of iatrogenesis, see Richard Taylor, *Medicine out of Control,* Melbourne: Sun Books, 1977. Also, Thomas Preston, *The Clay Pedestal.* Also, Geoffrey York, *The High Price of Health: A Patient's Guide to the Hazards of Medical Politics,* Toronto: Lorimer, 1987.

23. CMA, *Health: A Need for Redirection,* 1985, p. 45.

24. Taylor, *Medicine Out of Control,* pp. 69-70.

25. J.F. Burnam, "Medical Vampires," *NEJM,* 1986, 314:1250.

26. B.R. Smoller, M.S. Krusker, "Phlebotomy for diagnostic laboratory tests in adults: pattern of use and effect on transfusion requirements," *NEJM,* 1986, 314: 1233-35.

27. Fowkes, et al., "Trial strategy for reducing the use of laboratory tests," *BMJ* 1986, 292:883.

28. J.M. Eisenberg, S.V. Williams, "Cost containment and changing physicians practice behavior: Can the fox learn to guard the chicken coop?" *JAMA* 1981, 246: 2195-2201.

29. W. Rothstein, *American Physicians in the 19th Century,* Baltimore: Johns Hopkins Press, 1972, p. 262.

30. J.C. Le Guennec, H. Bard, F. Teasdale, B. Doray, "Elective delivery and neonatal respiratory distress syndrome," *CMAJ,* 1980, 122: 307-309.

31. Kenneth Flegel, Robert Oseasohn, "Adverse effects of diagnostic tests," *Archives of Internal Medicine,* May 1982, 142: 883.

32. For further information about the diagnostic accuracy of ultrasound for liver tumours, see D.J. Cave-Bigley, G.H.R. Lamb, "The value of pre-operative ultrasound of the liver in colonic and gastric neoplasia," *British Journal of Radiology,* 1985, 58: 13-14. Also, Thomas J. Smith, M. Kemeny, Paul H. Sugarbaker, et al., "A prospective study of hepatic imaging in the detection of metastatic disease," *Annals of Surgery,* 1982, 195: 486-491.

33. *Medical Letter on Drugs and Therapeutics,* 1987, 29: 41-42.

34. James P. Isbister, "Poker machine pathology: Are all those special investigations giving us better medicine?" *Medical Journal of Australia,* November 28, 1981, p. 609.

35. OECD, *Measuring Health Care.*

36. L.J. Opit, S. Greenhill, "Prevalence of gallstones in relation to differing treatment rates for biliary disease," *British Journal of Preventive and Social Medicine,* 1974, 28: 268-272.

37. David Ransohoff, et al. "Prophylactic cholecystectomy or expectant management for silent gallstones,"*Annals of Internal Medicine,* 1983, 99: 199-204.

38. N. Roos, M. Cohen, R. Danzinger, "Treatment of gallstone disease in Manitoba, Canada: a population-based study," *Proceedings of the Third Canadian Conference on Health Economics, 1986,* edited by John M. Horne, Winnipeg: University of Manitoba, 1987.

39. C.K. McSherry, H. Ferstenberg, F. Calhoun, et al., "The natural history of diagnosed gallstone disease in symptomatic and asymptomatic patients," *Annals of Surgery,* 1985, 202: 59-63.

40. Statistics Canada, *"Surgical Procedures and Treatments 1981-82, 1982-83,* Cat. No. 82-208 (1987).

41. F. Dyck, et al., "Effect of surveillance on the number of hysterectomies in the province of Saskatchewan," *NEJM,* 1977, 296: 1326.

42. The EC-IC Bypass Study Group, "Failure of extracranial-intracranial arterial bypass to reduce the risk of ischemic stroke: results of an international randomized trial," *NEJM,* 1985, 313:1191-1200.

43. American Neurological Association, Committee on Health Care Issues, "Does carotid endarterectomy decrease stroke and death in patients with transient ischemic attacks?" *Annals of Neurology,* 1987, 22: 72-76.

44. Aspirin has been proven more effective than no treatment at all at least in some trials, for some patients. See Canadian Cooperative Stroke Study Group, "A randomized trial of aspirin and sulfinpyrozone in threatened stroke,"*NEJM,* 1978, 299: 53-59. Also, M.J. Bousser, E. Eschwege, M. Haguenau, et al., "AICLA-controlled trial of aspirin and dipyridamole in the secondary prevention of athrothrombotic cerebral ischemia," *Stroke,* 1983, 14:5-14.

45. J.C. Grotta, "Current medical and surgical therapy for cerebrovascular disease," *NEJM,* 1978, 317: 1505-1516.

46. Preston, *The Clay Pedestal.*

47. Taylor, *Medicine Out of Control.*

CHAPTER 4

1. Alain Enthoven, *Health Plan, The Only Practical Solution to the Soaring Cost of Health Care,* Reading, Massachusetts: Addison-Wesley, 1980.

2. D. Feeney, G. Guyatt, P. Tugwell, eds., *Health Care Technology,* Montreal: IRPP, 1986, p. 17.

3. K.W. Brown, R.L. MacMillan, N. Forbath, et al., "Coronary unit: An Intensive Care Centre for Acute Myocardial Infarction," *Lancet,* 1963, 2: 349-352.

4. R.L. MacMillan, K.W. Brown, "Comparison of the Effects of treatment of Acute Myocardial Infarction in a coronary unit and on a general medical ward,"*CMAJ,* 1971, 105: 1037-1040.

5. H.G. Mather, N.G. Pearson, K.L.Q. Read, et al., "Acute myocardial infarction: home and hospital treatment," *BMJ,* 1971, 3: 334-338.

6. J.D. Hill, J.R. Hampton, J.R.A. Mitchell, "A randomized trial of home versus hospital management for patients with suspected myocardial infarction," *Lancet,* 1978, 2: 837-841. (The death rates were 11% in the hospital group and 13% in the home group; this difference could well have occurred by chance.)

7. S.C. Eggerton, A.O. Berg, "Is It Good Practice to Treat Patients with Uncomplicated Myocardial Infarction at home?"*JAMA,*1984, 251: 349-350.

8. L. Westrom, "Incidence, Prevalence and Trends of Acute Pelvic Inflammatory Disease and its Consequences in Industrialized Countries," *American Journal of Obstetrics and Gynecology,* 1980, 138: 880-892.

9. Ibid.

10. P.F. Brenner, S. Roy, D.R. Mishell, "Ectopic Pregnancy, a study of 300 consecutive surgically treated patients,"*JAMA,* 1980, 243: 673-676.

11. J.C. Hockin, A.G. Jessamine, "Trends in Ectopic Pregnancy in Canada," *CMAJ,* 1984, 131: 737-740.

12. J.A. Collins, W. Wrixon, L.B. Janes, E.H. Wilson, "Treatment-independent pregnancy among infertile couples," *NEJM,* 1983, 309: 1201-1206.

13. K. Luber, et al., "Results of micro-surgical treatment of tubal infertility and early second-look laparoscopy in patients: implications for *in vitro* fertilization," *American Journal of Obstetrics and Gynecology,* 1986, 154: 1264-70.

14. Anne Pappert, "The Business of Making Babies," *The Globe and Mail,* February 6-9, 1988.

15. *The Globe and Mail,* August 15,1987.

16. *The Globe and Mail,* May 24, 1988.

17. J.F. Burnam, "Medical Practice à la mode: How medical fashions determine medical care,"*NEJM,* 1987, 317: 1220-22.

18. E.A. Clarke, N. Kreiger, L.D. Marrett, "Cancer incidence, mortality, and treatment in Ontario," in *Cancer in Ontario,* Ontario Cancer Treatment and Research Foundation, Toronto, 1986.

19. Personal communication with Professors Gordon Guyatt and David Feeney.

20. *The Toronto Star,* June 29, 1987.

21. Ibid.

22. M. Dujovny, et al., "Aneurysm clip motion experimental study with metallurgical factor analysis," *Neurosurgery,* 1985, 17: 543-548.

23. Feeney, et al., eds., *Health Care Technology,* p. 8.

24. Ibid., p. 10.

25. Ibid.

26. John B. McKinlay, Sonja M. McKinlay, "From promising report to standard procedure: Seven stages in the career of a medical innovation," *Milbank Memorial Fund Quarterly,* 1981, 59: 374-411.

27. Feeney, et al., eds., *Health Care Technology,* p. 11.

28. Francis Notzon, Paul Placek, Thelma Taffel, "Comparisons of national Caesarean section rates," *NEJM,* 1987, 316: 386-389.

30. K. Leveno, F. G. Cunningham, Sheryl Nelson, Micki Roark, et al., "A prospective comparison of selective and universal electronic fetal monitoring in 34,995 cases," *NEJM,* 1986, 315: 615-619.

31. Ibid., p. 617.

32. Society of Obstetricians and Gynecologists of Canada, "Consensus statement on indications for Caesarean Section,"*NEJM,* 1986, 134: 1348-1352.

33. G. Prescia, H. Nguyen The, eds., *Chorionic Villi Sampling,* Basel: Karger, 1986.

34. G. Bjorn, " Miscarriage Rate in women aged 35 years or more," in Prescia and The, eds., *Chorionic Villi Sampling,* pp. 45-49.

35. Prescia and The, "Chorionic villi sampling: point of view of the medical geneticist," in *Chorionic Villi Sampling,* p. 59.

36. Henry Dunn, "Social aspects of low birthweight," *CMAJ,* 1984, 130: 1131-1140.

37. S. Saigal, P. Rosenbaum, B. Stoskopf, J.C. Sinclair, "The outcome of infants 500-1000 grams birth weight delivered to residents of the McMaster Health Region," *Journal of Pediatrics,* 1984, 105: 969-976.

38. M.H. Boyle, G.W. Torrance, J.C. Sinclair, S.P. Horwood, "Economic evaluation of neonatal intensive care of very-low-birthweight infants," *NEJM,* 1983, 308: 1330-1337.

39. O.L.Phelps, "Retinopathy of vision loss in the United States," *Pediatrics,* 1981, 67: 924-926.

40. B. Guyer, Lee Ann Wallach, S.L. Rosen, "Birthweight-standardized neonatal mortality rates and the prevention of low birthweight: How does Massachusetts compare with Sweden?" *NEJM,* 1982, 306: 1230-1233. *In vitro* fertilization is also implicated in the increasing incidence of low-birthweight children, as related to the prevalence of pre-term delivery, multiple births, and/or premature Caesarean delivery. J.C. Spensley, D. Mushin, M. Barreda-Hanson, "The Children of IVF Pregnancies: a cohort study," *Australian Paediatrics Journal,* 1986, 22: 285-289.

41. Feeney et al., eds., *Health Care Technology,* p. 17.

42. The Skull X-Ray Referral Criteria Panel, "Skull X-rays after head trauma," *NEJM,* 1987, 316: 84-89.

CHAPTER 5

1. Ruth Cooperstock, Penny Parnell, "Research on psychotropic drug use: a review of findings and methods,"*Social Science and Medicine,* 1982, 16:1180.

2. "Ranitidine," in. *Medical Letter on Drug Therapy,* 1982, 24: 111-113.

3. Personal communication with Dave Mussar, Syntax, Inc.

4. The literature on adverse drug reactions (ADRs) is large, complex, contradictory, and acrimonious. Studies report rates of hospital admissions due to ADRs ranging from less than one percent to as high as 20%. Some authors have found as many as 35% of hospitalized patients experience ADRs, while others report as few as one percent. Reported rates of fatal ADRs vary as well, from a low of 0.08% to 1.5% of all hospitalized patients. The proportion of all in-hospital deaths attributed to ADRs varies from one to eight percent. There are many pitfalls in per-

forming this kind of research properly. For example, it is well-known that if an investigator looks for ADRs, he is far more likely to find them. And certain reactions, such as fever and rash, or even death, can occur in people who are not taking drugs. What seems indisputable is that doctors have little knowledge about the proper use of drugs, and that ADRs do take a considerable toll on Canadians' health and health care costs. For further information, see F.E. Karch, L. Lasagna, "Adverse drug reactions: A Critical Review," *JAMA* 1975, 234: 1236-1241. Also, E.W. Gotti, "Adverse drug reactions and the autopsy: prevalence and perspective," *Archives of Pathology,* 1974, 97: 201-204. Also, D.A. Lane, "The Bayesian approach to causality assessment: an introduction," *The Drug Information Journal,* 1986. 20: 455-461.

5. Health and Welfare Canada, *Health Expenditures in Canada 1975-1985,* Policy, Communications and Information Branch, Ottawa, 1987.

6. *Report of the Commission of Inquiry on the Pharmaceutical Industry,*(Eastman Commission), Consumer and Corporate Affairs Canada, 1985, p. 422.

7. Joel Lexchin, *The Real Pushers: a critical analysis of the Canadian drug industry,* Vancouver: New Star Books, 1984, p. 19.

8. Cooperstock and Parnell, *Social Science and Medicine,* pp. 1179-1196.

9. S. Zisook, R.A. DeVaul, "Adverse behavioral effects of benzodiazepines," *Journal of Family Practice,* 1977, 5: 963-966.

10. Ruth Cooperstock, J. Hill, *The Effects of Tranquillization: Benzodiazepine Use in Canada,* Health and Welfare Canada, 1982.

11. Lexchin, *The Real Pushers,* p. 22.

12. D.G. Workman, D.G. Cunningham, "Effects of psychotropic drugs on aggression in a prison setting," *Canadian Family Physician,* 1975, 21: 63-66.

13. Eastman Commission, p. 177-183.

14. J.J. Misciwicz, R.E. Pounder, C.W. Venables, eds., *Diseases of the Gut and Pancreas,* London: Blackwell Scientific Publications, 1987.

15. Kevin W. Hall, Marie Behun, Janice Irvine-Meek, Nicolaas Otten, "Use of cimetidine in Hospital Patients,"*CMAJ,* 1981, 124: 1579-1585.

16. L. Kopola, "The use of cimetidine in hospitalized patients," *Canadian Family Physician,* 1984, 30: 69-72. (In 1985, Dr. Kopola published the results of a second study at her hospital, in the same journal, 1985, 31: 971-972. This time 58% of cimetidine prescriptions were deemed inappropriate.)

17. H. Diamond, et al., "Naproxen and aspirin in rheumatoid arthritis: a multicentre double-blind crossover comparison study," *Journal of Clinical Pharmacology,* April 1975, pp. 335-339.

18. J. Melton, et al., "Naproxen vs. aspirin in osteoarthritis of the hip and knee," *Journal of Rheumatology,* 1978, 5: 338-346.

19. Lexchin, *The Real Pushers,* p. 75.

20. David L. Sackett, R. Brian Haynes, Peter Tugwell, *Clinical Epidemiology: a basic science for clinical medicine,* Toronto and Boston: Little, Brown and Company, 1985, p. 150.

21. WHO, "Trial on Primary Prevention of ischaemic heart disease using clofibrate to lower serum cholesterol: Mortality Follow-up," (Report of the Committee of Principal Investigators), *Lancet,* 1980, ii:379.

22. Correspondents' Report, "Round the World: Clofibrate," *Lancet,* 1981, i:771.

23. Ontario Ministry of Health, *Drug Benefit Formulary,* Queen's Printer for Ontario, December 1986.

24. M.H. Frick, O. Elo, K. Haapa, et al., "Helsinki Heart Study: primary prevention trial with gemfibrozil in middle-aged men with dyslipidemia: safety of treatment, changes in risk factors, and incidence of coronary heart disease," *NEJM,* 1987, 317: 1237-1245.

25. Lipid Research Clinic's Program, "The Lipid Research Clinic's coronary primary prevention trial results: reduction in incidence of coronary heart disease," *JAMA,* 1984, 251: 351-364.

26. Based on 1981 census data, and cholesterol readings found in: Health and Welfare Canada, *The Health of Canadians: Report of the Canadian Health Survey,* Policy, Communications and Information Branch, Ottawa, 1981.

27. Cooperstock and Parnell, *Social Science and Medicine,* p. 1184-1185.

28. Lexchin, *The Real Pushers,* p. 155.

29. Vanna Schiralli, Marion McIntosh, "Benzodiazepines: Are We Overprescribing?" *Canadian Family Physician,* 1987, 33: 927-934.

30. L.E. Hollister, "Valium: a Discussion of current issues," *Psychosomatics,* 1977, 18: 44-58.

31. Ruth Cooperstock, Henry L. Lennard, "Role strains and tranquilizer use," in *Health and Canadian Society: Sociological Perspectives,* eds. David Coburn, Carl D'Arcy, Peter New, George Torrance, Toronto: Fitzhenry & Whiteside, 1981.

32. *The Globe and Mail,* August 13, 1985.

33. *The Globe and Mail,* September 21, 1987.

34. *The Globe and Mail,* May 30, 1987.

35. S. Asthana, V. Sood, "Prescribing for the elderly: one hospital's experience," *Geriatric Medicine (Canada),* 1987, 3: 113-117.

36. *The Globe and Mail,* May 30, 1985.

37. OECD, *Financing and Delivering Health Care: A comparative analysis of OECD countries,* Paris, 1987.

38. I.T. Borda, E. Napke, C. Stapleton, "Drug surveillance data in a Canadian Hospital," *CMAJ,* 1976, 114: 517-522.

39. Peter Lou, et al., "Drug adverse reactions in autopsy cases: a preliminary report," *Rx Bulletin,* 1974, 5:1.

40. J.L. Reynolds, "A survey of adverse drug reactions in family practice," *Canadian Family Physician,* January 1984, 30: 81-84.

41. Borda et al., *CMAJ.*

42. Ibid.

43. Stephen B. Soumerai, Jerry Avorn, "Efficacy and cost containment in hospital pharmacotherapy: state of the art and future directions,"*Milbank Memorial Fund Quarterly/Health and Society,* 1984, 62: 449.

44. Personal communication with Dr. Lexchin.

45. Ellen Ruppel Shell, "First, do no harm: Lack of understanding often results in the misprescription of drugs," *Atlantic Monthly,* May 1988.

46. J. Avorn, M. Chen, R. Hartley, "Scientific versus commercial sources of influence on the prescribing behaviour of physicians," *American Journal of Medicine,* 1982, 73: 4.

47. Editorial, "You and the Ads," *CMAJ,* 1970, 103: 329.

48. W.A. Parker, "The Compendium of Pharmaceuticals and Specialties as a Drug Information Resource for the Treatment of Acute Drug Overdose," *Canadian Family Physician,* 1979, 25: 211-212, 214-215.

49. R.H. Beill, J. Osterman, "The Compendium of Pharmaceuticals and Specialties: A critical analysis," *International Journal of Health Services,* 1983, 13: 107-118.

50. Eastman Commission, p. 223.

51. Martin Shapiro, *Getting Doctored,* Kitchener: Between the Lines, 1978, pp. 53-55.

52. Shell, *Atlantic Monthly.*

53. Lexchin, *The Real Pushers,* pp. 123.

54. R.G. McAuley, F. Little, "Junk Mail," *CMAJ,* 1983, 129: 1174-1176.

55. Symposium on Drugs, "Drug Information for the Health Care Team," McGill University, May 30/31, 1975. (Mimeograph of summary publication.)

56. Alan Klass, *There's Gold in Them Thar Pills,* United Kingdom: Penguin, 1975.

57. J. Pekkanen, "The Impact of Promotion on Physicians' Prescribing Patterns," *Journal of Drug Issues,* 1976, 6: 13-20.

58. Lexchin, *The Real Pushers,* p. 115.

59. Avorn, *AJM,* 73: 4-8.

60. *The Globe and Mail,* October 22, 1982.

61. Lexchin, *The Real Pushers,* p. 20.

62. The term bioequivalence means the drugs are "chemical equivalents which when administered to the same individuals in the same dosage regimen will result in comparable bioavailability." Bioavailability refers to the ability of a dosage form to deliver the active ingredients to its site of action in an amount sufficient to elicit the desired pharmacologic response. Chemical equivalence does not necessarily imply bioequivalence, inasmuch as differences in the excipients and manufacturing processes can lead to much faster or slower dissolution, absorption and distribution, or even to the absence of dissolution." Quoted from Brian L. Strom, "Special Article: Generic Drug Substitution Revisited," *NEJM,* 1987, 316: 1456.

63. *The Medical Post,* September 1986.

64. *The Globe and Mail,* August 13, 1985.

65. Ibid.

66. Eastman Commission, p. 223.

67. Martin F. Shapiro, Robert P. Charrow, "Scientific misconduct in investigational drug trials," *NEJM,* 1985, 312: 731-736.

68. *The Globe and Mail,* February 11, 1988.

69. WHO "Selection of Essential Drugs: Report of a WHO expert committee," *Technical Report Series,* No. 615, Geneva, 1977.

70. Eastman Commission, p. 410.

71. Lexchin, *The Real Pushers,* p. 45.

72. Eastman Commission, p. xix.

73. Eastman Commission, pp. xvii-xxxvi.

74. *The Toronto Star,* December 7, 1986.

75. *The Globe and Mail,* September 30, 1986.

76. John Sawatsky, Harvey Cashore, "Inside Dope: the multimillion-dollar sellout of Canada's generic drug industry," *This Magazine,* August-September, 1986, pp. 6-7.

77. *CMAJ,* 1978, 119: 1336.

78. J. Avorn, "Scientific versus commercial sources. . ."

79. *The Globe and Mail,* August 13, 1985.

80. *The Gazette,* (Montreal) October 26, 1982.

81. Shell, *Atlantic Monthly.*

CHAPTER 6

1. M.G. Taylor, H.M. Stevenson, A.P. Williams, *Medical Perspectives on Canadian Medicare,* Toronto: York University, 1984, p. 159.

2. CMA, "CMA policy summary: Health Care financing," *CMAJ,* 1986, 134: 656A.

3. R.G. Beck, John Horne, "Utilization of publicly insured health services in Saskatchewan before, during, and after copayment," *Medical Care,* 1980, 18: 787-806. Also Morris Barer, et al., *Controlling Health Care Costs by Direct Charges to Patients: Snare or Delusion,* Ontario Economic Council, Toronto, 1979.

4.Taylor, et al., *Medical Perspectives,* p. 151-152.

5. Leslie Hendeles, "Need for 'counter-detailing' antibiotics," *American Journal of Hospital Pharmacy,* 1976, 33: 918-924.

6. Howard Seiden, "The prescribing of antibiotics can be tricky business," *The Toronto Star,* January 21, 1988.

7. W.R. Best, "Chloramphenicol-associated blood dyscrasias,"*JAMA,* 1967, 201: 181. (Also, Howard Seiden column, note 6.)

8. Richard Allentuck, *Who Speaks for the Patient?: The Crisis in Canadian Health Care,*Toronto: Burns and MacEachern, 1978, p. 22.

9. David E. Rogers, "The Challenge of Primary Care," in *Doing Better Feeling Worse: Health in the U.S.,* J.K. Knowles, ed., New York: W.W. Norton and Co., 1977, pp. 90-91. Also, Cynthia Carver, *Patient Beware: Dealing with doctors and other medical dilemmas,* Scarborough: Prentice-Hall Canada Inc., 1984, p. 66.

10. For more on walk-in clinics, see the following: *The Medical Post,* October 13, 1987; *The Winnipeg Free Press,* January 5, 1986; *The Toronto Star,* November 1, 1986.

11. Andy Stergachis, "Use of a controlled trial to evaluate the impact of self-care on health services utilization,"*Journal of Ambulatory Care Management,* 1986, 9: 16.

12. Eugene Vayda, "Comparison of surgical rates in Canada and in England and Wales," *NEJM,* 1973, 289: 1224.

13. OECD, *Measuring Health Care,* Paris, 1985.

14. Heather Stockwell, Eugene Vayda, "Variations in surgery in Ontario," *Medical Care,* 1979, 17: 390-396.

15. J. Lomas, G. Anderson, "Regionalization and access to coronary artery bypass surgery: distance versus centre effects," 1988. (Submitted to *Medical Care* for publication.)

16. John Wennberg, et al., "Variations in medical care among small areas," *Scientific American,* 1982, 246: 120-133.

17. Ibid.

18. Robert G. Evans, "Finding the levers, finding the courage: Lessons from cost containment in North America," *Journal of Health Politics, Policy and Law,* Durham: Duke University, 1986, Vol.II, No. 4, 585-615.

19. A.R. Feinstein, D.M. Sosin, C.K. Wells, "The Will Rogers phenomenon: stage migration and new diagnostic techniques as a source of misleading statistics for survival in cancer," *NEJM,* 1985, 312: 1604-1608.

20. Anonymous, "Adjuvant therapy for lung cancer: now sits expectation in the air,"*BMJ,* January 22, 1977, pp. 187-188.

21. Ian Tannock, "Treating the patient, not just the cancer,"*NEJM,* 1988, 317: 1534-1535.

22. *The Medical Post,* December 8, 1987.

23. W. J. Mackillop, B.O. Sullivan, G.K. Ward, "Non-small cell lung cancer: how oncologists want to be treated," *International Journal of Radiation Oncology and Biological Physics,* 1987, 13: 929-934.

24. W.J. Mackillop, W.E. Stewart, A.D. Ginsburg, S.S. Stewart, "The Cancer Patients' Perceptions of their disease and its treatments," (in press) *British Journal of Cancer,* 1988.

25. Dennis Roch, et al., *Manitoba and Medicare: 1971 to the Present,* Manitoba Department of Health, 1985.

26. B.B. Roe, "The UCR boondoggle: a death knell for private practice," *NEJM,* 1981, 305: 41-45.

27. W.O. Spitzer, et al., "The Burlington randomized trial of the nurse practitioner," *NEJM,* 1974, 290: 251-256.

28. Marc Renaud, et al., "Practice settings and prescribing profiles: The simulation of tension headaches to general practitioners working in different practice settings in the Montreal area," *American Journal of Public Health,* 1980, 70: 1068-1073.

29. Renaldo Battista,"Adult prevention in primary care: Patterns of Practice in Québec," *American Journal of Public Health,*1983, 73: 1036-1039. Also, Renaldo Battista, et al., "Adult cancer detection in primary care: contrasts among primary care settings in Québec," *American Journal Of Public Health,* 1983, 73: 1040-1041.

30. Robert Allard, et al., "Delays in the primary immunization of children," *CMAJ,* 1985, 133: 108-110.

31. John Hastings, et al., "Prepaid group practice in Sault Ste. Marie, Ontario: Part I: analysis of utilization records," *Medical Care,* 1973, 11: 91-103.

32. Personal communication with Fred Griffith, executive director of the Sault Ste. Marie Group Health Centre.

33. Harold Luft, *Health Maintenance Organizations: Dimensions of Performance,* New York: John Wiley, 1981.

34. Health and Welfare Canada, *Health Sector in Canada Fact Sheets,* (mimeograph) Policy, Communications, and Information Branch, 1987. Also, Statistics Canada, *Current Demographic Analysis: Report on the Demographic Situation in Canada in 1986,* Cat. No. 91-524E, (1987).

35. Health and Welfare Canada, *Health Personnel in Canada 1986,* Supply and Services, Cat. No. H1-9/1-1986, (1987).

36. *The Globe and Mail,* February 13, 1987.

37. *The Winnipeg Free Press,* October 22, 1987,

38. John Horne, "Searching for Shortage: A population-based analysis of medical care utilization," in *Proceedings of the 3rd Canadian Conference on Health Economics,* ed. John Horne, Winnipeg: University of Manitoba Department of Social and Preventive Medicine, 1986.

39. Evans, "Finding the Levers," p. 600.

40. Robert G. Evans, "Hang Together, or Hang Separately: The Viability of a Universal Health Care System in an Aging Society," *Canadian Public Policy,* 1987, Vol. XIII, 2: 165-180.

41. Morris Barer, Robert Evans, Clyde Hertzman, Jonathan Lomas, "Aging and Health Care Utilization: New Evidence on Old Fallacies,"*Social Science and Medicine,* 1987, 24: 851-862.

42. Ibid.

43. Stanislaw Judek, *Royal Commission on Health Services: Medical Manpower in Canada,* Supply and Services, 1964.

44. Health and Welfare Canada, *Health Sector Fact Sheets.*

45. Ontario Council of Health, *Medical Manpower for Ontario,* Toronto; Queen's Printer for Ontario, 1983.

46. D.M. Steinwachs, et al., "A comparison of the requirements for primary care physicians in HMOs with projections made by the GMENAC," *NEJM,* 1986, 314: 217-222.

47. Jonathan Lomas, (untitled letter), *NEJM,* 1986, 315: 324-325.

48. Jonathan Lomas, et al., *Physician Manpower Planning: Lessons from the Macdonald Report,* Toronto: Ontario Economic Council, 1985.

49. Spitzer, et al., "The Burlington Randomized Trial."

50. Health and Welfare Canada, *Health Personnel in Canada 1986,* p. 114

51. Martin O'Malley, *Hospital: Life and Death in a Major Medical Centre,* Toronto: Macmillan of Canada, 1986.

52. *The Toronto Star,* February 2, 1987. Also, Noah M. Meltz, *Sorry, No Care Available due to Nursing Shortage*, Registered Nurses Association of Ontario, November, 1988.

53. T. Hilden, R. Raaschou, K. Iversen, M. Schwartz, "Anticoagulants in acute myocardial infarction," *Lancet,* 1961, ii: 327-331. Also, United Kingdom, Medical Research Council Working Party on Anticoagulant Therapy in Coronary Thrombosis, "Assessment of short-term anticoagulant administration after cardiac infarction," *BMJ,* 1969, 1: 335-342. Also, L. Goldman, E.F. Cook, "The decline in ischemic heart disease mortality rates: An analysis of the comparative effects of medical interventions and changes in lifestyle," *Annals of Internal Medicine,* 1984, 101: 825-836.

54. Taylor, *Medical Perspectives.*

55. Milton Roemer, "Bed supply and hospital utilization: a natural experiment," *Hospitals* (the journal of the American Hospital Association), 1961, 35: 36-42.

56. Paul Griner, "Treatment of acute pulmonary edema: conventional or intensive care?" *Annals of Internal Medicine,* 1972, 77: 501-506.

57. Daniel Singer, et al., "Rationing intensive care—physician responses to a resource shortage," *NEJM,* 1983, 309: 1155-1160.

58. Bernard S. Linn, et al., "Do dollars spent relate to outcomes in burn care?" *Medical Care,* 1979, 17: 835-843.

59. Health and Welfare Canada, *Health Care Sector Fact Sheets.*

60. Luft, *Health Maintenance Organizations.* Also, Willard Manning, et al., "A controlled trial of the effect of a pre-paid group practice on use of services," *NEJM,* 1984, 310: 1505-1510. Also, John Ware, et al., "Comparison of health outcomes at a health maintenance organization with those of fee-for-service care,"*Lancet,* 1986, i: 1017-1022.

61. Roch, *Manitoba and Medicare.*

62. CMA, *Health: A Need for Redirection,* Ottawa, 1985.

63. Ann Silversides, "Elderly Waiting in Hospital are Treated Like Refugees," *The Globe and Mail,* March 21, 1987.

64. *The Medical Post,* June 2, 1987.

65. Ibid.

66. *The Globe and Mail,* June 6, 1987.

67. Chris Wood, "The Transplant Revolution," *Macleans,* November 30, 1987.

68. Dorothy Lipovenko, "Need surgery, medical tests? Go to the end of the line," *The Globe and Mail,* May 28, 1988.

CHAPTER 7

1. Thomas McKeown, *The Role of Medicine: Dream, Mirage, or Nemesis?* Princeton: Princeton University Press, 1979, p. 29.

2. Ibid., p. xi-xii.

3. G.L. Siler Wells, F.M. Garcia, S.F. Jackson, *Planning for Health: A Guide to Creating Strategies for Ontario's Health Care System,* Ontario Council of Health, 1983.

4. Ibid.

5. T. Reves, "Declining fertility in England and Wales as a major cause of the 20th century decline in mortality," *American Journal of Epidemiology,* 1985, 122: 112-126.

6. E. Nicolls, C. Nair, L. MacWilliam, et al., *Cardiovascular Disease in Canada,* Supply and Services, Ottawa, 1986.

7. Gary E. Fraser, *Preventive Cardiology,* New York and Oxford: Oxford University Press, 1986, p. 3.

8. Nicolls, *Cardiovascular Disease in Canada.*

9. Fraser, *Preventive Cardiology,* pp. 4-5.

10. Nicolls, *Cardiovascular Disease in Canada.*

11. Ibid.

12. Ibid.

13. S. Pell, W.E. Fayerweather, "Trends in the incidence of myocardial infarction and in associated mortality and morbidity in a large employed population, 1957-1983," *NEJM,* 1985, 312: 1005-1011.

14. Pell reports on the incidence and mortality from myocardial infarction in the employed population of Dupont Corporation from 1957 to 1983. He classifies mortality as either within 24 hours of the onset of symptoms or between 24 hours and 30 days of the onset of symptoms. From Pell's data, one may calculate the effects of decreasing incidence of disease and decreasing case fatality rates on the number of deaths observed. If one assumes that medical care had no effect on incidence and little effect on 24-hour case fatality rates (most of these deaths occurred within minutes and were classified as "sudden deaths"), then medical care was responsible for only about one-quarter of the reduction in death rates, at most. A full explanation of this point is available by writing to the authors.

15. Fraser, *Preventive Cardiology,* pp. 16-17.

16. Nicholls, *Cardiovascular Disease in Canada,* pp. 69-70.

17. G. Fraser, *Preventive Cardiology,* p. 16. Also, Roslyn Lindheim, S. Leonard Syme, "Environments, people, and health," *Annual Review of Public Health* 1983, 4: 335-359.

18. Canadian Cancer Society and Statistics Canada, *Canadian Cancer Statistics 1987,* Ottawa: Canadian Cancer Society, 1987.

19. John C. Bailar III, Elaine M. Smith, "Progress Against Cancer?" *NEJM,* 1986, 314: 1226-1232.

20. Unless otherwise specified, all further data on cancer comes from M.P. Vessey, Marie Gray, *Cancer, Risks and Prevention,* New York and Oxford: Oxford University Press, 1985; and/or M. Kurihara, K. Aoki, and S. Tominaga, eds., *Cancer Mortality Statistics in the World,* Nagaya: University of Nagaya Press, October 1984.

21. Health and Welfare Canada, *Mortality Atlas of Canada, Volume I: Cancer,* Ottawa, 1980.

22. Radio broadcast, *As It Happens,* May 15, 1987, produced by CBC, Toronto.

23. Bailar and Smith, "Progress Against Cancer?"

24. Ibid., p. 1227.

25. Neil Collishaw, Gordon Myers, "Dollar estimates of the consequences of tobacco use in Canada, 1979," *Canadian Journal of Public Health,* 1984, 75: 192-199.

26. In 1986 there were 744 work-related deaths for which compensation was paid. (Personal communication from Rick Farmer, Labour Canada, March 25, 1988.)

27. Walter Willett, Adele Green, Meir Stampfer, et al., "Relative and absolute excess risks of coronary heart disease among women who smoke cigarettes," *NEJM,* 1987, 317: 1303.

28. Statistics Canada, *Report of the Canadian Health and Disability Survey 1983-84,* Cat. No. 82-55E, (1986).

29. For a further discussion of the search for cause and effect, see David Sackett, R. Brian Haynes, and Peter Tugwell, *Clinical Epidemiology,* Chapter 9, Toronto: Little Brown and Company, 1985.

30. Richard Doll, Richard Peto, "Mortality in relation to smoking: 20 years observations on male British doctors," *BMJ,* 1976, 2: 1525-1536. Also, see a study of nearly 200,000 men conducted by the American Cancer Society: E.C. Hammond, D. Horn, "Smoking and death rates: reports on 44 months of follow-up of 187,783 men," *JAMA,* 1958, 166: 1159.

31. With information from Doll and Peto, "Mortality in relation to smoking," and Canadian Cancer Society, *Canadian Cancer Statistics, 1987.*

32. Russell Wilkins, Owen Adams, *Healthfulness of Life,* Montreal: IRPP Montreal, 1983.

33. *Rapport de la Commission d'enquête sur les services de santé et les services sociaux,* (Rochon Commission), Publications du Québec, 1988, p. 73. Original source: J. O'Loughlin, J. F. Boivin, "Indicateurs de santé, facteurs de risque liés au mode de vie et utilisation du système de soins dans la région centre-ouest de Montréal, Rapport déposé à la CESSS," Publications du Québec, 1987.

34. Wayne Millar, Donald Wigle, "Socio-economic disparities in risk factors for cardiovascular disease," *CMAJ,* 1986, 134: 127-132.

35. Ken Battle, *Poverty Profile 1988: A report by the National Council of Welfare,* National Council of Welfare, 1988. Also, *Transitions, Report of the Social Assistance Review Committee,* prepared for the Ontario Ministry of Community and Social Services, Toronto, 1988.

36. B. Postl, "Native Health — a Continuing Concern,"*Canadian Journal of Public Health,* 1986, 77: 253-254. Also, T. Kue Young, "The Canadian North and the Third World: Is the Analogy Appropriate?" *Canadian Journal of Public Health,* 1983, 74: 239-241.

37. Yang Mao, H. Morrison, R. Semenciw, D. Wigle, "Mortality on Canadian Indian Reserves 1977-1982," *Canadian Journal of Public Health,* 1986, 77: 263-268.

38. Ibid., p. 267.

39. W. McDermott, K.W. Deuschle, C.R. Barnett, "Health care experiment at Many Farms," *Science,* 1972, 175: 23-31.

40. *The Globe and Mail,* January 23, 1987.

41. Dr. Shah is a professor of preventive medicine at the University of Toronto. He made these remarks at a presentation to the Social Assistance Review Committee, which was investigating Ontario's social assistance system.

42. John Berg, et al., "Economic status and survival of cancer patients," *Cancer,* 1977, 39: 467-477. Also M. Bassett, N. Krieger, "Social class and black-white differences in breast cancer survival," *American Journal of Public Health,* 1986, 76: 1400-1403.

43. John Silins, Robert Semenciw, Howard Morrison, et al., "Risk factor for perinatal mortality in Canada," *CMAJ,* 1985, 133: 1214-1219.

44. Henry Dunn, "Social aspects of low birthweight," *CMAJ,* 1984, 130: 1131-1140.

45. Yolande Pelchat, Russel Wilkins, "Report on Births: certain sociodemographic and health aspects of mothers and newborns in Region 6A (metropolitan Montreal), 1979-1983," Association of Community Health Departments of Metropolitan Montreal, April 1987.

46. Personal communication with Horst Stiebert, Statistics Canada, March 21, 1988.

47. OECD, *Living Conditions in OECD Countries: a Compendium of Social Indicators,* Paris, 1986.

48. Christopher Waddell, "Beyond McJobs," *Report on Business Magazine,* June 1988.

49. Arthur Donner, "Economic shift leaves wage earners behind," *The Toronto Star,* May 30, 1988.

50. W. Eugene Broadhead, B. Kaplan, S. James, et al., "The epidemiologic evidence for a relationship between social support and health," *American Journal of Epidemiology,* 1983, 117: 521-537.

51. R. Lindheim, L. Syme, "Environments, people, and health," *Annual Review of Public Health,* 1983, 4: 335-359.

52. "Domestic murders: police need help,"*The Toronto Star,* February 27, 1988.

53. *The Toronto Star,* February 7, 1988.

54. Linda MacLeod, *Battered but not Beaten: Preventing Wife Battering in Canada,* Canadian Advisory Council on the Status of Women, Ottawa, 1987.

55. Nedra Belloc, Lester Breslow, "Relationship of physical health status and health pracices," *Preventive Medicine,* 1972, 1: 409-421. Also, Nedra Belloc, "Relationship of health practices and mortality," *Preventive Medicine,* 1973, 2: 67-81.

56. S. Leonard Syme,"Social determinants of health and disease," in *Maxcy-Rosenau: Public Health and Preventive Medicine,* ed. John Last, 12th edition, Norwalk (Connecticut): Appleton-Century-Crofts, 1986.

57. D. Offord, et al., *Ontario Child Health Study,* Ministry of Community and Social Services, Toronto, 1986. Also "The Ontario Child Health Study, parts I and II," *Archives of General Psychiatry,* 1987, 44: 826-836. Also, D. Cadman, et al., "Chronic illness, disability, and mental and social well-being: findings of the Ontario Child Health Study," *Pediatrics,* 1987, 79: 805-813. Also D. Offord, et al., "Psychiatric disorder and poor school performance among welfare children in Ontario," *Canadian Journal of Psychiatry,* 1987, 32: 518-525.

58. Lindheim and Syme, "Environments, people, and health."

CHAPTER 8

1. From a speech by Professor George Albee at the Prevention Congress III, held in Waterloo, Ontario, May 1987.

2. G.N. Jenkins, "The recent fall in dental cavities incidence," *Ontario Dentist,* 1984, 61: 29-32.

3. S. Leonard Syme, "Social determinants of health and disease," in: *Maxcy-Rosenau: Public Health and Preventive Medicine,* ed. John Last, 12th edition, Norwalk, Connecticut: Appleton-Century-Crofts, 1986.

4. *The Globe and Mail,* November 20, 1987.

5. *The Toronto Star,* January 21, 1988.

6. Louise Russell, *Is Prevention Better Than Cure?* Washington: The Brookings Institute, 1986.

7. Michael B. Gregg, B.M. Nkowane, "Poliomyelitis," in Last (ed.), *Maxcy-Rosenau.*

8. Russell, *Is Prevention Better than Cure?*

9. A.L. Cochrane, W.W. Holland, "Validation of screening procedures," *British Medical Bulletin,* 1971, 27: 3-8.

10. Several screening trials for lung cancer have shown that screening does not increase life expectancy. See J. C. Bailar III, "Screening for lung cancer — where are we now?" *American Review of Respiratory Disease,* 1984, 130: 541-542. Also, Robert Fontana, D.R. Sanderson, L.B. Woolner, et al., "Lung cancer screening: The Mayo program," *Journal of Occupational Medicine,* 1986, 28: 746-750.

11. D. Cadman, L.W. Chambers, L.W. Smith, D.L. Sackett, "Assessing the effectiveness of community screening programs,"*JAMA,* 1984, 251: 1580.

12. J.W. Frank, "Occult blood screening for colorectal carcinoma: the benefits, the risks, and the yield and the costs," *The American Journal of Preventive Medicine,* 1985, Vol. I, No. 3: 3-9, No. 4: 25-32, No. 5: 18-24. Also, Anonymous, "Questions about occult-blood screening for cancer," *Lancet,* 1986, i: 22.

13. R. Gnauck, "Occult-blood screening," *Lancet,* 1986, i: 444. Also, J. Kettner, J.M.A. Northover, (letters to the Editor) *Lancet,* 1986, i: 562-563.

14. Louise Russell, *Is Prevention Better than Cure?* Also, Herman Tyroler, "Hypertension," in, Last (ed.), *Maxcy-Rosenau.*

15. I.K.Zola, "Helping — does it matter?: The problems and prospects of mutual aid groups," 1970. (Address to the United Ostomy Association.)

16. In a presentation at the 1987 annual meeting of the Canadian Public Health Association in Halifax, Nova Scotia.

17. William Haddon, Jr., "Advances in the epidemiology of injuries as a basis for public policy," *Public Health Reports,* 1980, 95: 411-421.

18. In a speech at the Prevention Congress III, held in Waterloo, Ontario, May, 1987.

CHAPTER 9

1. John Naisbitt, Patricia Aburdene, *Re-inventing the Corporation,* New York: Warner Books, 1985.

2. InterStudy, *Interstudy Edge*, Excelsior, Minnesota, fall issue, 1988.

3. Harold Luft, *Health Maintenance Organizations: Dimensions of Performance,* New York: John Wiley and Sons, 1981.

4. Ibid.

5. Alain Enthoven, "An Overview of the U.S. Health Care Economy," *Introduction to Health Economics,* Kaiser Foundation, February 1, 1987. p. 39.

6. Luft, *Health Maintenance Organizations.*

7. An HMO alternative to the PPG is the Individual Practice Association or IPA, sometimes known as a "fee-for-service solo-practice HMO." In an IPA, the doctor continues a traditional private office

practice, billing the plan on fee-for-service even though the patient pays a fixed premium. In return for a guaranteed referral of patients from the plan, the physician must submit to a number of controls, such as a fee schedule and utilization reviews, imposed by the plan. Overall, IPAs are not as cost-effective as PPGs, primarily because they haven't had much impact on lowering the use of outpatient services.

8. Scott Fleming, Douglas Gentry, "A Perspective on Kaiser-Permanente Type Health Care Programs; The Performance Record, Criticisms and Responses," Kaiser Foundation, January 1979, pp. 4-5.

9. The overall economic results are found in Willard Manning, et al., "A controlled trial of the effect of a prepaid group practice on use of services," *NEJM,* 1984, 310: 1505-1510.

The clinical results are found in: John Ware, et al., "Comparison of health outcomes at a health maintenance organization with those of fee for service care," *Lancet,* 1986, i: 1017-1022.

10. Dennis Roch, et al., *Manitoba and Medicare: 1971 to the present,* Manitoba Department of Health, 1985.

11. R.G. Evans, "We have seen the future and they is us; Health care and the greying of Canada," (mimeograph) University of British Columbia, Department of Economics, 1983.

12. CMA, *Health: A Need for Redirection,* Ottawa, 1985. (A Task Force on the Reallocation of Health Care Resources.)

13. L.I. Stein, L.J. Genser, "The dollar follows the patient: Wisconsin's system for funding mental health services," *New Directions for Mental Health Services,* No. 18 June, 1983. Also, L.I. Stein, M.A. Test, "Alternative to mental hospital treatment: I. Conceptual model, treatment program, and clinical evaluation," *Archives of General Psychiatry,* 1980, 37: 392-397. Also, B.A. Weisbrod, M.A. Test, L.I. Stein, "Alternative to mental hospital treatment: II. Economic benefit-cost analysis." *Archives of General Psychiatry,* 1980, 37: 400-405. Also, M.A. Test, L.I. Stein, "Alternative to mental hospital treatment: III. Social cost," *Archives of General Psychiatry,* 1980, 37: 409-412.

14. Foothills Hospital, "The V.I.P. at Foothills Hospital," (mimeograph), Calgary, 1986.

15. *Commission d'enquête sur la santé et le bien-être social,* (Castonguay-Nepveu Commission), Publications du Québec, 1970.

16. *Rapport de la commission d'enquête sur les services de santé et les services sociaux,* (Rochon Commission), Publications du Québec, 1988.

17. *Rapport du Comité de réflections et d'analyse des services dispensés par les CLSC,* (Brunet Committee), Ministère de la santé et des services sociaux, Publications du Québec, 1987.

18. Ibid.

19. J. Roy, *Bilan du maintien à domicile dans les CLSC: I Problématique des services, II problématique des ressources,* Fédération des CLSCs du Québec, 1986.

20. Ibid.

21. Personal communication with Fred Griffith, executive director of SSMGHC.

22. David Sackett, Brian R. Haynes, P. Tugwell, *Clinical Epidemiology: A Basic Science for Clinical Medicine,* Boston and Toronto: Little, Brown and Company, 1985.

CHAPTER 10

1. George Rosen, *A History of Public Health,* New York: MD Publications Inc., 1976, pp. 42-43.

2. Ibid, p. 206.

3. The Health and Morals of Apprentices Act, 1802, in Rosen, *A History of Public Health,* p. 207

4. Edwin Chadwick, et al., *Report on an Inquiry into the Sanitary Condition of the Labouring Population of Great Britain,*1842, in Rosen, *A History of Public Health,* p. 211.

5. Ibid, p. 215.

6. Dr. Southwood Smith, "An Address to the Working Classes of the United Kingdom on their Duty in the Present State of the Sanitary Question, 1847, in Rosen, *A History of Public Health,* p. 220.

7. John Snow, "On the Mode of Communication of Cholera," in *Snow on Cholera,* London: Oxford University Press, 1936.

8. Rosen, *A History of Public Health,* pp. 226-27.

9. Peter Taylor, *Smoke Ring: the Politics of Tobacco,* London: The Bodley Head, 1984.

10. James I, *Counterblaste to Tobacco,* 1608, in Taylor, *Smoke Ring.*

11. Daniel Stoffman, "Where there's smoke. . .there are profits," *The Globe and Mail Report on Business Magazine,* September, 1987.

12. Neil Collishaw, Byron Roger, "Tobacco in Canada,"*Canadian Pharmaceutical Journal,* April, 1984.

13. Ibid.

14. Daniel Stoffman, "Where There's Smoke. . .

15. Michael Daube, "Ethical and Political Issues in Smoking Control," in *Strategies for a smoke-free world,* ed. Jan Skirrow, The Alberta Alcohol and Drug Abuse Commission, Edmonton, 1986.

16. Peter Taylor, *Smoke Ring.*

17. For more information about effective actions against smoking, see, Gail Frankel, "Reducing tobacco consumption: public policy initiative for Canada," *CMAJ,* 1988, 138: 419-423. Also, The Ontario Task Force on Smoking, *Smoking and Health in Ontario: A Need for Balance,* The Ontario Council of Health, Toronto, 1982.

18. John Luik, "Bad Prescription for Good Health," *The Globe and Mail,* February 22, 1988.

19. For recent reviews on the health effects of lead, see K. Hare, *Lead in the Canadian Environment: Science and Regulation, Final report of the Royal Society of the Canada Commission on Lead in the Environment,* Toronto: Royal Society of Canada, 1986. Also, The United States Environmental Protection Agency, *Air Quality Criteria for Lead,* Research Triangle Park, North Carolina, 1986.

20. Hare et al., *Lead in the Canadian Environment.* Also, EPA, *Air Quality.*

21. Jerome O. Nriagu, "Saturnine gout among Roman aristocrats: Did lead poisoning contribute to the fall of the Empire?" *NEJM,* 1983, 308: 660-663.

22. For an interesting historical summary about the politics of TEL see David Rosner and Gerald Markowitz, "A 'Gift of God'?: the public health controversy over leaded gasoline during the 1920's" *American Journal of Public Health,* 1985, 75: 344.

23. Ibid.

24. Hare, *Lead in the Canadian Environment.* Also, EPA, *Air Quality.*

25. EPA, *Air Quality.*

26. H.L. Needleman, C. Gunnoe, A. Leviton, et al., "Deficits in psychologic and classroom performance of children with elevated dentine levels," *NEJM,* 1979, 300: 689-695.

27. This topic is covered elegantly in a seminal article by the reknowned British epidemiologist, Geoffrey Rose, in "Strategy of Prevention: lessons from cardiovascular disease," *BMJ,* 1981, 282: 1847-1851.

28. J.W. Farquhar, *The American Way of Life Need Not Be Hazardous to Your Health,* New York: Norton, 1978. Also, J. W. Farquhar, P.D. Wood, H. Breitrose, et al., "Community education for cardiovascular health," *Lancet,* 1977, i: 1192.

29. G. Fraser, *Preventive Cardiology.* Also, P. Puska, J. Tuomilehto, J. Salonen, et al., "Changes in coronary risk factors during a comprehensive five-year community program to control cardiovascular diseases (North Karelia Project),"*BMJ,* 1979, 2: 1173. Also, J. Salonen, P. Puska, T. Kottke, et al., "Changes in smoking, serum cholesterol, and blood pressure levels during a community-based cardiovascular disease prevention program — the North Karelia Project," *American Journal of Epidemiology,* 1981, 114: 81. Also, J. Salonen, P. Puska, T. Kottke, et al., "Decline in coronary heart mortality in Finland from 1969 to 1979" *BMJ,* 1983. 286: 1857.

30. Linda MacLeod, *Battered, But Not Beaten: Preventing Wife Battering in Canada,* Canadian Advisory Council on the Status of Women, Ottawa, 1987.

31. P.G. Jaffe, J.K. Thompson, M.J. Paquin, "Immediate family crisis intervention as preventative mental health: the family consultant service," *Professional Psychology,* November, 1978, 551-560.

32. P. Jaffe, S. Wilson, D.A. Wolfe, "Promoting changing in attitudes and understanding of conflict resolution among child witnesses of family violence," *Canadian Journal of Behavioural Science,* 1986, 18: 356-366.

33. P. Jaffe, D. Wolfe, S.K. Wilson, L. Zak, "Family violence and child adjustment: a comparative analysis of girls and boys behavioral symptoms," *American Journal of Psychiatry,* 1986, 143: 74-77.

34. J. Waller, "Prevention of Premature Death and Disability due to injury" in: *Maxcy-Rosenau, Public Health and Preventive Medicine,* ed. John Last, Norwalk, Connecticut: Appleton-Century-Crofts, 1986.

35. Ibid.

36. Ibid.

37. Holly Johnson, "Homicide in Canada," *Canadian Social Trends,* Statistics Canada, Winter 1987.

38. J. Naisbitt, P. Aburdene, *Re-inventing the Corporation: Transforming your job and your company for the new information society,* New York: Warner Books, 1985, p. 9.

CHAPTER 11

1. CMA, *Health: A Need for Redirection,* Ottawa, 1985.

2. John R. Evans, et al., *Toward a Shared Direction for Health in Ontario: Report of the Ontario Health Review Panel,* Toronto: Ontario Health Review Board, June, 1987.

3. *Rapport de la Commission d'enquête sur les services de santé et les services sociaux,* (Rochon Commission), Publications du Québec, 1988.

4. Things are moving swifty in this area, but for a recent review of anti-coagulants and heart attack, see Victor Marder, Sol Sherry, "Thrombolytic therapy: current status," *NEJM,* 1988, 318: 1512-1520.

5. There are many possible models for developing the capitation rate. The British National Health Service uses a formula that combines factors such as age, sex, marital status, fertility rates, and mortality rates, as well as referral patterns. For further information on this see: Victor Rodwin, *The Health Planning Predicament,* Berkeley: Univerity of California Press, 1984.

6. Almost all quality control and utilization review activities focus on process, not outcomes. For example, the Canadian Council on Hospital Accreditation ensures that operating rooms are sterile, but the council has no mechanism for ensuring that the operations performed within are really necessary. For a recent review of this topic, see Michael Rachlis, Catherine Fooks, "Utilization analysis: current initiatives across Canada," paper presented to the First Annual Policy Conference of the Centre for Health Economics and Policy Analysis at McMaster University, Hamilton, May 27, 1988.

7. Health and Welfare Canada, *Health Sector in Canada Fact Sheets,* (mimeograph), Policy, Communications, and Information Branch, November 1987.

8. Hugh Scully, "Ontario's evolving health-care system," *Ontario Medical Review,* 1988, 55: 14-16.

9. Malcolm G. Taylor, H. Michael Stevenson, A. Paul Williams, *Medical Perspectives on Canadian Medicare: Attitudes of Canadian Physicians to Policies and Problems of the Medical Care Insurance Program,* Toronto: York University, 1984, p. 119.

10. Russell Wilkins, Owen Adams, *Healthfulness of Life,* Montreal: IRPP, 1983.

11. Estimates for institutional rates among seniors living in Australia and the United States from CMA, *Health: A Need for Redirection.*

12. W.O. Spitzer, et al., "The Burlington randomized trial of the nurse practitioner," *NEJM,* 1974, 290: 251-256.

13. *Report of the Task Force on the Implementation of Midwifery in Ontario* (chaired by Mary Eberts), Ontario Ministry of Health, Toronto, 1987.

14. U.S. Surgeon General, *Healthy People,* Washington: Department of Health and Human Services, 1979.

15. U.S. Public Health Service, *Promoting Health, Preventing Disease: Objectives for the Nation,* Washington: Department of Health and Human Services, Fall 1980.

16. For example, see the National Centre for Health Statistics, *Health United States,* 87-1232, Public Health Service, Washington, 1986. Also, D.R. Shopland, C. Brown, "Toward the 1990 objectives for smoking: measuring the progress with 1985 NHIS data," *Public Health Reports,* 1987, 102: 68-73. Also, M.M. Silverman *et al., "*Control of stress and violent behaviour: mid-course review of the 1990 health objectives,"*Public Health Reports,* 1988, 103: 38-49.

17. *Objectif: santé. Rapport du comité d'étude sur la promotion de la santé,* Conseil des affaires sociales et de la famille, Québec, August 1984.

18. "Gallup National Omnibus Attitudes toward smoking restrictions," (A poll conducted by Gallup for the Canadian Cancer Society.) October 1987.

19. Marshall Jones, "The benefits of beneficence,"*Social Service Review,* 1987, 6: 183-217.

20. In 1987, there were 230 shelters for women fleeing abusive relationships, with an average funding of $173,000. (Linda MacLeod, *Battered But Not Beaten.)* And there were about 60 rape crisis and sexual assault centres, some of which had no government funding at all. Even the best-endowed operate with government grants of less than $100,000, (Personal communications with Esther Ignagni, Toronto Rape Crisis Centre, and Diane Guilbault, Vancouver Rape Relief and Women's Shelter.)

21. Gail Siler-Wells, "An implementation model for health system reform," *Social Science and Medicine,* 1987, 24: 821-832.

Index